Frontiers in PEDIATRIC NEUROLOGY

Frontiers in PEDIATRIC NEUROLOGY

Editor

TM Ananda Kesavan
MD DNB MNAMS FIAP FIAMS PGDDN

Additional Professor
Department of Pediatrics
Government Medical College, Thrissur
Nodal Officer
Institutional Research Committee
Government Medical College (GMC), Thrissur
Chairman
Institutional Ethics Committee, GMC
Palakkad, Kerala, India
Editor-in-Chief
Indian Academy of Pediatrics (IAP) Textbook of Pediatric Radiology
National President 2017
IAP Neurology Chapter

Foreword
MKC Nair

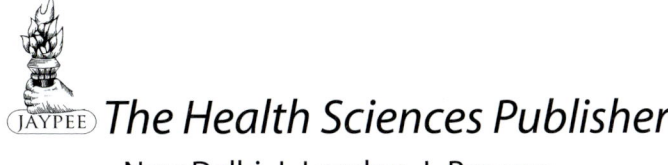

The Health Sciences Publisher
New Delhi | London | Panama

Jaypee Brothers Medical Publishers (P) Ltd.

Headquarters
Jaypee Brothers Medical Publishers (P) Ltd.
4838/24, Ansari Road, Daryaganj
New Delhi 110 002, India
Phone: +91-11-43574357
Fax: +91-11-43574314
E-mail: jaypee@jaypeebrothers.com

Overseas Offices

J.P. Medical Ltd.
83, Victoria Street, London
SW1H 0HW (UK)
Phone: +44-20 3170 8910
Fax: +44(0) 20 3008 6180
E-mail: info@jpmedpub.com

Jaypee Brothers Medical Publishers (P) Ltd.
17/1-B, Babar Road, Block-B, Shaymali
Mohammadpur, Dhaka-1207
Bangladesh
Mobile: +08801912003485
E-mail: jaypeedhaka@gmail.com

Jaypee-Highlights Medical Publishers Inc.
City of Knowledge, Bld. 235, 2nd Floor, Clayton
Panama City, Panama
Phone: +1 507-301-0496
Fax: +1 507-301-0499
E-mail: cservice@jphmedical.com

Jaypee Brothers Medical Publishers (P) Ltd.
Bhotahity, Kathmandu, Nepal
Phone: +977-9741283608
E-mail: kathmandu@jaypeebrothers.com

Website: www.jaypeebrothers.com
Website: www.jaypeedigital.com

© 2017, Jaypee Brothers Medical Publishers

The views and opinions expressed in this book are solely those of the original contributor(s)/author(s) and do not necessarily represent those of editor(s) of the book.

All rights reserved. No part of this publication may be reproduced, stored or transmitted in any form or by any means, electronic, mechanical, photocopying, recording or otherwise, without the prior permission in writing of the publishers.

All brand names and product names used in this book are trade names, service marks, trademarks or registered trademarks of their respective owners. The publisher is not associated with any product or vendor mentioned in this book.

Medical knowledge and practice change constantly. This book is designed to provide accurate, authoritative information about the subject matter in question. However, readers are advised to check the most current information available on procedures included and check information from the manufacturer of each product to be administered, to verify the recommended dose, formula, method and duration of administration, adverse effects and contraindications. It is the responsibility of the practitioner to take all appropriate safety precautions. Neither the publisher nor the author(s)/editor(s) assume any liability for any injury and/or damage to persons or property arising from or related to use of material in this book.

This book is sold on the understanding that the publisher is not engaged in providing professional medical services. If such advice or services are required, the services of a competent medical professional should be sought.

Every effort has been made where necessary to contact holders of copyright to obtain permission to reproduce copyright material. If any has been inadvertently overlooked, the publisher will be pleased to make the necessary arrangements at the first opportunity.

Inquiries for bulk sales may be solicited at: jaypee@jaypeebrothers.com

Frontiers in Pediatric Neurology

First Edition: **2017**
ISBN: 978-93-86261-75-5
Printed at: Samrat offset Pvt. Ltd.

Dedicated to

Late TMK Vishnu Nambisa (My father)
Every single word in this book has been written with the endless support of my father
who had been my mentor in my journey throughout...
More than a father, he was my teacher and my friend....

Contributors

Anoop Verma MD FIAP
Consultant Pediatrician
Swapnil Nursing Home and Research Center
Raipur, Chhattisgarh, India

Ciju Ravindranath MD (Pediatrics)
Assistant Professor
Department of Pediatrics
Jubilee Mission Medical College
and Research Center
Thrissur, Kerala, India

D Kalpana MD DM (Neurology) DNB (Neuro)
Additional Professor
Department of Pediatric Neurology
Sree Avittom Thirunal (SAT) Hospital
Government Medical College
Thiruvananthapuram, Kerala, India

G Kumaresan MD DCH DM (Neuro)
Retired Professor
Department of Pediatric Neurology
Madras Medical College
Consultant Pediatric Neurologist
Kanchi Kamakoti CHILDS Trust Hospital
Chennai, Tamil Nadu, India

Jitendra Kumar Sahu MD DM (Pediatric Neurology)
Associate Professor
Child Neurology Division
Department of Pediatrics
Postgraduate Institute of Medical Education and
Research (PGIMER)
Chandigarh, India

Kavita Srivastava MD (Pediatrics)
Fellowship in Pediatric Epilepsy
Associate Professor and Specialist in Pediatric
Epilepsy and Neurology
Bharati Vidyapeeth Deemed University
Medical College
Pune, Maharashtra, India

Ketan H Shah MD (Pediatrics)
Consultant Pediatrician
Ketan Children Hospital
Surat, Gujarat, India

KP Sarabhai MD FCGP
Director
Sarabhai Polyclinic
Raipur, Chhattisgarh, India

Latika Nayar
MD (Ped) FHM (Fellowship in HIV Medicine)
Associate Professor
Department of Pediatrics
Government Medical College
Thrissur, Kerala, India

M Madhusudanan DM (Neurology)
MD (Medicine)
Professor and Head
Department of Neurology
Pushpagiri Medical College
Thiruvalla, Kerala, India

Mallika OU MS DO DNB MNAMS
Professor
Department of Ophthalmology
Government TD Medical College
Alappuzha, Kerala, India

Mary Iype MD DM (Neurology) MNAMS
(Neuro) FIMSA FRCPCH (Lon)
Additional Professor
Department of Pediatric Neurology
SAT Hospital, Government Medical College
Thiruvananthapuram, Kerala, India

Naveen Jain MD DM (Neonatology)
Professor
Department of Neonatology
Kerala Institute of Medical Sciences
Thiruvananthapuram, Kerala, India

PA Mohammed Kunju MD DM WHO
Fellowship in Pediatric Neurology
Professor and Head
Department of Pediatric Neurology
SAT Hospital
Government Medical College
Thiruvananthapuram, Kerala, India

S Mini MD (Pediatrics) DNB (Pediatrics)
DM (Neurology) Fellowship (EEG and Epilepsy)
Additional Professor
Department of Pediatric Neurology
SAT Hospital
Government Medical College
Thiruvananthapuram, Kerala, India

Shaji Abraham MD (Medicine) DM (Neurology)
Head
Department of Neurology
Government Medical College
Thrissur, Kerala, India

Sumeet R Dhawan MD
Senior Resident (DM)
Child Neurology Division
Department of Pediatrics
PGIMER, Chandigarh, India

Susan Uthup MD DNB (Ped) DM DNB (Nephro)
Professor and Head
Department of Pediatric Nephrology
SAT Hospital, Government Medical College
Thiruvananthapuram, Kerala, India

TA Sheela MD
Associate Professor
Department of Pediatrics
Government Medical College
Thrissur, Kerala, India

TM Ananda Kesavan
MD DNB MNAMS FIAP FIAMS PGDDN
Additional Professor
Department of Pediatrics
Government Medical College, Thrissur
Nodal Officer
Institutional Research Committee
Government Medical College (GMC), Thrissur
Chairman
Institutional Ethics Committee, GMC
Palakkad, Kerala, India
Editor-in-Chief
Indian Academy of Pediatrics (IAP) Textbook of
Pediatric Radiology
National President 2017
IAP Neurology Chapter

V Viswanathan
DCH MRCP PhD (Pediatric Neurology)
Consultant Pediatric Neurologist
Kanchi Kamakoti CHILDS Trust Hospital and
Apollo Children's Hospital
Chennai, Tamil Nadu, India

Vinayan KP MD (Pediatrics) DM
Professor and Head
Division of Pediatric Neurology
Amrita Institute of Medical Sciences
Kochi, Kerala, India

VT Haridas
MD DNB (Gen Med) DNB (Neuro) DM (Neuro)
Head
Department of Neurology
Elite Mission Hospital
Thrissur, Kerala, India

Yeeshu Singh Sudan MD
Fellow in Pediatric Neurology
Consultant Pediatric Neurologist
Medanta—The Medicity Hospital
Gurugram, Haryana, India

Foreword

It is indeed a matter of great pleasure for me to write a foreword to *Frontiers in Pediatric Neurology* brought out by my erstwhile student, TM Ananda Kesavan, an astute clinician, an academician and a sincere teacher. Neurological problems in children are a leading cause for morbidity, and sometimes mortality in India, and other middle-income countries. The book meant for postgraduate students in pediatrics and pediatric neurology, practicing pediatricians and faculty from teaching hospitals, is a welcome addition to the available literature on pediatric neurology.

The topics covered by eminent pediatricians and pediatric neurologists include common and practical problems such as febrile seizure, epilepsy, hypoxic-ischemic encephalopathy, cerebral palsy, etc. It has given much importance to relevant clinical examinations, particularly, in chapters such as pitfalls in neurological examination, ataxia and muscle disorders. Each chapter has been given emphasis on latest developments in pediatric neurology and management strategies available in developing countries.

I am confident that the book would satisfy a growing need for such a comprehensive book to guide the postgraduate students and practicing pediatricians. I have no hesitation to recommend this book to all healthcare personnel involved in taking care of children with neurological diseases.

MKC Nair
Vice Chancellor
Kerala University of Health Sciences
Founder Director
Child Development Centre
Kerala, India
National President of IAP (2004) and
National Neonatology Forum (NNF) (2011–12)

Preface

Diseases of the nervous system are quite common in children in the developing countries. They are one of the main causes of morbidity and mortality in our children. Unfortunately, many of these problems are not satisfactorily addressed in countries such as India and other middle-income countries.

My idea in writing this book is to provide a proper perspective to the pediatricians, postgraduates in pediatrics and neurology, practicing pediatricians and teaching faculties to understand the important neurological diseases that they may come across in their practice. Many topics discussed in *Frontiers in Pediatric Neurology*, are not available in the recently published pediatric Neurology books.

Chapters in the book include topics ranging from the problems arising from clinical examinations, infectious diseases, autoimmune problems, various aspects of epilepsy, electrolytes imbalance to brain death.

I believe that the book would contribute to a better understanding and effective management of children with neurological diseases.

TM Ananda Kesavan

Acknowledgments

I acknowledge the help of all contributors from all over the world, without whose help, this textbook would not have become a reality.

I acknowledge the constant support and encouragement provided by Professors PA Mohammed Kunju and KK Purushothaman. I would also like to thank Professor MKC Nair who was gracious enough to write a foreword for this book.

I would like to thank Dr Sujatha Anand, Aditya Anand and Akash Anand for helping me to prepare this book in many ways. I also thank M/s Jaypee Brothers Medical Publishers (P) Ltd, New Delhi, India, for showing interest in publishing the book.

Contents

1. **Pitfalls in Neurological Examination of Children** — 1
   G Kumaresan
   History 1 • Examination 2 • Cranial Nerves 3
   Significance and Use of the Neurodevelopmental Reflexes in Pediatric Practice 8

2. **Malformations of the Central Nervous System** — 11
   TM Ananda Kesavan
   Etiology 11 • Classification 11

3. **Perinatal Hypoxic-ischemic Encephalopathy** — 23
   Naveen Jain
   Etiology 23 • Clinical Features 23 • Investigations 24
   Neurodevelopment Disability due to Hypoxic-ischemic Encephalopathy 24

4. **Approach to Neurodegenerative Disorders** — 27
   PA Mohammed Kunju
   Clinical Clues of Neurodegenerative Disorders 27 • Inheritance 28
   Organic Acid Disorders 30 • Urea Cycle Defects 32 • Investigations 35

5. **Neural Tube Defects: Prevalence, Predisposing Factors and Prevention** — 42
   TM Ananda Kesavan, Ciju Ravindranath
   Prevalence 42 • Embryology 42 • Classification 42
   Predisposing Factors 43 • Prevention 44

6. **Cerebral Palsy** — 47
   PA Mohammed Kunju
   Etiology 47 • Classification 47
   Terminologies Used in Topographic Definition of Cerebral Palsy 48

7. **Neuronal Migration Disorders** — 54
   TM Ananda Kesavan
   Mechanism of Neuronal Migration 54 • Radial Migration 55
   Tangential Migration 55 • Others Modes of Migration 55
   Neurotrophic Hypothesis 55 • Etiology 55 • Clinical Features 56

8. **Acute Disseminated Encephalomyelitis** — 59
   Ciju Ravindranath
   Causes of Acute Disseminated Encephalomyelitis 59
   Pathogenesis 60 • Clinical Presentation 60 • Investigation 60
   Treatment and Management 62 • Outcome and Prognosis 63

9. Guillain-Barré Syndrome   64
Shaji Abraham

Epidemiology *64* • Pathogenesis *64* • Clinical Features *65* • Diagnosis *65*
Management *66* • Immunotherapy *67* • Plasmapheresis *68* • Corticosteroids *68*
Miller Fisher Syndrome *68* • Treatment of Patients who Deteriorate in Spite of Therapy *68*
Vaccination and GBS *69* • Prognosis *69*

10. Autoimmune Encephalitis in Children   71
V Viswanathan

Acute Disseminated Encephalomyelitis *71* • NMDA Receptor-associated Encephalitis *72*
Rasmussen's Encephalitis *73* • Hashimoto's Encephalitis *74*
Voltage-gated Potassium Channel Antibody Limbic Encephalitis *74*

11. Tuberculous Meningitis in India   76
Jitendra Kumar Sahu, Sumeet R Dhawan

Pathogenesis *76* • Pathology *77* • Diagnosis of Tubercular Meningitis *77*
Complications and Sequelae *81* • Treatment of Tubercular Meningitis *81* • Outcome *84*

12. Cerebrospinal Fluid Examination in Bacterial Meningitis: Common Pitfalls   87
TM Ananda Kesavan

Cerebrospinal Fluid in Bacterial Meningitis *87*
Diagnostic Dilemmas in Cerebrospinal Fluid Examination *88*
When to do Repeat Lumbar Puncture? *90*

13. Cerebral Malaria   92
Ketan H Shah

About Pathogen *92* • Treatment *94*

14. Neurocysticercosis   97
Anoop Verma

The Indian Facts *97* • Classification of NCC *98* • Clinical Features *98*
Solitary Cerebral Cystic Granuloma *98* • Diagnosis *99* • Concepts of Treatment *100*

15. Neurological Manifestations in Human Immunodeficiency Virus Infection   103
Latika Nayar

Pathogenesis *103* • HIV Encephalopathy *104*
Opportunistic Infections of Nervous System *104*

16. Febrile Seizures   110
KP Sarabhai

How Common are Febrile Seizures? *110* • Pathophysiology *110* • Genetics *111*
Types of Febrile Seizures *111* • Risk Factors *112* • Lab Studies *112*
Imaging Studies *112* • Electroencephalogram *112* • Lumbar Puncture *112*
Treatment *113* • Prophylaxis *113* • Risk Factors for Recurrent Febrile Seizure *113*
Prognosis *114* • Risk Factors for Epilepsy *114* • Parental Anxiety *114*
Analysis of Intellectual Ability of Children with Febrile Seizure *114*
What Research is being done on Febrile Seizures? *114*

17. Epileptic Syndromes — 116
Mary Iype

Neonatal Epileptic Syndromes *116*
Epileptic Syndromes seen after the Neonatal Period *117*

18. Treatment of Childhood Epilepsy — 123
M Madhusudanan

When to Start Treatment? *123* • Which Drug to Choose? *124*
Which Drug for Initial Treatment? *125* • Drug Interactions *127*
When to Stop the Treatment? *128*

19. Newer Antiepileptic Drugs in Treatment of Childhood Epilepsy — 130
Kavita Srivastava

Individual Drugs: Pharmacology, Indications, Efficacy and Tolerability *130*
Practical Considerations: Place of Newer Drugs in Management of Pediatric Epilepsy *137*

20. Practical Management of Status Epilepticus — 143
Yeeshu Singh Sudan, Vinayan KP

Classification of Status Epilepticus *143* • Management *144* • Investigations *145*
Pharmacologic Management *145* • Management Protocol *147*

21. Role of Ketogenic Diet in Management of Pediatric Epilepsy — 151
Kavita Srivastava

Overview of Ketogenic Diet *15* • Mechanism of Action: How does it Work? *151*
Efficacy of Ketogenic Diet *152* • Indications and Contraindications *152*
Prediet Evaluation *153* • Initiation of Diet *154*
Classical/Johns Hopkins Hospital Protocol *154*
Modifications to Johns Hopkins Hospital Protocol *154*
Adverse Effects of the Ketogenic Diet *155* • Discontinuation of Ketogenic Diet *156*
Recent Advances in Ketogenic Diet *156* • More Liberal Ketogenic Diets *156*

22. Neurological Dysfunctions in Iron Deficiency Anemia — 160
TM Ananda Kesavan

Pathophysiology *160* • Neurologic Sequelae of Iron Deficiency in Children *162*

23. Cerebral Edema — 167
S Mini

Basic Physiology *167* • Definition *167* • Types of Cerebral Edema *168*
Pathophysiology *168* • Clinical Features *169* • Herniation Syndromes *170*
Imaging Features of Cerebral Edema *170* • Monitoring of Intracranial Pressure *170*
Management of Patient with Raised Intracranial Pressure *173*

24. Sodium Dysequilibrium and the Brain Disorders in Children — 179
Susan Uthup

Physiology of Sodium and Water Balance *179* • Disorders of Sodium Balance *180*
Impact of Sodium Balance Disorders on Brain *180*
Hyponatremia *181* • Hypernatremia *183*

25. Muscle Disorders: A Practical Approach 185
D Kalpana

Clinical Evaluation *185* • Differential Diagnosis *188*
Investigations *190* • Management *192*

26. Ocular Movement Disorders in Children 193
M Madhusudanan

Childhood Patterns of Nystagmus *198*

27. Approach to a Child with Ataxia 203
TM Ananda Kesavan

Pitfalls in the Recognition of Ataxia *203* • How to Approach to Child with Ataxia? *203*
History *204* • Investigations *206*

28. Eye: A Window to Neurological Disorders 210
Mallika OU

Pediatric Neuro-ophthalmology Examination *210*
Anterior Segment Anomalies of Neuro-ophthalmic Significance *211*
Posterior Segment Abnormalities of Neuro-ophthalmological Significance *213*
Optic Atrophy *214* • Phakomatosis *216*
Metabolic and Neurodegenerative Diseases of Ophthalmological Significance *217*
Optic Atrophy *218* • Corneal Involvement *218*
Abnormal Ocular Movements of Neuro-ophthalmic Significance *219*
Maternal Infections of Neuro-ophthalmic Significance *220*

29. An Approach to Children with Neurogenic Bladder Dysfunction 223
VT Haridas

Basic Neuroanatomy and Physiology *223* • Evaluation *226*
Urodynamic Study of Bladder *227* • Common Pediatric Neurourologic Conditions *229*

30. Brain Death in Children 232
TA Sheela

Evolution of Criteria for Brain Death *232* • Definition of Brain Death *232*
Process for Brain Death Determination *233* • Demonstration of Absent Cerebral Function *233*
Assessment of Brainstem Reflexes *233* • Apnea Test *234* • Interval Observation Period *235*
Number of Examinations, and Examiners *236* • Confirmatory Tests (Ancillary Studies) *236*
Special Consideration for Term Newborns Babies *239* • Certification of Brain Death *239*
Medical Record Documentation *239* • Supportive Care *241*

Index *245*

Plate 1

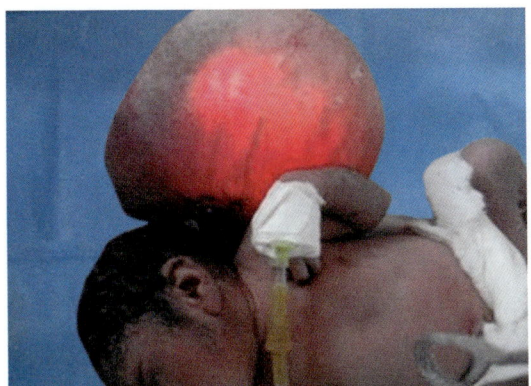

Figure 2.1 *Occipital meningocele:* Transilluminant sac contain minimal brain tissue

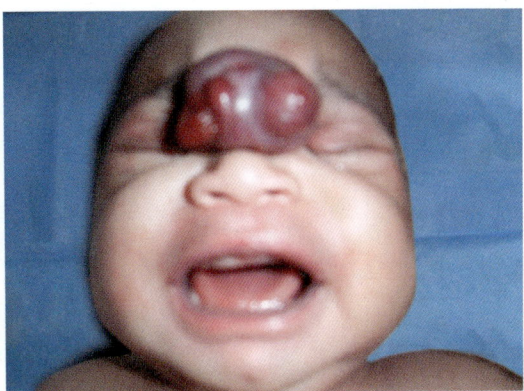

Figure 2.3 Nasal meningoencephalocele

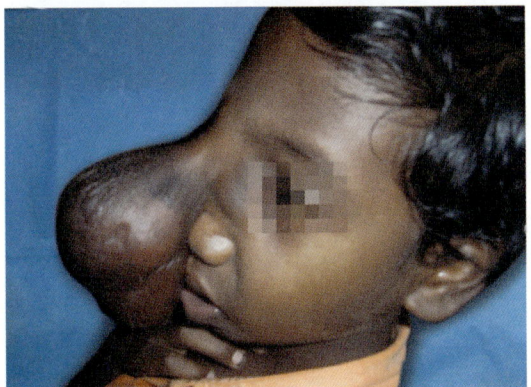

Figure 2.2 A rare case of large frontonasal meningoencephalocele

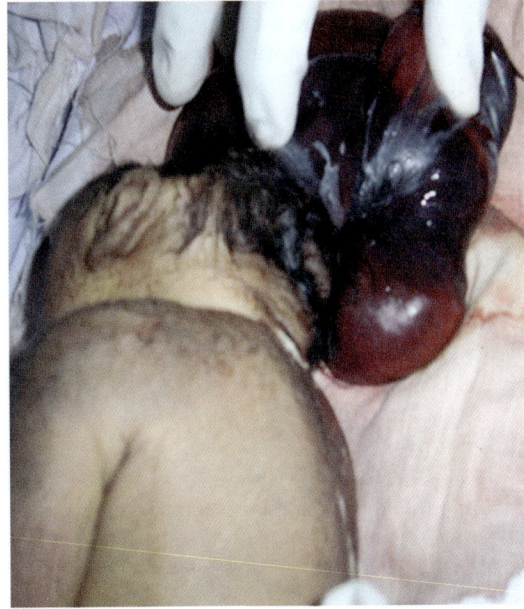

Figure 2.4 *Anencephaly:* Cranial vault defective and brain contents are inside the sac

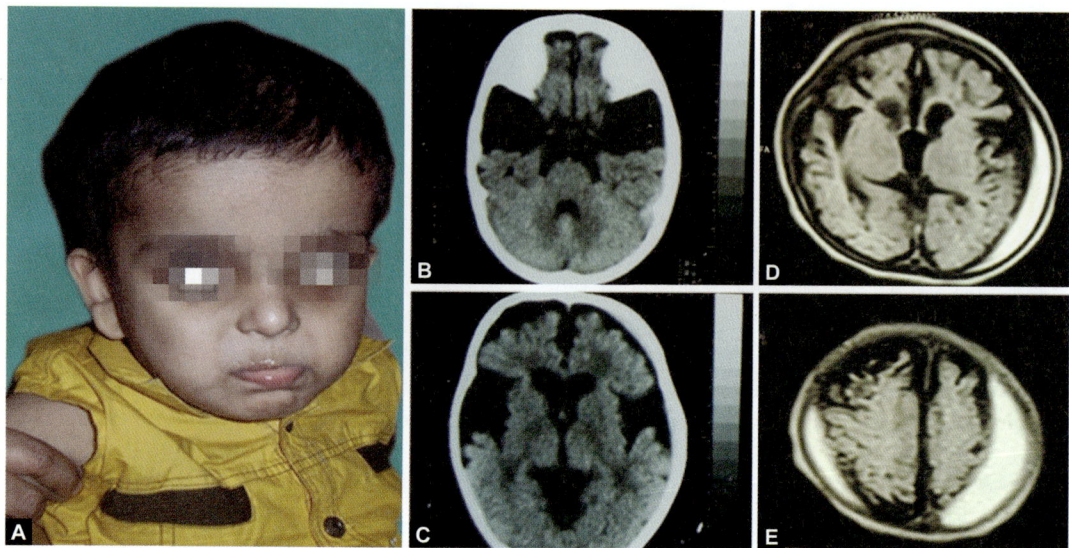

Figures 4.1A to E *Glutaric acidemia type I:* (A) Macrocephaly; (B and C) Dilated Sylvian fissure (Bat-wing appearance); (D and E) Nontraumatic subdural hematoma

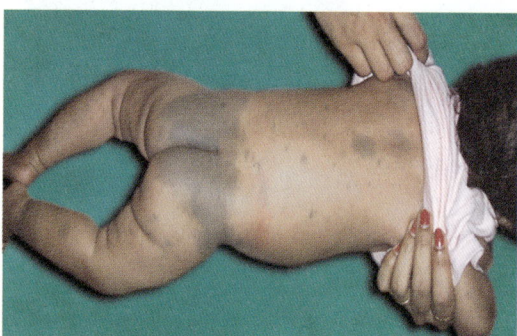

Figure 4.4 Extensive and persistent Mongolian blue spots may be an indicator of gray matter disorders like GM1 gangliosidosis or mucopolysaccharidosis

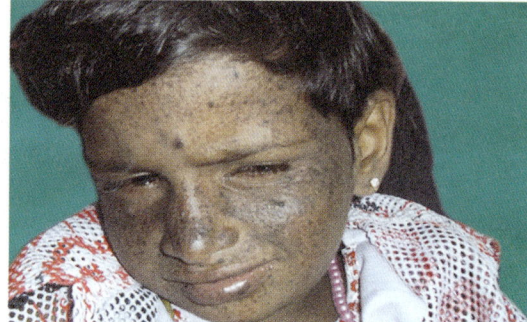

Figure 4.5 A subtle skin change to severe photo-dermatitis can be seen in xeroderma pigmentosa. This child had severe mental retardation (*DeSanctis-Cacchione syndrome*)

Plate 3

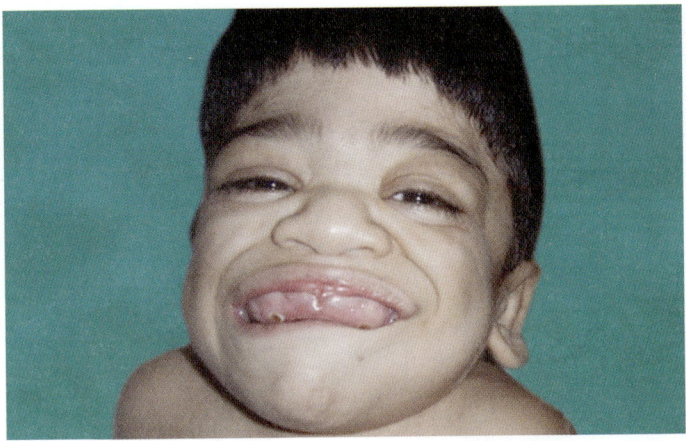

Figure 4.6 Role of facies
- High forehead, puffy eyelids, epicanthal folds
- Flat nasal bridge, anteverted nares, long philtrum
- Gingival hypertrophy, macroglossia—diagnostic of mucolipidosis type 1 (sialidosis I)

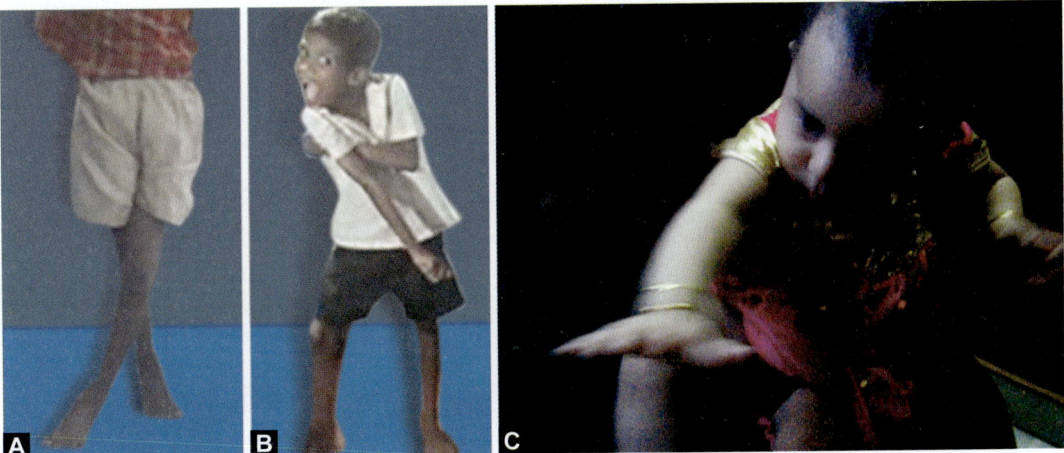

Figures 6.1A to C Types of cerebral palsy: (A) Diplegic CP—notice the scissoring; (B) Choreoathetotic CP—notice the twisted posturing; finger posturing; (C) Ataxic CP—early evidence of incoordinated approach

Plate 4

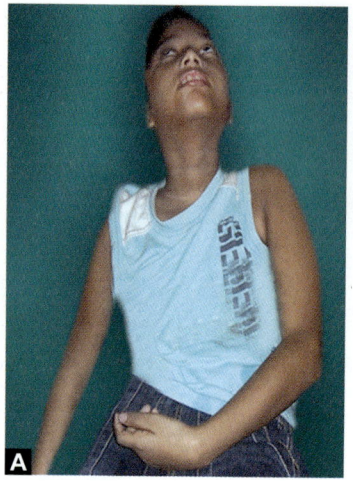

Figure 6.2A (A) Left hemiplegic CP

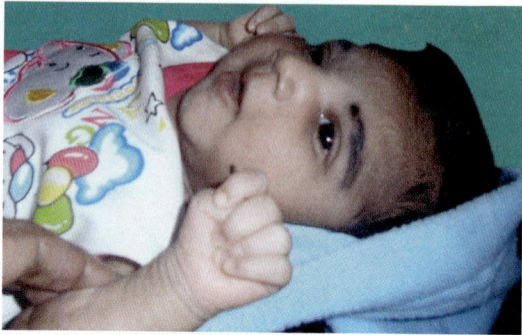

Figure 6.5 Persistent fisting

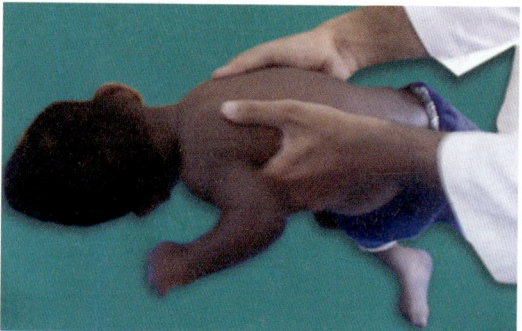

Figure 6.4 An early sign of cerebral palsy. On ventral suspension abnormal head and shoulder retraction; stiff extension of lower limbs

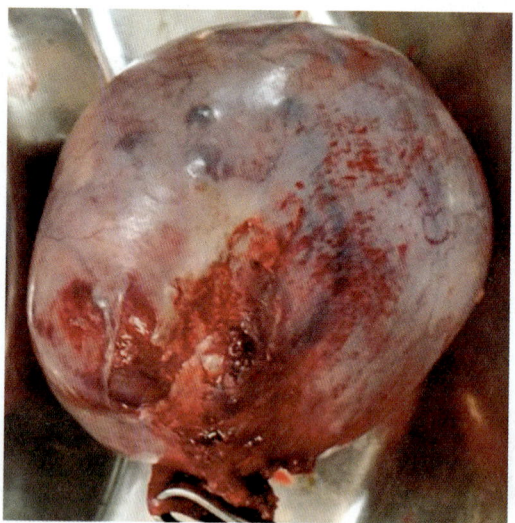

Figure 10.2 Ovarian tumor removed from a girl presented with encephalitis
Courtesy: CHILDS Trust Medical Research Foundation and Apollo Hospitals, Chennai

Plate 5

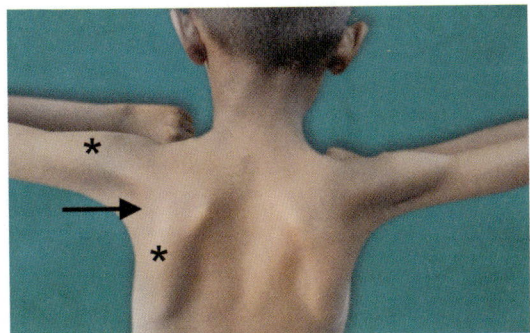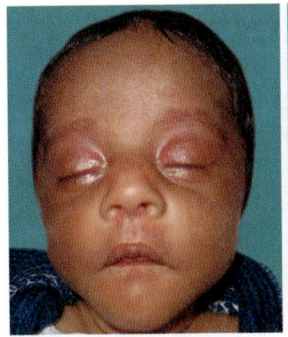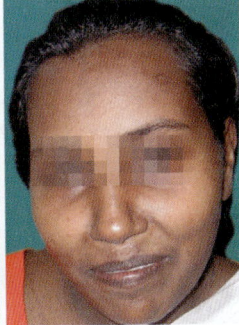

Figure 25.2: Valley sign in DMD. Note the valley (arrow) between hypertrophied deltoid and infraspinatus

Figure 25.3 Baby with congenital myotonic dystrophy, note the myopathic facies, also note the frontal baldness of mother, she was short (148 cm) and had myotonia, previous baby was still born

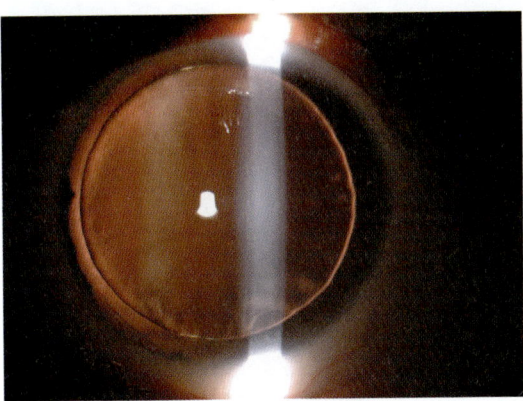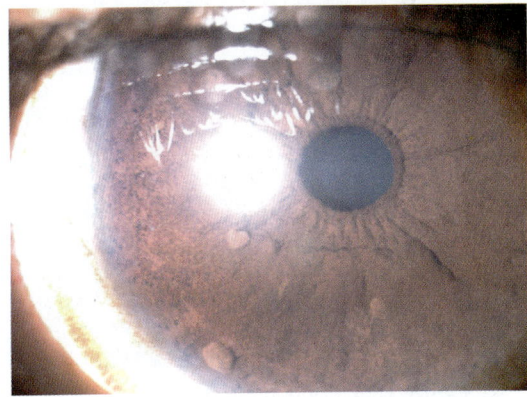

Figure 28.1 Aniridia

Figure 28.3 Lisch nodules

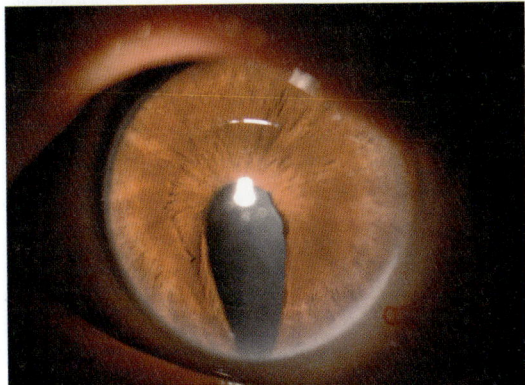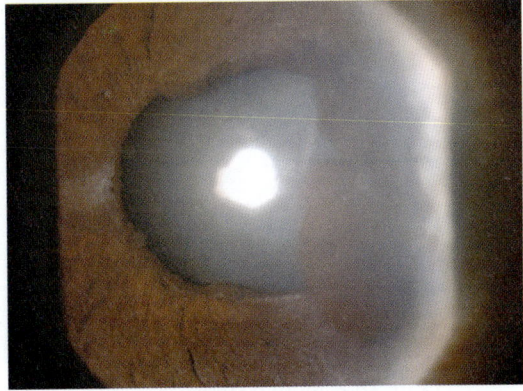

Figure 28.2 Iris coloboma

Figure 28.4 Congenital ectropion uvea with iris nodule

Plate 6

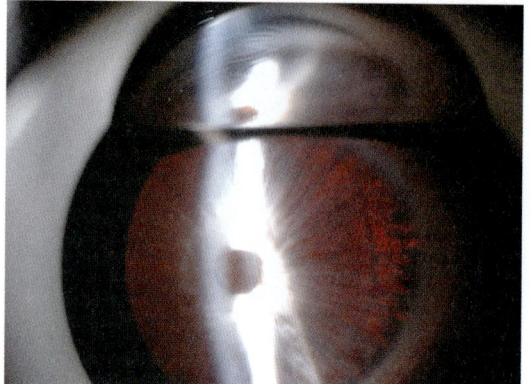

Figure 28.5 Iris transillumination defect

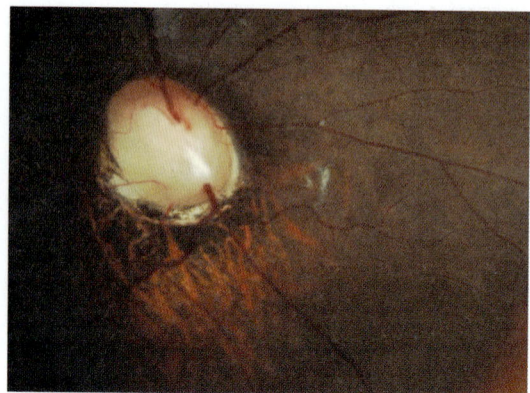

Figure 28.8 Coloboma of the optic nerve head

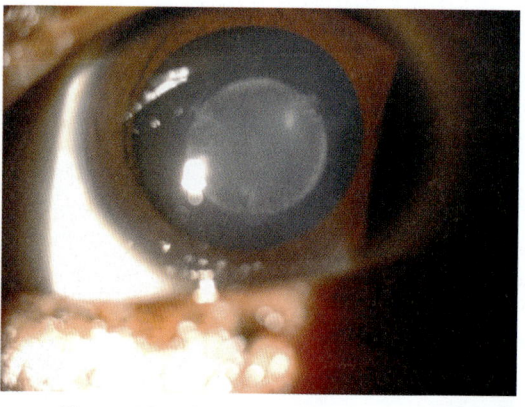

Figure 28.6 Congenital zonular cataract

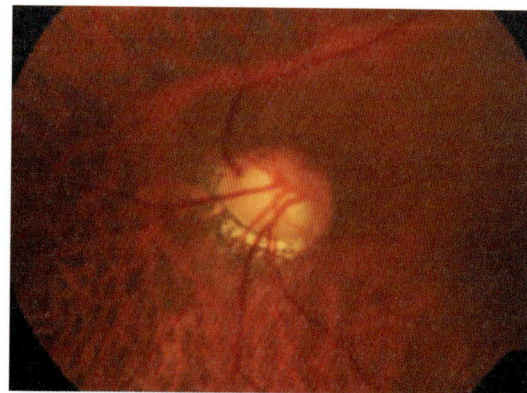

Figure 28.9 Tilted disc

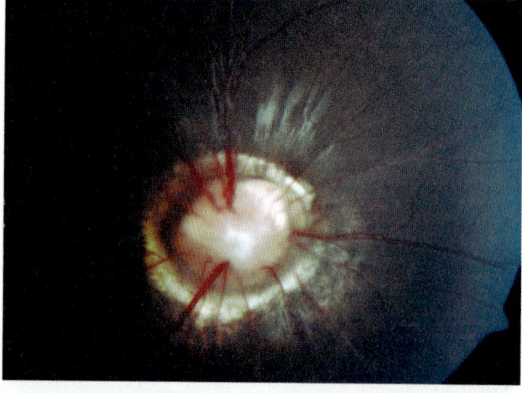

Figure 28.7 Morning glory syndrome

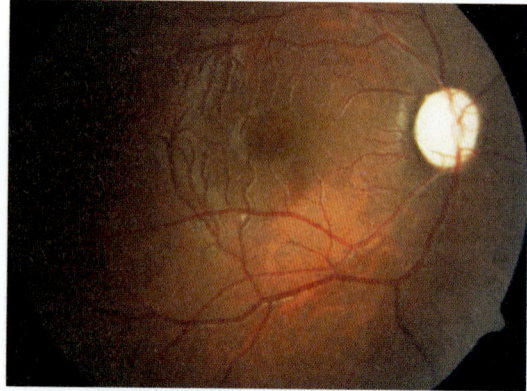

Figure 28.10 Primary optic atrophy

Plate 7

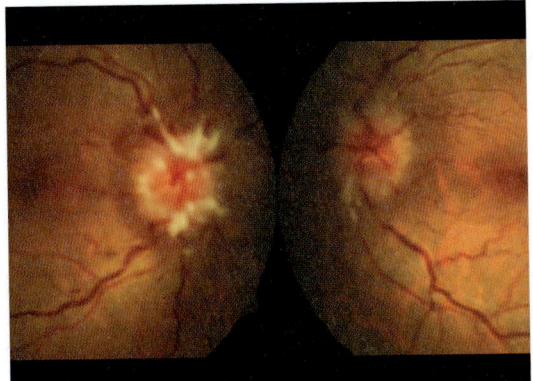

Figure 28.11 Papilledema

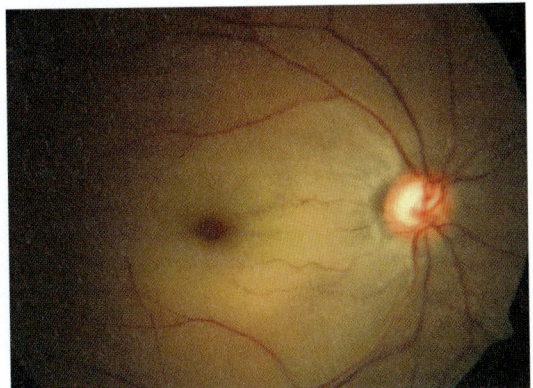

Figure 28.14 Cherry red spot

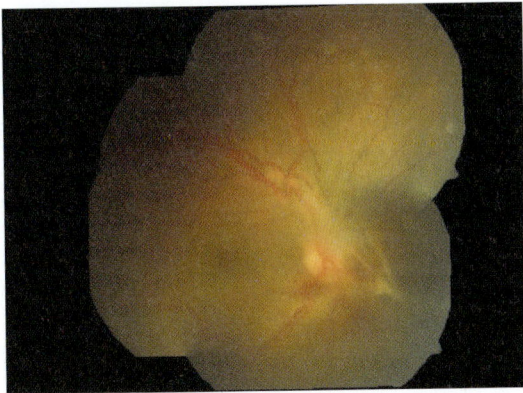

Figure 28.12 Retinal angioma in Von Hippel-Lindau's disease

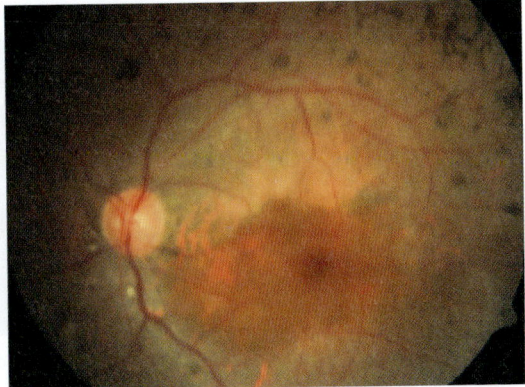

Figure 28.15 Retinitis pigmentosa

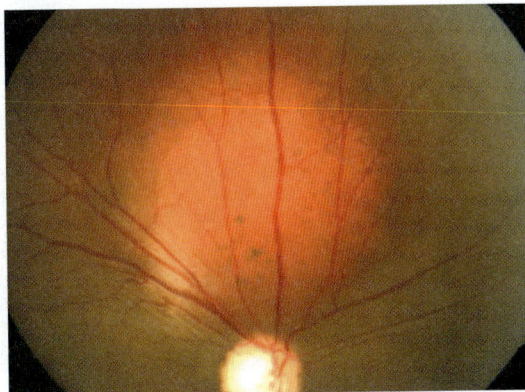

Figure 28.13 Circumscribed choroidal hemangioma

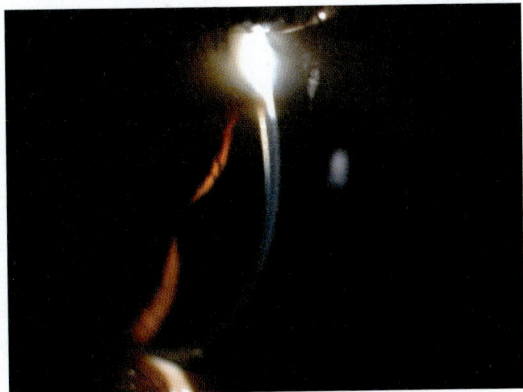

Figure 28.16 Kayser–Fleischer ring

Plate 8

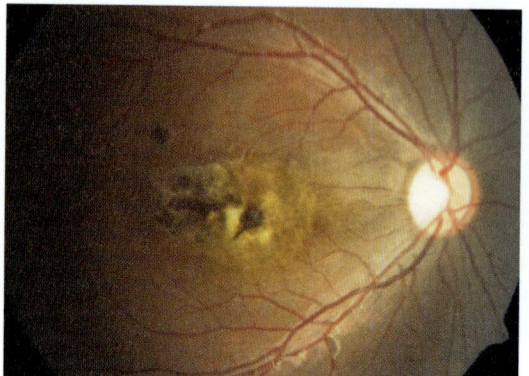

Figure 28.17 Toxoplasma scar at macula

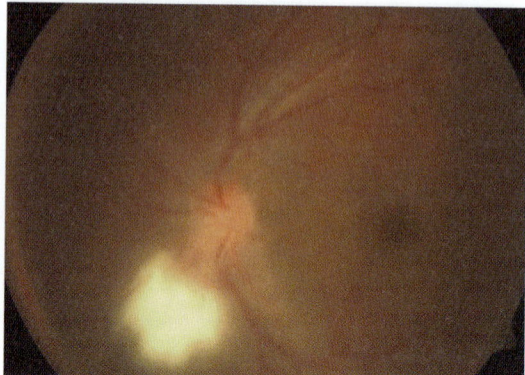

Figure 28.18 Active toxoplasma retinochoroiditis with headlight in fog appearance

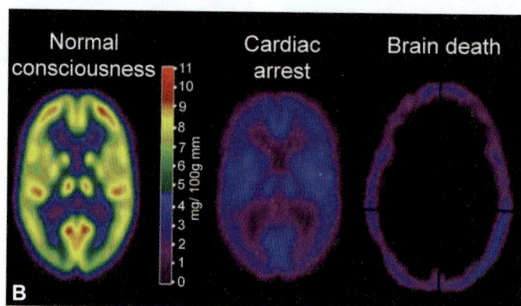

Figure 30.3B The hollow skull phenomenon of nuclear brain scanning

CHAPTER 1

Pitfalls in Neurological Examination of Children

G Kumaresan

INTRODUCTION

There is no need to feel tense in examining a child suspected to have a neurological ailment. It is easy when conducted systematically.

Examination will give a clue to plan further evaluation to confirm the diagnosis.

HISTORY

This will answer the following questions:
"A good history is often more informative than examination, especially in pediatric neurology" and should encourage the parents to record their statement verbatim, avoiding substituting medical terms. For example, the term vertigo or unconsciousness are vague terms and need more detailed description. At the end of examination, the clinician should be able to answer the following questions:[1]

- *Is there an illness*?
  Primary neurological or is it a complication of a systemic illness or nonorganic illness
- *Where is the lesion*?
  The localization can be of different types.
  - It can be a discrete localization
  - Multiple sites or diffuse lesion
  - Maybe related to a system—for example, disorder of extrapyramidal system. This is achieved mainly on the basis of physical signs.
- *What is the lesion*?
  History will give clue to pathology. For this mode of onset and the evolution is important.
  Onset can be:
  - Acute
  - Subacute
  - Chronic.

Evolution may be:
- Improving
- Deteriorating
- Static
- Recurrent illness.

The difficulties may arise because of parents poor recall, misconceptions and level of understanding. Parents may fail to recognize previous subtle symptoms and attribute acute exacerbation with intercurrent infection as acute onset.

For example, failure to recognize prior mild weakness may lead one to think of acute polymyositis whereas it may, in reality, be a muscular dystrophy brought to light by intercurrent infection. This is common in many chronic neurodegenerative illnesses. Similarly, failure to elicit past history of similar illness may lead to errors.

Example—wrong diagnosis of Guillain-Barré syndrome instead of periodic paralysis.

Hence while analyzing the history, care must be taken to clearly establish up to what point of time the child was completely normal. Was he normal in studies? Or was there a perceptible drop in academic performance? Did he actively participation in games or was a mere spectator in the ground. But mother will say he goes to play unless these details are specifically sought. Slight fall in school performance prior to onset of myoclonus is another example often overlooked in cases of SSPE.

The so-called acute onset has always been used to analyze as to whether it was in minutes or hours or over days. To give an example, acute onset of hemiplegia in minutes indicates hemorrhage or embolism whereas, over hours, indicates thrombosis or demyelination and, over days, may indicate space-soccupying lesion.

Similarly, while eliciting developmental milestones, parents may find it difficult to recall correctly. Certain milestones like walking or uttering first word are recalled more easily than others. Asking the parents to compare the development with previous sibling or relative's children may be useful. Once a clue to a probable pathology is suspected, history should include elucidation of corroborative symptoms like fever in infective pathology, symptoms of headache, vomiting, visual symptoms when intracranial hypertension is suspected. Remember that fundamental pathologies can overlap in certain illnesses. For example, symptoms of raised intracranial tension may coexist along with infective pathology.

Neurological examination is assisted greatly by developmental history. The examiner must be familiar with the developmental milestones at various ages.

It gives important information as to up to which point was the child normal, giving clue as to age at which the abnormality appeared helping to differentiate early onset static lesions from later onset acquired pathologies. However, it should be remembered that developmental history is not a substitute for a detailed neurological examination. Developmental history is based on the twin foundations of history and physical examination.

Edward Brett in his textbook[2] of pediatric neurology lists the pitfalls in the developmental history:

- Defects in communication
- Mothers are usually right—they are not bad observers and neglecting to take note of their observation you will assuredly repent later. This is true. Examples for this are plenty. When the grand mother told me that her grandchild admitted for fever is a good child and never cries when injections are given, I ignored it to miss the diagnosis of hereditary sensory neuropathy. When the mother was definite that the child moved the upper limb well on day one of life this will alert the diagnosis against of Erb's palsy and suspect osteomyelitis.

Parents misconceptions may also lead to difficulties in diagnosis. For example, early neck control due to rigidity may mask the diagnosis of cerebral palsy. Similar wrong impression may lead to doubts about static encephalopathies.

- Failure to recognize normal variations may lead to mistakes in development. Familiarity with Trivandrum developmental scale is important
- Adverse testing conditions—environment, mother, child and doctor
- Social, cultural and ethical factors.

Remember that history taking is not a mere collection of data and each detail collected should be analyzed simultaneously in the mental computer.

Family History

Pedigree charts in appropriate situations is needed. Examination of family photos may give important clue to certain familial conditions like myotonia dystrophica showing many mildly affected not overtly symptomatic persons.

EXAMINATION

General Examination

There may be many clues in general and system examination.

Broadly one may divide general examination findings into:
- Ocular signs
- Cutaneous signs
- Visceromegaly-enlarged liver

- Involvement of other systems like renal, lung, heart
- Skeletal abnormalities.

Dysmorphological Examination

It is gaining more importance. Many clinical conditions like chromosomal syndromes and metabolic disorders may show these features are classified as major and minor abnormalities. Major abnormality indicates disorders that need medical or surgical therapy. Minor abnormalities do not need them except for cosmetic reasons. Three or more minor abnormalities may be associated with one major abnormality or dysmorphic syndrome. More complete list can be obtained from London dysmorphic database or diagnostic dysmorphology.

Neurological examination should be complete covering:
- Higher functions
- Cranial nerves
- Spinomotor system
- Reflexes
- Sensory system
- Examination of spine and cranium.

Neurological examination should be a pleasant and enjoyable process for the child. The examiner should not be stiff but flexible and not too demanding. Much information can be gained by observing the child while eliciting the history and observing it play on the floor with his siblings.

In children, the examination can be carried out in three stages:
1. Observing the child as history is being taken.
2. Observing the child at play.
3. Examination needing restriction of the child.

Information collected by these though not in the order of conventional examination should be complete.

Higher function—up to two to three years of age, developmental milestones give a good information about mental development and the use of Trivandrum developmental scale which is a part of health cards is useful.

Evaluation of development in all domains of development will help to recognize pure motor delays, delay in visual, social and language development and will help to differentiate between neuromuscular disorders, pervasive developmental disorders and peripheral sensory defects. In older children, performance in school-academic, play activities and social behavior gives valuable clues. Nonverbal memory testing is simple by hiding an object in the presence of the child and asking him to find it after a few minutes.

Observe the emotion and behavior of the child. There can be three types of response when the child enters the doctor's room—he can be pleasant and smiling indicating a normal child or he may be afraid and cry—also a normal behavior. He may be hyperactive snatching the doctor's spectacle or stethoscope indicating behavior disorders. At the same time, his agility gives a good index of motor power. The third, child may ignore the doctor totally, not consider him as a living person but explore the environment. This behavior should alert the possibility of autistic spectrum.

Speech development has to be evaluated by observing the child's ability to recognize and name familiar objects, body parts, obeying commands and spontaneous speech.

In school going child's reading and writing also should be evaluated. At the end of a medical diagnosis as to -is it a peripheral defect like dysarthria, spastic or dystonic speech or central speech defect involving reception, and or expression of spoken and writing skills.

In older children mini mental scale as in adults can be used in addition to evaluation of academic achievements. While formal figures of IQ tests are useful, they are associated with fallacies and less importance is given to them. However, in one situation they are important. Good IQ and poor academic performance—a discrepancy between "ability and achievement" may indicate specific learning disability.

CRANIAL NERVES (FIG. 1.1)[3]

Olfactory nerve testing is not routinely done. It may be useful in unilateral proptosis or unilateral visual loss wherein unilateral anosmia may be seen. Children may recognize but not able to name them. Changes in facial expression may indicate recognition of smell.

Recognizing the mother by voice and not by seeing will alert about visual defects. Visual assessment below two years of age is done by STYCAR testing using tiny balls of different sizes.

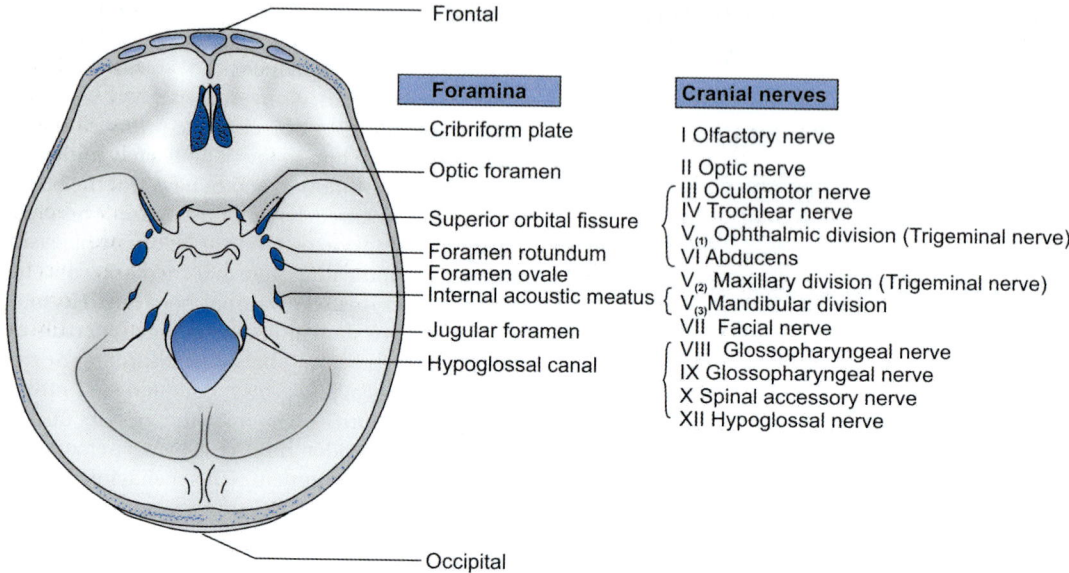

Figure 1.1 Foramina through which cranial nerves leave the skull[3]

Table 1.1 Appearance of optic fundus in three important clinical conditions			
	Papilledema	*Papillitis*	*Optic atrophy*
Depth	Elevated disc Physiological cup obliterated	Elevated disc Physiological cup obliterated	Shallow
Edge	Blurred edge	Blurred edge	Very sharp
Vessels	Engorged	Engorged	Narrow/few
Color	No venous pulse Hyperemia	Absent venous pulsations	Pallor
Vision	Good or enlarged blind spot	Poor vision or loss of central vision	Reduced vision

Between 3 years and 4 years, ability to recognize familiar items of different sizes and colors may be used. Beyond four years, E-test may be used.

Examination of pupil is important to differentiate peripheral versus cortical blindness. In unilateral visual loss, consensual light reflexes may obscure afferent visual defect and closing the other eye will bring about the pupillary asymmetry.

The torch used should have a central beam and not a diffuse light. Unless acute in onset, unilateral visual loss may remain unrecognized until the other eye is accidently closed. Look specifically for red or white reflex with the torch light. Fundus examination, though difficult, must be done. Pinching the back of neck gently elicits celiospinal reflex and dilates the pupil and may make examination easy. Do not make the child to focus a bright light as it will constrict the pupil. In younger children, defer fundus examination towards the end. First show the light beam on the hand or on the mother to make it comfortable. The color of disc may be grayish in infants. Every pediatrician should be confident of recognizing papilledema, pseudopapilledema and different types of optic atrophy (**Table 1.1**). Absence of venous pulsation is an early sign of papilledema.

Cover test is a simple bedside test to evaluate for squint. Slight divergent squint will alert about visual defects. Position of eyes at rest, range of movements in all directions should be evaluated (**Table 1.2**).

Gaze palsies and nystagmus give valuable localizing signs.

Pitfalls in Neurological Examination of Children

Table 1.2 Extraocular muscle paralysis (position at eye at rest)

Inferior oblique	III	Down and out
Inferior rectus	III	Up and in
Lateral rectus	VI	Medial
Medial rectus	III	Lateral
Superior oblique	IV	Upward and outward (head tilted)
Superior rectus	III	Down and in

Care should be taken not to mistake a few jerks at extremes of gaze (endpoint nystagmus) as abnormal. Type of nystagmus gives useful clue to the structure involved—rotary, pendular, gaze evoked and vertical are a few examples. Superior and inferior oblique muscle are tested in with eyes in the adducted position **(Figs 1.2A and B)**. Gaze palsies, Duane retraction syndrome, internuclear ophthalmoplegia, Cogen apraxia are easily recognizable. Looking at the bite marks on a biscuit is a good sign to test fifth motor functions. Corneal and conjunctival reflex share same reflex pathway

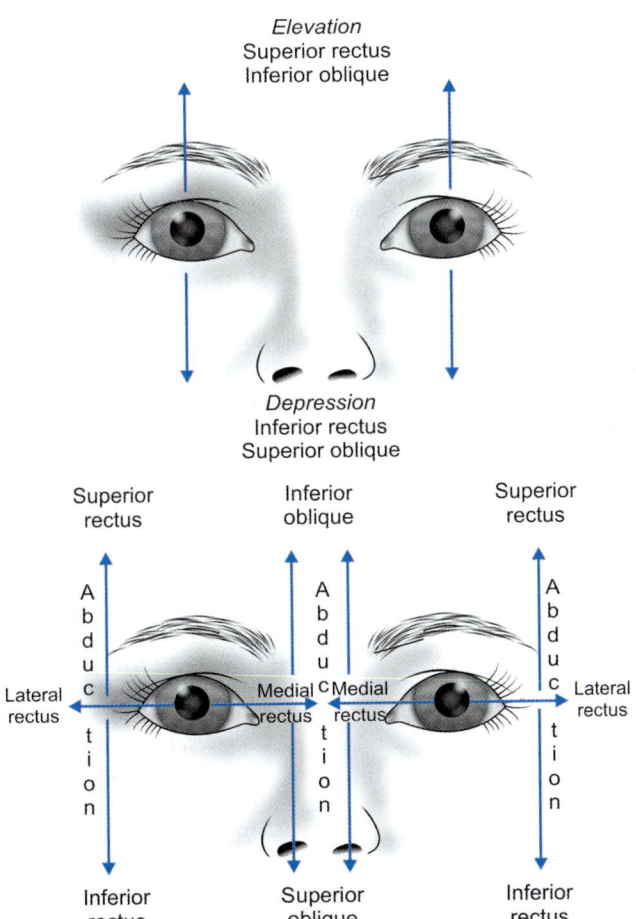

Figures 1.2A and B Extraocular muscle movement: (A) In primary position; (B) In aduction and adduction[4]

but the difference is in the receptor. Corneal reflex is mediated by free nerve endings carrying pain sensations whereas conjunctival reflex is mediated through touch receptors. Selective loss of corneal reflex occurs in high cervical cord lesions and selective loss of conjunctival reflex in pontine lesions affecting chief sensory nucleus.

Care must be taken to differentiate facial palsy from agenesis of depressor anguli oris (cardio-facial syndrome) wherein the angle of the mouth is deviated up as against down in facial palsy. Inability to bury the eyelashes on one side may be seen in unilateral facial palsy. Preserved emotional response, preserved corneal reflex and brisk jaw jerk will help to differentiate bilateral facial palsy of upper motor neuron versus lower motor neuron lesions. If bulbar palsy is suspected change in voice, nasal regurgitation and difficulty in swallowing liquids should be asked for. Palatal reflex, jaw jerk and emotional liability will help to differentiate bulbar versus pseudobulbar palsy. Power of hypoglossal nerve may be tested using a lollypop or asking to push the examiner's finger. *While localizing the cranial nerve signs, one should also remember about false localizing signs such as:*
- Sixth nerve palsy
- Visual field effects
- Foster-Kennedy syndrome
- Ocular bobbing
- Fifth nerve palsy
- Papilledema
- Trigeminal sensory loss.

Cranial Nerve Signs in High Cervical Cord Lesions

- Absent corneal reflux
- Nystagmus
- Papilledema
- Lower cranial nerve palsies.

However, certain combination of signs will alert to localization of level in serious situations of cerebral herniation.

Transtentorial Brain Herniation[5]

Diencephalic Stage

- Regular or Cheyne–stokes respiration (**Fig. 1.3**)
- Small, reactive pupils

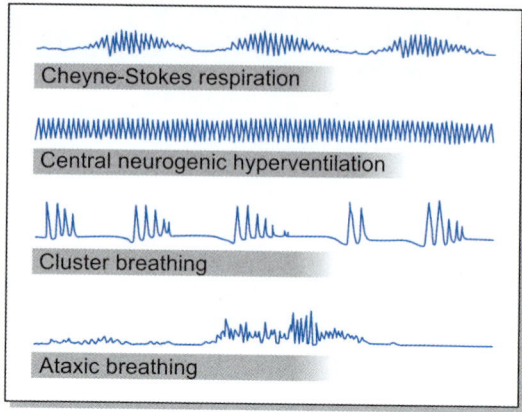

Figure 1.3 Patterns of respiration frequently observed in comatose patients

- Reflex ocular movements present
- Hypertonicity, decorticate rigidity.

Midbrain—Pontine Stage

- Regular or increased respiration (**Fig. 1.3**)
- Mid position, fixed pupils
- Eye movements conjugate or dysconjugate or absent
- Hypertonicity, decerebrate rigidity.

Medullary Stage

- Slow, irregular, and gasping respiration (**Fig. 1.3**); apnea
- Mid position or dilated, fixed pupils
- Reflex ocular movements absent
- Flaccidity.

Points to Remember—Cranial Nerves

- Unilateral visual loss may go unnoticed
- Unilateral anosmia is more important
- Diplopia indicates LMN paralysis of ocular muscles
- Diplopia in long distance indicates sixth nerve palsy
- Early visual loss in proptosis indicates optic nerve glioma
- In unilateral third nerve palsy test opposite side superior rectus (nuclear palsy)

- Facial sensation and palatal reflex are not routinely tested
- Onion peel sensory loss in the face occurs in brain stem lesion
- Reverse of UMN facial palsy (upper half affected) is seen in branch paralysis
- Unilateral deafness indicates peripheral lesions
- In fifth and twelfth nerve paralysis deviation occurs on the paralyzed side whereas in seventh and tenth nerve deviation is to the normal side.
- Trepezius and sternomastoid muscles are supplied by both cranial and spinal nerves.

Spinal Motor System Examination

The spinal motor system examination should cover the following five domains:
1. Nutrition
2. Power
3. Tone
4. Coordination
5. Involuntary movements.

If abnormalities are noted in-coordination cerebellar signs should be looked for. If abnormal involuntary movements are noticed in extrapyramidal system and the type of involuntary movements, their absence in sleep should be taken note of. In lower motor neuron lesions, look for fasciculation. Tone should be examined by palpation, resistance to passive movements, typical postures and various angles signs like Scarf sign, popliteal angle. Spasticity is velocity-dependent (clasp knife) and gives way, whereas in rigidity the resistance is uniform (lead pipe). Power can be tested using MRC chart in older children but in young children best observed power and looking for asymmetry will be informative **(Table 1.3)**.

Examination of the child at play or on walking on outer border of feet may bring out signs of minor degrees of weakness, example—Fog sign. Posture of the child may give you characteristic clue, examples Erbs' palsy, claw hand, decorticate or decerebrate posture or unilateral persistent fist **(Fig. 1.4)**.

While testing the reflexes, the child can be seated in mother's lap and examining the mother's reflex first will make the child cooperative.

Abdominal reflexes absence on one side is usually seen in recent pyramidal lesions and hence may be preserved in congenital hemiplegia.

Soft neurological signs indicate minor degrees of incoordination or involuntary movements persistent beyond 5–6 years of age. This may be seen in children with learning disabilities. However, this has no significant localizing value.

In the presence of one abnormal sign, look for other signs of that system involvement.

For example, if spasticity is noted, look for other signs of pyramidal dysfunction but all the signs may not be present in the same child **(Table 1.4)**.

Cerebellar Signs

Nystagmus, finger-nose incoordination, staccato speech, titubation, rebound, dysdiadochokinesia,

Table 1.3 Code for grading muscle power (MRC Gradez)[6]

Grade	Characteristic	Muscle power (%)
0	No muscular contraction	0
1	Trace, visible contraction without motion of joint	10
2	Movement at joint but not against gravity	25
3	Full movement at joint against gravity, variable resistance	50
4	Resists opposing force of moderate strength	75
5	Maximal resistance	100

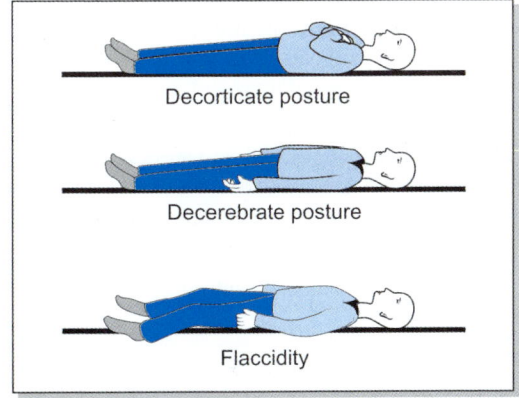

Figure 1.4 Postural motor abnormalities frequently observed in comatose patients[6]

dysmetria, truncal ataxia, pendular knee jerk, heel knee incoordination toe heel test stance and gait abnormalities.

Reflexes—this gives a more objective evaluation than many other signs always include.

Superficial Reflexes (Table 1.5)

The spinal levels involved in some cutaneous reflexes.

While eliciting abdominal reflexes, it should be stroked towards the umbilicus.

Deep Tendon Reflexes (Table 1.6)

The spinal levels involved in the more important deep tendon reflexes.
- Visceral reflexes—Bladder and bowel control
- Bladder reflexes atonic, automatic, autonomous
- Reflexes—Anal and bulbo cavernous.

Primitive and Postural Reflexes

Developmental reflexes are described well in clinical methods in pediatric diagnosis by Balu H Athreya indicating there localizing and clinical significance **(Table 1.7)**.

SIGNIFICANCE AND USE OF THE NEURODEVELOPMENTAL REFLEXES IN PEDIATRIC PRACTICE

- Abnormal responses of these categories suggest brain damage (e.g. Cerebral palsy, head injury, and meningitis).
- Persistence of reflexes mediated by the brain stem and spinal cord after four to six months of age signifies brain damage.
- Delay in the appearance of reflexes mediated at the midbrain and cortical level after appropriate age signifies brain damage.
- Asymmetric responses (such as lack of parachute response on one side only and unilateral Moro) signify hemiplegia.
- These reflexes may mature at a slower pace in children with cerebral palsy (e.g. Landau reflex may appear only at age two).

Table 1.4 Signs of upper motor neuron (UMN) lesions[1]

Signs of pyramidal dysfunction	Signs of extra pyramidal dysfunction
Spasticity	Rigidity
Deep tendon jerks exaggerated	Normal or difficult to elicit
Absent superficial reflexes	No change
Distribution of weakness	
Distal more than proximal (exception exist)	Facial expression, trunk muscles Limb muscles (generally proximal more)
Plantar extensor	Flexors
Clonus	No clonus but tremors, dystonia chorea

Table 1.5 Superficial reflexes[4]

Reflex	Spinal segment
Superficial abdominal reflexes	Thoracic 7–12
Cremasteric reflex	Lumbar 1
Plantar response	Sacral 1
Anal reflex	Sacral 4 and 5

Table 1.6 Deep tendon reflexes[4]

Reflex	Spinal segment	Peripheral nerve
Biceps jerk	Cervical 5 and 6	Musculocutaneous
Supinator or brachioradialis jerk	Cervical 5 and 6	Radial
Triceps jerk	Cervical 6 and 7	Radial (Musculospiral)
Knee jerk	Lumbar 2, 3 and 4	Femoral
Ankle jerk	Sacral 1	Tibial

Table 1.7 Primitive and postural reflexes[1]

Group	Reflex	Level
Group 1	Flexor withdrawal Extensor thrust Crossed extensor	Spinal cord level
Group 2	Asymmetric tonic neck Symmetric tonic neck Positive supporting Negative supporting Tonic labyrinthine	Brainstem level
Group 3	Neck correcting body Labyrinthine correcting body Optical correcting body	Midbrain
Group 4	Various balancing reflexes	Cortical/cerebellar
Group 5	Moro reflex	Stretch receptors of the neck
Group 6	Parachute reflex Landau reflex	? semicircular canals

- Older children with head injury and infectious brain insult lose their advanced reflexes and regress back to spinal cord and brain stem level soon after the cerebral insult. They then go through the various stages during the recovery period.
- These reflexes are useful as indicators of prognosis in walling for children with cerebral palsy, for example, strong asymmetric tonic reflex, crossed—extensor reflex, and Moro, together with absence of parachute response, give a poor prognosis for walking
- These reflexes can be useful in physical therapy. For example, rolling an infant over a large beach ball will elicit a parachute response if present. This will help open spastic fisted thumb, since opening of the palm and extension of fingers is part of this response. A child with severe tonic labyrinthine reflex may get equinus deformity if he is in supine position most of the day, since extensor tone is increased in this position. If this child is treated in prone position most of the day, flexor tone is accentuated as part of the same reflex.

Associated Movements

A normal child has freely swinging arms during walking. In the presence of pyramidal or extrapyramidal disease, this movement is lost. A paralyzed upper arm also does not move and swing.

Forgetting one of them in certain situation will lead to errors in localization.

Sensory Examination

This is often overlooked. History of absence of crying while injections are given, presence of trophic changes and nonhealing ulcers will alert to sensory abnormalities. While examining for pain sensation, always test the area of suspected loss first without the child seeing you. Normal rooting reflex indicates normal facial sensation.

When muscle disease is suspected do not forget to look for myotonia.

When peripheral nerve disease is suspected do not forget to look for thickened nerves.

Gait abnormalities like hemiplegic gait, fisted thumb gait, diplegic scissoring gait, ataxic gait, high stepping gait and slow shuffling gaits are spotters to be picked up.

Points to Remember— Spinomotor System

- Differential weakness of muscles of the same dermatome indicates anterior horn cell involvement
- Distribution of hypertrophied muscles help in the differential diagnosis of muscle diseases
- Limb Girdle syndrome can occur in anterior horn cell disease, myopathies, polymyositis and myasthenia

- Myotonia and thickened peripheral nerves are usually missed
- Foot drop in pyramidal weakness is not dependent on gravity
- Peripheral nerve diseases can be purely motor, purely sensory or purely autonomic
- Muscle weakness with preserved deep tendon jerks are seen in metabolic myopathies
- Painful muscle indicates inflammatory or metabolic muscle disease.

Head and spine examination should not be forgotten. Care should be taken to measure head circumference and repeating it to avoid errors in serial recording on follow-up. Give the other end of the tape to the child or first measure head size of the parent to win the child's co-operation."Head circumference is the direct reflection of head growth and may be the first index of underlying abnormality". It is measured 1-2 cm above the glabella anteriorly and most prominent part of the occiput posteriorly. Head circumference is influenced by skull shape for example dolichocephalic head has a larger volume. Always compare the head size with other anthropo metric values to rule out small head proportionate to small stature (proportionate microcephaly).

Remember the head growth of pre-term infants is higher and hence should not be mistaken for progressive macrocephaly.

At the end of examination core signs consistent with the diagnosis is considered first followed by signs and symptoms that does not fit with this be looked into as to an alternate diagnosis or additional sites of involvement in the same disease process. Even then some signs may remain unexplained which will have to be followed.

REFERENCES

1. Gorden N. Pediatric neurology for the clinician. Spastic International Medical Publication. The Lavenham Press Limited, Suffolk; 1976.
2. Brett EM. Pediatric neurology. Churchill Livingstone. New York; 1983.
3. Farmer TW. Pediatric neurology. 3rd edn. Harper and Row Publishers. Philadelphia; 1983.
4. Swaiman KF. Pediatric neurology-principles and practice. Mosby, Elsevier.
5. Neurologic emergencies in infancy and childhood. Pellock JM, Myer EC. Harper and Row Publishers; 1984.
6. Atherya BH. Clinical methods in pediatric diagnosis. CBS Distributors, New Delhi, 2000.

CHAPTER 2

Malformations of the Central Nervous System

TM Ananda Kesavan

INTRODUCTION

Congenital brain malformation is a major group of neurological disorders associated with high morbidity and mortality. During last few years, due to better supportive care and multidisciplinary approach, the survival of children suffering from congenital brain malformation has improved. Improvement in antenatal detection, availability of newer diagnostic modality and counseling of parents—all urge a need for better understanding about congenital brain malformation in children.

Incidence: The incidence varies in different populations. A study conducted in Chennai, found an incidence of brain malformations to be 2.4 per 1000 births. 74% of fetal deaths have brain malformations and one-third of all major anomalies involve central nervous system.[1]

ETIOLOGY

In majority (60%) the exact etiology is not known. Genetic factors responsible for 27.5% of cases, chromosomal factors for 6% and environmental factors for 3.5%.

The timing of antenatal insult is more important than the nature of the teratogen in inducing a malformation. Teratogen exposure in the first trimester causes the most severe malformations. Main etiological agents are:

- *Intrauterine infection*: Rubella, varicella, CMV, mumps, *Toxoplasma gondii*, HIV, CMV, HSV.
- *Maternal metabolic derangements*: Phenylketonuria, overt diabetes mellitus, toxemia, malnutrition especially folic acid deficiency.
- *Physical agents*: Trauma, fetal position, crowding, hyperthermia, radiation.
- *Toxins and drugs*: CO, alcohol, vitamin excess or deficiency, antimetabolite, AEDs.
- Genetic and chromosomal factors.

CLASSIFICATION

Classification of congenital brain malformation has been done by several and different systems and most of them are according to the major developmental stages of human brain. A commonly used classification is followed here.[2]

- Disorder of neurulation.
- Midline malformation of the forebrain.
- Disorder of neuronal migration.
- Disorder of cerebellar development.
- Hypertrophic dysplasia of the brain.
- Disorder of ventricular system.
- Vascular and other malformation.

Disorder of Neurulation

The defects due to disorder of neurulation occurs in the first 4 weeks of gestation. It is the most common type of CNS malformation. There is incomplete or defective formation of neural tube from neural placode e.g. anencephaly, cephalocele.

- *Cephalocele*: It is a skull defect in association with herniation of intracranial content. The sac may contain leptomeninges and CSF (menigocele) or leptomeninges, CSF and brain (meningoencephalocele). In atretic cephalocele skin covered by subcutaneous tissue consists of meningeal or CNS tissue. The 90% of the cases involve the midline. Most often in occipital region (**Fig. 2.1**), followed by frontal (**Figs 2.2 and 2.3**), parietal, nasal and transsphenoidal. Prognosis depends on presence or absence of brain tissue in the herniated sac and associated other anomalies.
- In anencephaly cranial vault is defective and structures above brainstem are incomplete.

The incidence is 1 in 1000 live. The insult occurs between 16 days and 26 days. It is 4–7 times more common in females with lowest incidence in Asia. The cranial vault is defective (**Fig. 2.4**); frontal, parietal and occipital lobes are partially absent. Forebrain structures including pituitary do not develop. Only vascular tangles of remnant tissue is seen above brainstem. It is a lethal condition

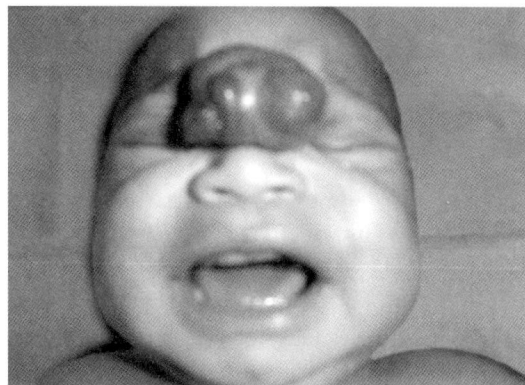

Figure 2.3 Nasal meningoencephalocele
(For color version, see Plate 1)

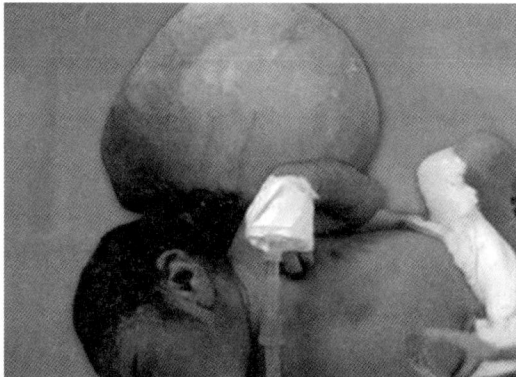

Figure 2.1 *Occipital meningocele:* Transilluminant sac contain minimal brain tissue
(For color version, see Plate 1)

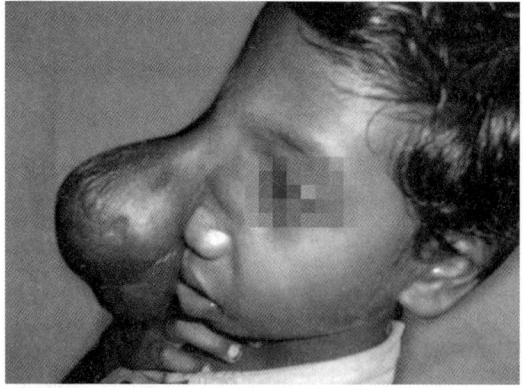

Figure 2.2 A rare case of large frontonasal meningoencephalocele
(For color version, see Plate 1)

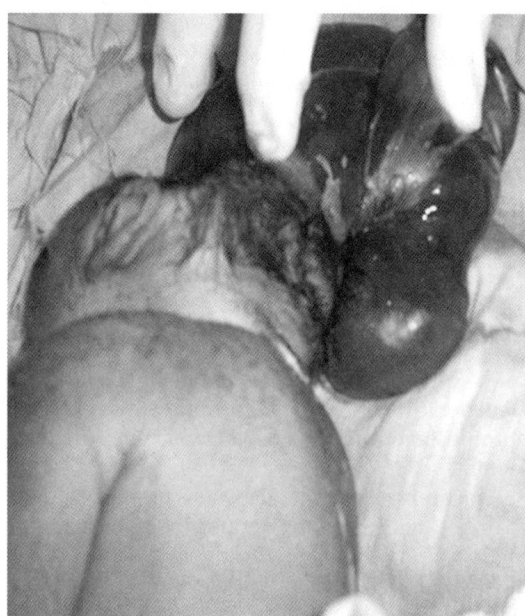

Figure 2.4 *Anencephaly:* Cranial vault defective and brain contents are inside the sac
(For color version, see Plate 1)

and most children are still born. Antenatal USG supported by high alpha-feto protein (AFP) will help in diagnosis.

Midline Malformation of the Forebrain

Malformation occurs due to intrauterine insult during 4–8 weeks of gestation. Major malformations under this category include: Holoprosencephaly, arhinencephaly, septo-optic dysplasia and agenesis of corpus callosum.

Holoprosencephaly: Here there is failure of separation of prosencephalon into symmetrical cerebral hemispheres. Clinical features include: delayed development, spastic quadriplegia, seizures, failure to thrive and neuroendocrine dysfunction. Majority of them exhibit midline facial dysplasia ranging from hypertelorism to midline facial aplasia with single median eye. About one third have other system malformations. More common in children of diabetic mothers and in chromosomal anomalies (Trisomy-13,18, triploidy).

There are three types of holoprosencephaly:
1. *Alobar*: Brain consist of a single lobe and single ventricle **(Fig. 2.5A)**
2. *Semilobar*: Incomplete interhemispheric fissure
3. *Lobar*: Mildest form with absent corpus callosum and septum pellucidum **(Fig. 2.5B)**.

Agenesis of corpus callosum: It may be complete or partial. Clinical features are mental retardation, learning disabilities, exotropia, epilepsy, hypertelorism. Also associated with other CNS malformations like heterotopias, microgyria, etc. EEG is characterized by interhemispheric asynchrony.[3]

Characteristic imaging features of corpus callosum agenesis are:
- High riding 3rd ventricle open superiorly **(Fig. 2.6A)**
- Radial spoke like orientation of gyri
- Parallel nonconverging lateral ventricles-medial margin concave
- Colpocephaly–enlarged occipital horn **(Fig. 2.6B)**.

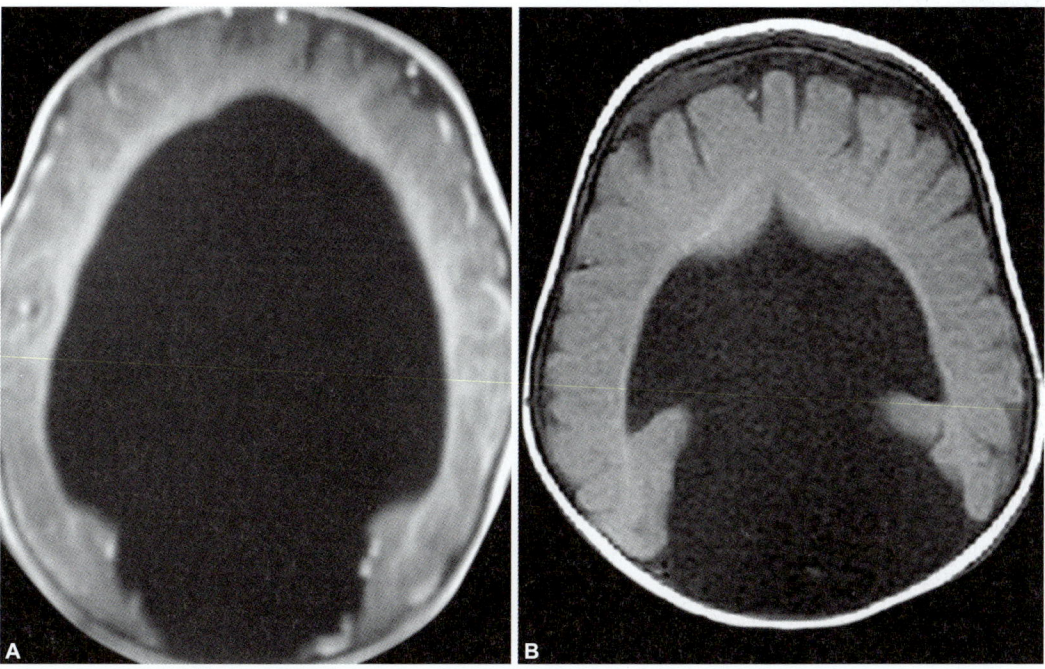

Figures 2.5A and B (A) *Alobar holoprosencephaly:* Brain showing a single lobe and single ventricle; (B) *Lobar holoprosencephaly:* Mild form with partial separation of ventricle

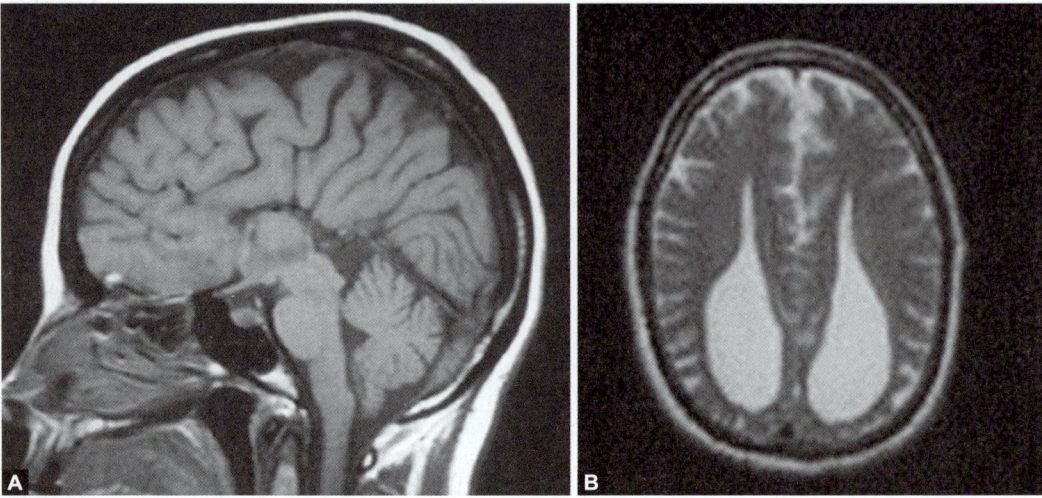

Figures 2.6A and B (A) *Agenesis of corpus callosum:* High riding 3rd ventricle open superiorly and radial spoke like orientation of gyri; (B) Parallel nonconverging lateral ventricles (medial margin concave) and colpocephaly

Andermann's syndrome (AR, Agenesis of CC with MR and peripheral neuropathy) and Aicardi syndrome (X-LD only in females, mental retardation, chorioretinal, vertebral anomalies, myoclonus) are associated with corpus callosum agenesis.

- *Corpus callosum lipoma*: It is due to persistence of meninx primativa, not a true neoplasm
  - *Two types*: Anterior-bulky, tubulonodular, associated with forebrain and rostral callosal anomalies and posterior curvilinear seen with near normal corpus callosum. In 50% of corpus callosum agenesis have lipoma.
- *Septo-optic dysplasia*: The association of absent of septum pellucidum with hypoplasia of optic nerve, corpus callosum and anterior commissure is called septo-optic dysplasia. Clinical manifestations are mainly due to endocrine dysfunction and visual impairment
- *Arhinencephaly*: There is absence of olfactory bulbs, tracts and tubercles, usually accompanied by holoprosencephaly and septo-optic dysplasia.

Disorder of Neuronal Migration

Neuronal migration disorder (NMD) is a group of brain malformations resulting from interference in normal neuronal migration at the time of brain development (8–20 weeks of gestation). The migrating neurons fail to reach their intended destination.

Neuronal migration is very important stage in brain development. Cerebral gyri and sulci are formed due to migration of the neuron. If there were no gyri and sulci, the brain will be so large that a normal delivery would not be possible.

Clinical Features

They are in order of frequency: Seizure—64%, delayed development—42%, mental retardation—25%, motor deficit—42% and others—dysmorphic features, poor schooling. Some of them may be normal also. Clinical features also depends on the associated conditions.

Common migration disorders are lissencephaly, schizencephaly, heterotopia, and cortical dysplasia.

Lissencephaly: The word Lissos (Gk) means—smooth. It is the most common migration disorder. It occurs due to insult to fetal brain occur during 8–14 weeks gestation. Characteristic feature is paucity of gyral and sulcal formation. In lissencephaly cortex shows 4 layers (layer III and IV missing). It is associated with deletion and mutation in LISI on 17p.

Clinical features of lissencephaly are intractable seizures, mental retardation, microcephaly, delayed development. Lissencephaly broadly divided in 2 types.

Type I is classical Agyria—pachygyria spectrum. It is classically seen in Miller-Dieker syndrome (microcephaly, long philtrum, narrow temples, anteverted nares, wide spaced eyes, etc.) and lissencephaly with cerebellar hypoplasia.

Type II lissencephaly has disorganized cluster of neurons with haphazard orientation and no definitive layer or pattern (cobblestone lissencephaly) associated with Walker-Warburg syndrome, muscle-eye disease and Fukuyama congenital muscular dystrophy.

MRI in lissencephaly is very characteristic. It shows smooth brain with thick, broad cortex **(Fig. 2.7)**. Shallow vertically oriented sylvian fissures giving an overall figure of eight (8) appearance in axial imaging.

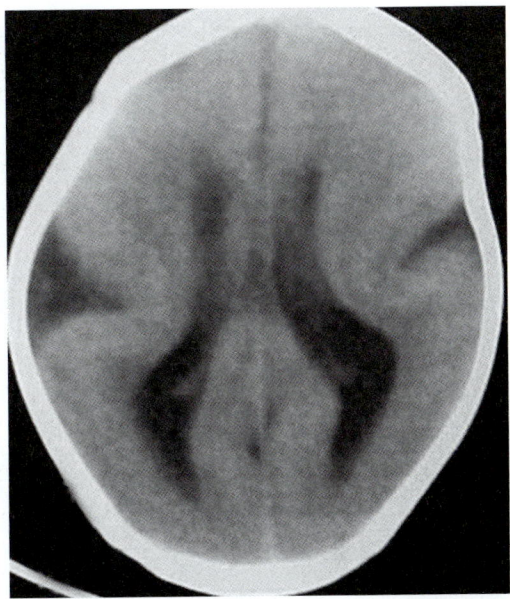

Figure 2.7 *Lissencephaly:* Smooth brain, thickened cortex with figure of 8 appearance. Also note shallow vertically oriented sylvian fissure

Schizencephaly: Gray matter lined clefts extend from subarachnoid space to lateral ventricle (Schiz Greek-cleft). It is caused by defect in neuronal migration in fourth month of gestation. Two types are described:

Closed lip schizencephaly where no connection of the cleft to the ventricle and present with hemiparesis or motor delay. In minor deformity child may asymptomatic.

Open lip schizencephaly where clefts are filled with CSF. It may be unilateral or bilateral and common clinical features are: hemiplegia, epilepsy, mental retardation. The 80–90% is associated with absent septum pellucidum.

In schizencephaly MRI will show the sides of cleft touching and lined by dysplastic cortex **(Fig. 2.8A)** or clefts that may be open and filled with CSF **(Fig. 2.8B)**.

- *Heterotopia*: It is another form of NMD in which there is focal collection of ectopic neurons in cerebral hemispheres. Three types of heterotopias are: 1) Subependymal (nodules develop from subependymal region to ventricular system), 2) Focal: gray matter (mass lesion) in deep sub-cortical white matter, 3) Diffuse (underlying band of gray matter and white matter in band manner— band heterotopias or double cortex syndrome **(Figs 2.9 and 2.13)**. It is commonly associated with corpus callosum agenesis also.[4]
- *Cortical dysplasia*: Disorder in which developing neurons complete the initial phase of neuronal migration, i.e. to the cortex, but fail to organize themselves in a six layered cortical pattern.

Different types:
- *Focal*: Irregular inner and outer surface of sulci and gyri
- *Diffuse*: Bilatral involvement
- *Bilateral perisylvian syndrome*: Insular, opercular and perisylvian dysplasia and underdeveloped sylvian fissures.

Disorder of Cerebellar Development

From 32 days of gestation to 1 year postnatally. *Main malformations under this category are:*
1. Cerebellar agenesis.
2. Joubert syndrome.
3. Chiari malformations.
4. Dandy-Walker syndrome.

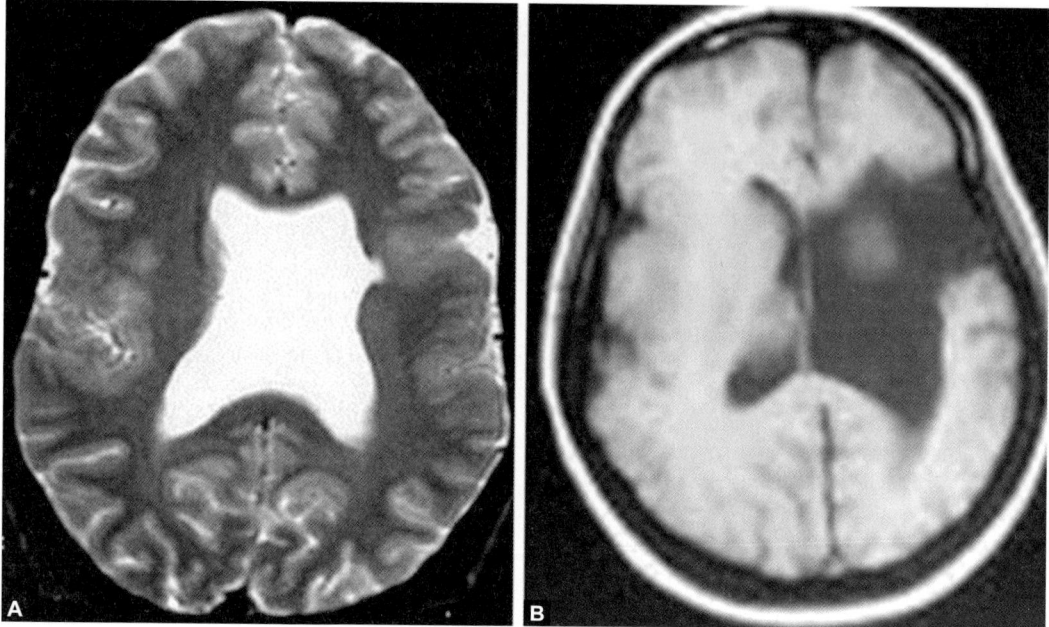

Figures 2.8A and B *Schizencephaly:* Gray matter lined clefts extend from subarachnoid space to lateral ventricle. (A) Type I-close lip; (B)Type II-open lip schizencephaly

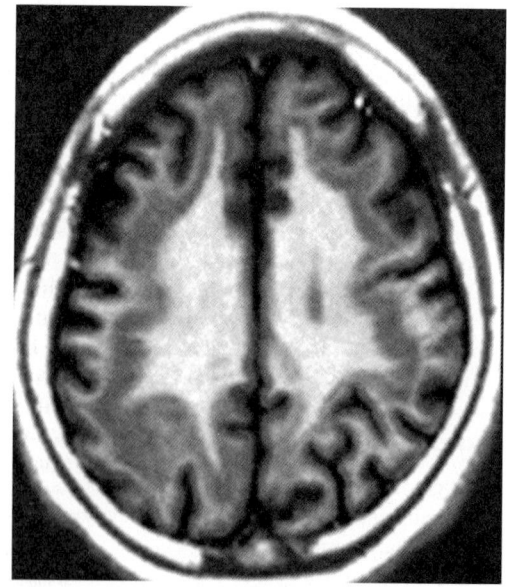

Figure 2.9 *Double cortex syndrome:* Alternate bands of gray and white matter

- *Cerebellar aplasia*: Isolated agenesis of cerebellum is uncommon and often asymptomatic. It may be partial or complete and may be associated with trisomy 13 and 18. When symptomatic, patients show hypotonia, incoordination, tremor, ataxia and delayed motor development.
- *Joubert syndrome*: Autosomal recessive trait with agenesis of cerebellar vermis. In infancy presents with generalized hypotonia and diminished DTR; later delayed motor milestones and truncal ataxia are characteristic. Rarely they present with alternating periods of apnea and hyperpnea. The respiratory abnormality improves with maturation. Neuroimaging shows enlarged fourth ventricle and dilated cistern magna (Molar tooth appearance) **(Figs 2.10A and B)**.
- *Chiari malformation*: First described by Hans Chiari (Austria) and Dr Julius Arnold, later contributed to the definition. Students of Dr Arnold suggested the term "Arnold-Chiari

Malformations of the Central Nervous System

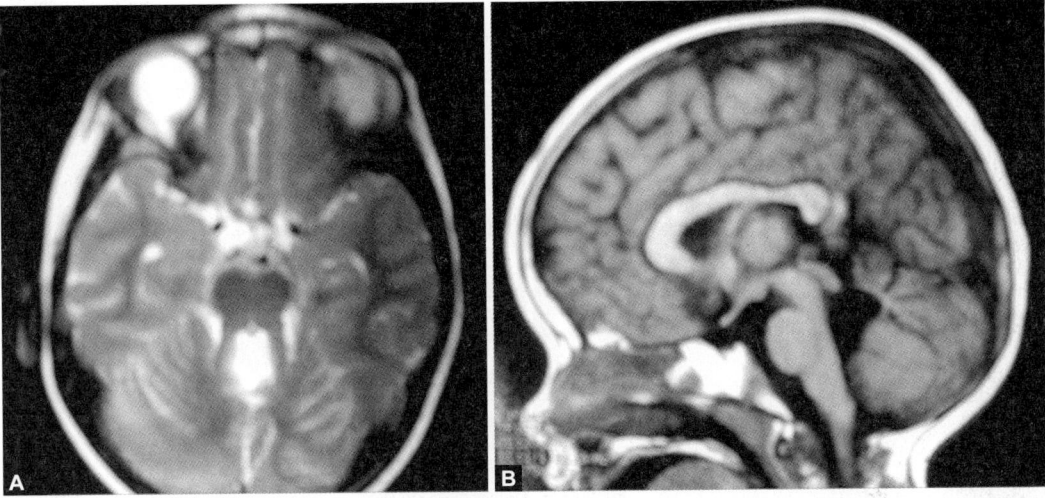

Figures 2.10A and B *Joubert syndrome:* (A) Classical molar tooth appearance; (B) Hypoplasia of cerebellum and peduncle

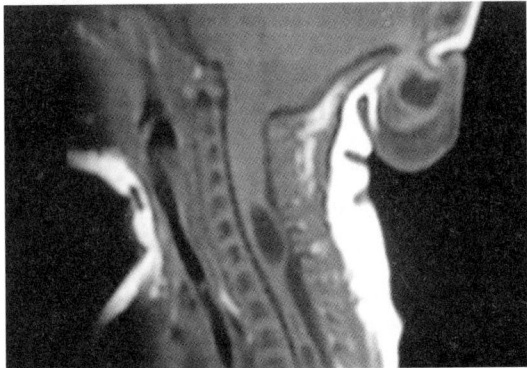

Figure 2.11 Chiari malformation-type III. Note the occipital encephalocele and downward displacement cerebellum. A rare association of syrinx also seen in cervical region

malformation". Many researchers use "Chiari malformation" to describe four specific grades, reserving the term "Arnold-Chiari" for type II only.
- *Type I*: Isolated herniation of cerebellar tonsils and medulla in to the cervical canal
- *Type II (ACM)*: Most common complex anomaly of skull, dura, brain, cord and spine (myelomeningocele, syrinx)
- *Type III*: Type II plus encephalocele (Fig. 2.11)
- *Type IV*: Severe cerebellar hypoplasia.
- *Chiari malformation is associated with conditions like*: Hydrocephalus, syringomyelia, spinal curvature, tethered spinal cord syndrome, platybasia, basal invagination and atlanto axial assimilation. Also associated with connective tissue disorders such as Ehlers-Danlos syndrome and Marfan syndrome.
- *Clinical features*: In ACM the brainstem, cranial nerves, and the lower portion of the cerebellum may be stretched or compressed. Therefore, any of the functions controlled by these areas may be affected. ACM is often associated with headaches, sometimes mistaken for migraines. Headaches due to ACM usually include intense pain in the back of the head, aggravated by Valsalva maneuvers, such as yawning, laughing, crying, coughing, sneezing or straining. Clinical features also include muscle weakness, facial pain, hearing problems, and extreme fatigue. ACM can cause insomnia, cycles of sleep deprivation followed by inability to remain awake. 15% of patients with adult Chiari malformation are asymptomatic.

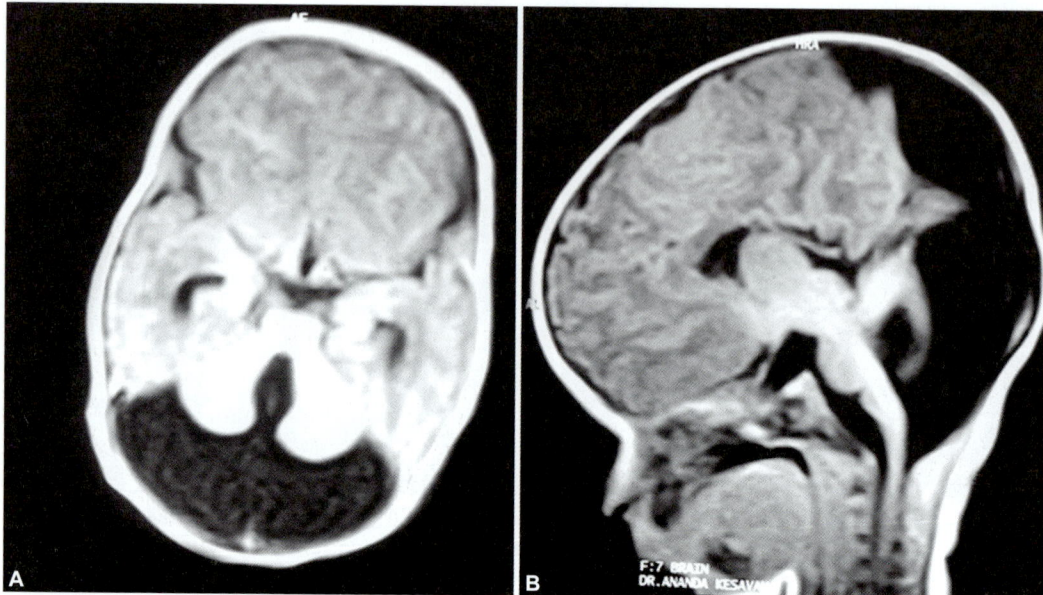

Figures 2.12A and B Dandy-Walker malformation; features include partial agenesis of the vermis, cystic dilatation of the fourth ventricle (A) and enlarged posterior fossa (B)

- *Dandy-Walker malformation*: The malformations most likely originates at around 32 days when fourth ventricle is formed.

  It is a triad of:
  - Complete or partial agenesis of the vermis
  - Cystic dilatation of the fourth ventricle
  - Enlarged posterior fossa.

Clinical Features

Present in infancy with delayed motor milestones, hydrocephalus, nystagmus, spasticity, titubation, apnea, etc. There is prominent occiput.

Imaging will show cystic enlargement of fourth ventricle with hypoplasia of cerebellar vermis and hydrocephalus **(Figs 2.12A and B)**.

Associated CNS anomalies are seen in 70% of children. It include—Dysgenesis of corpus callosum, lipoma of corpus callosum, holoprosencephaly (25%), porencephaly, dysplasia of cingulate gyrus (25%), schizencephaly, polymicrogyria and heterotopia (5–10%).

Hypertrophic Dysplasia of the Brain

Hemimegalencephaly is a rare malformation of the brain with over development of one cerebral hemisphere. Opposite hemisphere is normal **(Fig. 2.13)**. Features include macrocephaly, delayed global development, contralateral hemiparesis, hemianopsia and intractable seizures.

Disorder of Ventricular System

- *Porencephaly*: Porencephaly is the presence of cysts or cavities within the brain that result from developmental defects or acquired lesions, including infarction of tissue. True porencephalic cysts are most commonly located in the region of the sylvian fissure and typically communicate with the subarachnoid space, the ventricular system, or both **(Fig. 2.14)**. They represent developmental abnormalities of cell migration and are often associated with other malformations of the brain, including microcephaly, abnormal patterns of adjacent

Malformations of the Central Nervous System

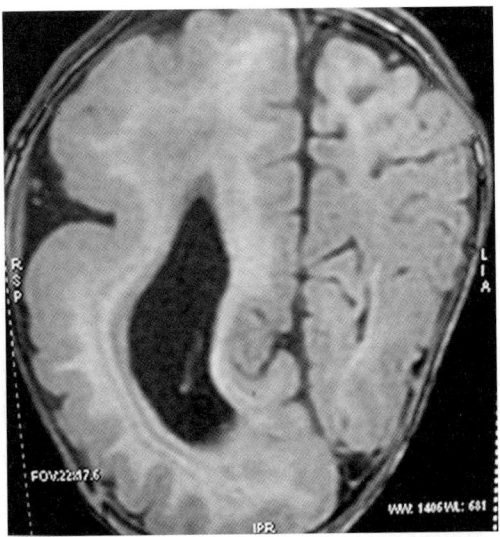

Figure 2.13 *Hemimegalencephaly:* MRI showing enlarged cerebrum involving right lobe, thickened cortex, band heterotopia, asymmetry of ventricle and subdural hygroma

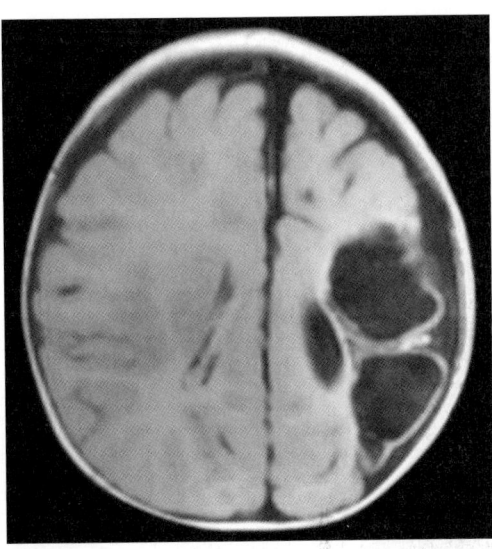

Figure 2.14 *Porencephalic cysts:* In the region of the sylvian fissure, communicating with the subarachnoid space

gyri, and encephalocele. Affected infants tend to have many problems, including mental retardation, spastic hemiparesis or quadriparesis, optic atrophy, and seizures.
- Several risk factors for porencephalic cyst formation have been identified including: hemorrhagic venous infarctions, various thrombophilias such as protein C deficiency and factor V Leiden mutations, perinatal alloimmune thrombocytopenia, von Willebrand's disease, congenital infections, trauma such as amniocentesis.
- Pseudoporencephalic cysts characteristically develop during the perinatal or postnatal period and result from abnormalities (infarction, hemorrhage) of arterial or venous circulation. These cysts tend to be unilateral, do not communicate with a fluid-filled cavity, and are not associated with abnormalities of cell migration or CNS malformations. Infants with pseudoporencephalic cysts present with hemiparesis and focal seizures in the 1st year of life.
- *Hydrancephaly*: It is a devastating CNS malformation consisting of nearly complete absence of cerebral hemisphere. Compromised blood flow in carotid arteries and intrauterine infections will predispose.

The child may appear to be normal at birth but then shows spasticity, myoclonic seizure and enlarging head circumference. Transillumination is readily demonstrable **(Figs 2.15A and B)**.
- *Aqueductal stenosis*: It may be secondary to intrauterine infection or caused by X-linked recessive gene. There is progressive enlargement of the head with bulging fontanellae. Lethargy, vomiting, opisthotonus, spastic lower extremities due to stretching of corticospinal fibers around the lateral ventricle, sixth nerve palsy are other clinical findings. Bilateral corticobulbar disruption may cause pseudobulbar palsy.

Neurosonogram and MRI are diagnostic. MRI show dilatation of lateral and third ventricle with normal sized fourth ventricle **(Fig. 2.16)**.

Arachnoid cyst: They are benign cysts that contain spinal fluid and occur within the arachnoid membrane. They are mostly asymptomatic, but may present with features of compression of both the brain and calvaria. If it enlarges, then patient may present with headache, seizure, focal enlargement of skull and signs of raised intracranial tension and focal signs.

Hallmark on imaging **(Fig. 2.17)** its tendency to form straight, flat surface against the brain.

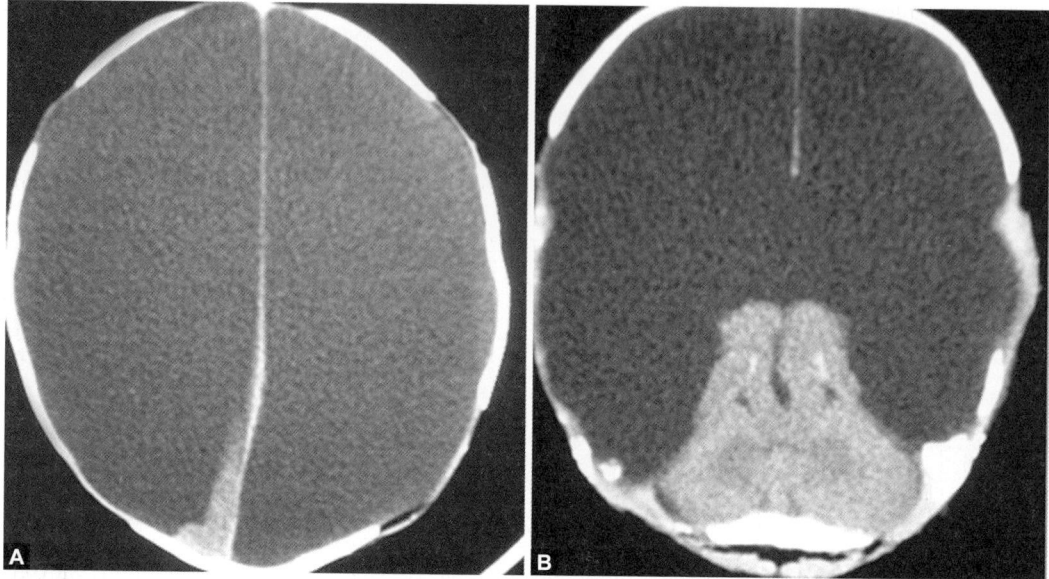

Figures 2.15A and B *Hydrancephaly:* (A) Fluid replacing the cerebral tissue; (B) Few parts of brainstem and cerebellum are seen
(*Courtesy*: Dr Jayakumar PR, Kottayam)

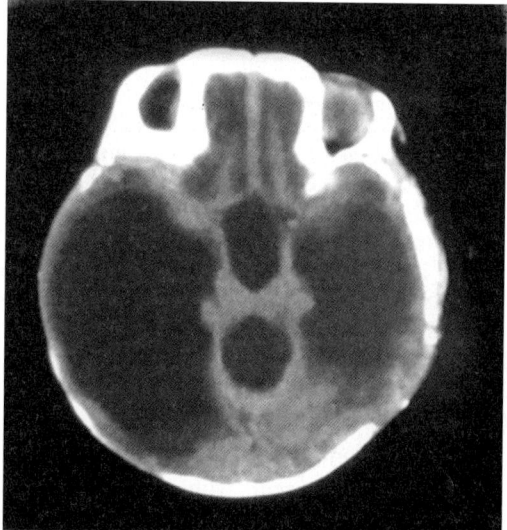

Figure 2.16 *Aqueductal stenosis:* Enlarged lateral and third ventricles

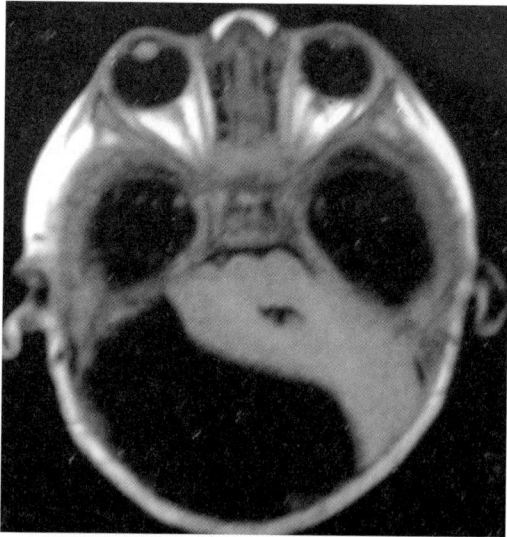

Figure 2.17 *Arachnoid cyst:* Cystic space in posterior fossa, not communicating with fourth ventricle and no cerebellar hypoplasia

An important differential diagnosis in the posterior fossa is Dandy-Walker variant.

Vascular Malformation

It includes vein of Galen malformations (VGM), arteriovenous malformations including Sturge-Weber syndrome, cavernous hemangioma and venous angioma.

Vein of Galen malformations: VGM develops during weeks 6-11 of fetal development as a persistent embryonic prosencephalic vein. The great vein of Galen receive flow from the internal cerebral veins and the basal veins of Rosenthal. It is a large vein, that in turn drains into the straight sinus. The vein of Galen is unsupported by surrounding tissue, lacks a fibrous wall, and is instead free within the fluid of the quadrigeminal plate cistern. Any increase in venous pressure results in a dilatation of the vein—often converting its normal cylindrical shape into a sphere—hence the nickname "vein of Galen *Aneurysm*".

They may present with high-output heart failure in the newborn. Cerebral ischemic changes such as strokes or steal phenomena that result in progressive hemiparesis. Hemorrhage from the

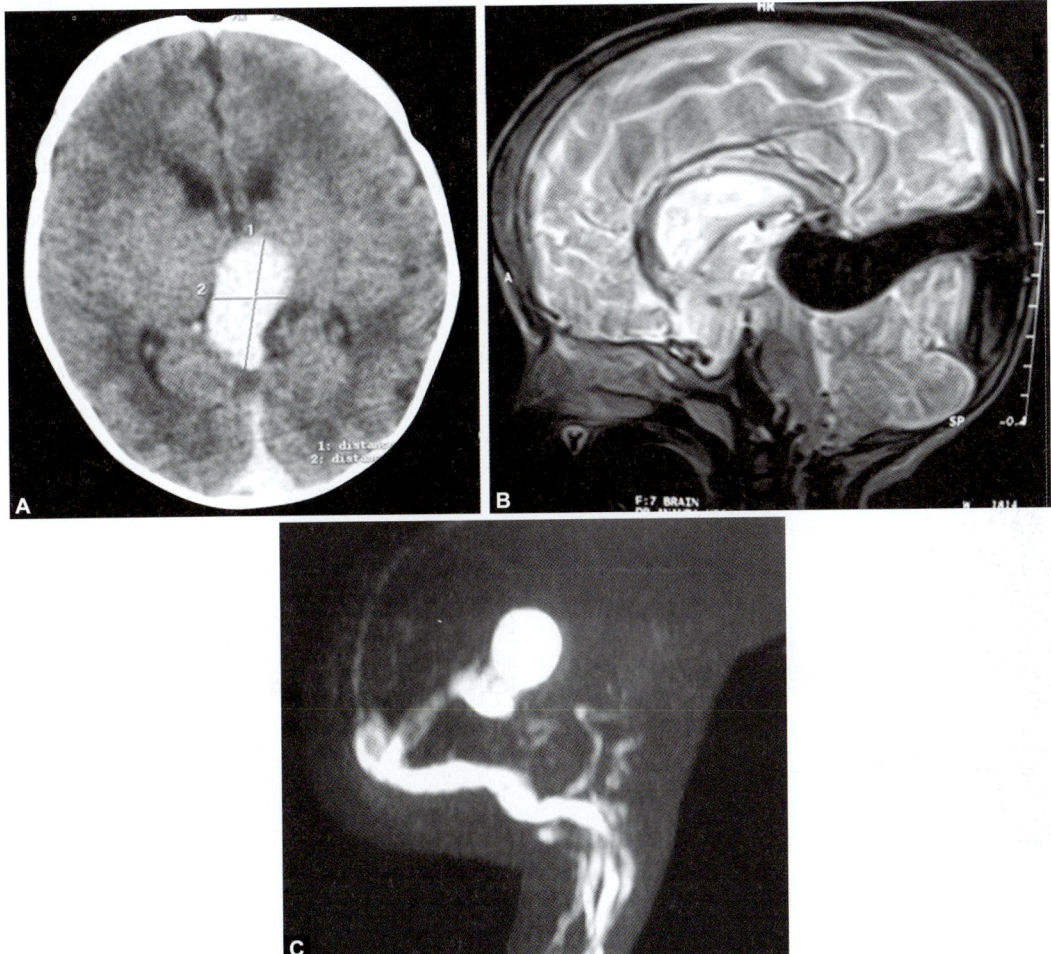

Figures 2.18A to C Vein of Galen malformations: (A and B) Dilated vein ('aneurysm'); (C) MRA showing dilated vein

malformation can occur. Features also include progressive neurological impairment due to mass effect, hydrocephalus and developmental delay.

Cranial ultrasound (Doppler) studies can help further to understand the hemodynamics of the lesion. Cranial MRI will demonstrate vein of Galen **(Figs 2.18A and B)** and MR angiography **(Fig. 2.18C)** is diagnostic.

Treatment of Congenital Brain Malformations

No definite treatment. Symptomatic and supportive treatment (management of seizure, Physiotherapy, etc.) will improve the quality of life. Surgical intervention is useful in conditions like VGM, arachnoid cyst. CSF shunt will help in many situations where hydrocephalus is a prominent.

Prevention

Antenatal diagnosis and genetic counseling possible in many situations. Peri-conceptional folic acid will help to reduce neural tube defects. MMR vaccination and avoidance of precipitating factors will help to decrease the malformations.

REFERENCES

1. Kinsman SL, Johnston MV. In: Kliegman, Stanton, Behrman (Eds). Congenital anomalies of the central nervous system in Nelson textbook of pediatrics, 19th edn. Elsevier; 2011. pp. 1998-2005.
2. Sarnat HB, Sarnat LF. In: Bradley WG, Fenichel GM, Daroll WB (Eds). Developmental anomalies of the brain in neurology in clinical practice, 5th edn. Elsevier; 2008. pp.1711-38.
3. Gupta AK. Congenital malformation of the brain. In: Talukdar B (Ed). Essentials of pediatric neurology. New Age Publications, New Delhi; 1997. pp. 54-64.
4. Gleeson JG, Dobyns WB, Plawnev L, Ashwal S. In: Swaiman K, Ashwal S, Ferriero DM, Schor NF (Eds). Congenital structural defects in Swaiman's pediatric neurology principles and practice, 5th edn. Saunders Publication; 2006. pp. 648-90.

CHAPTER 3

Perinatal Hypoxic-Ischemic Encephalopathy

Naveen Jain

INTRODUCTION

Hypoxic-ischemic encephalopathy (HIE) accounts for one-fourth of the 4 million neonatal deaths worldwide. Approximately 50% of survivors of moderate–severe HIE have motor and cognitive disability.

ETIOLOGY

Brain injury (encephalopathy) is a part of systemic hypoxia—ischemia due to varied causes like pregnancy-induced hypertension (PIH), abruption placentae, cord events, prolonged labor etc. The smooth transition from healthy placenta circulation to effective pulmonary gas exchange at first cry at birth does not happen, resulting in hypoxia, hypercarbia and mixed respiratory and metabolic acidosis.

Critical hypoxia-ischemia (HI) causes cell death. Uptake of excitotoxic amino acids (EAA) from synaptic junction is impaired, resulting in their accumulation; N-methyl-D-aspartate (NMDA), α-amino-3-hydroxy-5-methyl-4-isoxazolepropionic acid (AMPA) and kainite receptors are activated causing influx of sodium and calcium. This causes cytotoxic edema and cell death. A secondary phase of neuronal injury starts off after reoxygenation and reperfusion.

- Release of reactive oxygen and reactive nitrogen species cause secondary neuronal injury.
- Activation and migration of microglia—the inflammatory cells of brain, infiltration of peripheral macrophages into the brain, that phagocytose both injured and noninjured neurons; they also release cytokines. Cytokines promote migration of inflammatory cells and necrosis.
- Apoptosis (programmed cell death) is an important cause of secondary neuronal injury.

CLINICAL FEATURES[1]

- Fetal distress—some pointers to fetal hypoxia-ischemia are fetal heart rate disturbances, decreased fetal movements, meconium stained liquor, antepartum hemorrhage, abnormal Dopplers, abnormal non-stress test (NST), etc.
- Need for extensive resuscitation at birth [prolonged positive pressure ventilation (PPV) for poor respiratory efforts beyond 10 minutes of life, chest compression, medications] is necessary to establish an association between death/neurological handicap and perinatal asphyxia.
- Multiorgan injury due to hypoxia–ischemia.
  - Renal involvement is most common and manifests as oliguria, hematuria, pus cells in urine, proteinuria
  - Gastrointestinal tract involvement presents as abdominal distension, gastrointestinal (GI) bleed, frequent passage of meconium

due to autonomic effects, raised alanine aminotransferase (ALT) due to liver involvement (may be evident at end of 1 week of life)
- *Cardiac involvement*: Bradycardia, electrocardiography (ECG) changes, elevated cardiac enzymes, shock
- *Hematological manifestations*: Thrombocytopenia, leucopenia
- *Pulmonary*: Pulmonary hypertension, pulmonary infarct, secondary surfactant deficiency, pulmonary hemorrhage
- *Neonatal encephalopathy*: Poor activity or irritability, poor cry, suck, inability to swallow milk, poor spontaneous movements, depressed neonatal reflexes, depressed tone, poor seizures, respiratory effort requiring ventilation.[2] Severity of neonatal encephalopathy can be done one of the following:
  - Sarnat and Sarnat staging
  - Modified Levene's
  - Thomsons score.

INVESTIGATIONS

- Umbilical artery (cord) arterial blood gas (ABG) or at least ABG within one hour of birth: low pH < 7.0 and high base deficit > 12–16, raised lactate
- Neuroimaging (MRI) to rule out other pathology like cerebral malformations, intracranial hemorrhage, stroke as cause of encephalopathy. apparent diffusion coefficient (ADC) (diffusion weighted MRI sequence can detect and predict HIE severity very early (within hours of injury)

Typical finding of brain injury in HIE
- *Severe acute hypoxia-ischemia*: Typical areas of injury—lateral thalami and posterior putamen
- *Mild chronic hypoxia-ischemia*: Para-saggital and sub-cortical white matter in water shed zone

- *Magnetic resonance spectroscopy (MRS)*: Good biomarker for HIE, currently a research tool
- *Electroencephalography/amplitude-integrated electroencephalography (EEG/aEEG)*
  - Standard EEG can diagnose seizures
  - aEEG can be used to identify/monitor severity of encephalopathy
- Lumbar puncture—rule out meningitis as cause of neonatal encephalopathy
- Placenta histopathology.

NEURODEVELOPMENT DISABILITY DUE TO HYPOXIC-ISCHEMIC ENCEPHALOPATHY

- Motor—cerebral palsy (CP)–most consistent manifestation of brain injury in HIE spastic quadriplegia or dyskinetic cerebral palsy, other forms of CP are less likely due to HIE.
- Seizure disorder—common in babies with moderate to severe HIE, never occurs in isolation as epilepsy, CP always is present.
- Hearing impairment
- Cognitive, learning problems, behavioral problems—need not be always present. Motor deficits dominate HIE.

Predicting Neurodevelopmental Disability

- Need for resuscitation/APGAR—need for chest compressions, delay in onset of respiration as long as 30 minutes increase risk of death/disability. Low extended APGAR at 15–20 minutes predicts death/disability
- MRI[2]
  - Diffusion weighted imaging—is very sensitive and has high negative predictive value, i.e. a normal MRI predicts good outcomes.
  - Magnetic resonance imaging (MRI)—involvement of basal ganglia, "posterior limb of internal capsule not visualized" are associated with severe cerebral palsy.

Feature	Mild	Moderate	Severe
Consciousness	Irritable	Lethargy	Comatose
Tone	Hypotonia	Marked hypotonia	Severe hypotonia
Seizures	No	Yes	Prolonged
Sucking/respiration	Poor suck	Unable to suck	Unable to sustain spontaneous respiration

- MRS—high levels of choline and lactate levels predict death/disability. Biomarkers are of great relevance in studying neuroprotective strategies, and serve as reliable surrogates for long-term follow-up.
- Ultrasound Dopplers can study flow (resistive index), this has reasonable predictive ability.
- Staging of HIE—Sarnat and Sarnat, Thomsons have reasonable predictive ability
- Neuro examination at discharge—a normal neurological examination by 2 weeks of life/when baby is ready for discharge is associate with good prognosis.

Treatment

Labor Room

- *Effective resuscitation*: All deliveries should be attended by personnel capable of initiating resuscitation and all high risk deliveries must be attended by trained personnel capable of performing extensive resuscitation including chest compressions and medications. Functioning equipment like self inflating bag, suction catheters, appropriate size tubes and laryngoscopes must be readily available at all deliveries.
- *Room air resuscitation*: Normal babies requiring no resuscitation also achieve saturations of 100% only 10 minutes after birth; they require no supplemental oxygen. Well planned studies have demonstrated the benefit of initiating resuscitation in term born babies without use of oxygen (room air). Room air resuscitation is associated with faster response to resuscitation and decrease in neurodevelopmental disability (NDD) possibly because of decrease in free radical injury. If baby's heart rate remains below 60 despite effective resuscitation for 90 seconds, oxygen may be used.
- *Avoid hyperthermia*: If baby needs resuscitation at birth, the radiant warmer may be switched off and hyperthermia must be prevented in labor room and during transfer to NICU; hyperthermia increases the risk of disability.

Care in Neonatal Intensive Care Unit

- *Recent advance in HIE management*: Therapeutic hypothermia[3,4] is the only therapy that is associated with definite decrease in death/disability after asphyxia and is the standard of care in facilities where it can done safely—therapeutic cooling (rectal temperature 33–34°C) initiated early within 6 hours of life and continued for 72 hours is associated with decrease in death and disability. Cooling may be either whole body cooling or head cooling alone. Ideal control of temperature in a tight range is necessary and hence, one must ideally use servo-controlled devices for cooling. In resource limited regions cooling with ice gel packs, cold water bottles and phase change material have been used effectively and safely. Adverse effects of cooling include hypotension, thrombocytopenia, pain, skin effects, etc. close monitoring of all vitals besides rectal temperature is critical.
- *Ventilation*: Baby may require ventilation for poor respiratory efforts (HIE 3) or pulmonary involvement (hemorrhage, surfactant deficiency, persistent pulmonary hypertension (PPHN)
  - Avoid hypoxia and hyperoxia increase risk of brain injury.
  - Avoid hypocarbia and hypercarbia—if baby requires mechanical ventilation, monitoring by blood gas is essential to avoid over-ventilation and hypocarbia; it can cause serious cerebral ischemia.
- *Shock*: Monitor for signs of hypoperfusion like poor activity, increased heart rate, poor capillary refill, core peripheral temperature difference, decrease in blood pressure, metabolic acidosis, a maximum of one saline bolus of 10 mL/kg over 30 minutes must be given. If perfusion does not improve, inotropes may be necessary. Ionized calcium and hemoglobin must be normal.
- *Hypoglycemia*: Coexisting hypoglycemia increases risk of brain injury and death. Blood sugars must be monitored frequently to maintain levels between 75 and 125.
- *Fluid management*: Excess fluid cannot be excreted by the sick asphyxiated neonate due to decreased glomerular filtration rate (GFR), syndrome of inappropriate antidiuretic hormone (SIADH). Fluids must be restricted only if the baby has low urine output. Monitor sodium to guide fluid therapy. There is no role

for use of mannitol or diauretics for cerebral edema.
- *Seizures*: Long standing seizure can itself increase risk of brain injury and must be controlled by antiepileptic drug (AED). But all AED have serious effects on developing newborn brain. Hence, AED must be stopped as early as possible, if neurologic examination is normal. EEG/aEEG monitoring can identify electric seizures having that may/may not have visible clinical correlate. The need to treat them is not clear.

Experimental Neuroprotective Strategies

Erythropoietin, Melatonin, Allopurinol, Xenon.

SUMMARY

Asphyxia accounts for a large proportion of neonatal mortality and preventable morbidity. Prevention by appropriate antenatal and intrapartum care, resuscitation at birth by NRP trained personnel, therapeutic cooling and supportive care can decrease the burden.

REFERENCES

1. Executive summary: Neonatal encephalopathy and neurologic outcome, 2nd edn. Report of the American College of Obstetricians and Gynecologists' Task Force on Neonatal Encephalopathy. Obstet Gynecol. 2014;123:896.
2. Barnette AR, Horbar JD, Soll RF, et al. Neuroimaging in the evaluation of neonatal encephalopathy. Pediatrics. 2014;133:e1508.
3. Papile LA, Baley JE, et al. Hypothermia and neonatal encephalopathy. Pediatrics. 2014;133:1146.
4. Higgins RD, Raju TN, Perlman J, et al. Committee on fetus and newborn, hypothermia and perinatal asphyxia: executive summary of the National Institute of Child Health and Human Development Workshop. J Pediatr. 2006;148:170.

CHAPTER 4

Approach to Neurodegenerative Disorders

PA Mohammed Kunju

INTRODUCTION

Most genetic causes of neurodegenerative disorders in childhood are due to neurometabolic disease. There are over 200 disorders including amino acidopathies, creatine disorders, mitochondrial cytopathies, peroxisomal disorders and lysosomal storage disorders.[1] However, diagnosis can pose a challenge to the clinician when patients present with non-specific problems such as epilepsy, developmental delay, autism, dystonia and ataxia.

Usually, neurodegenerative disorders are suspected when there is a decline in the neurological function or there is a regression of developmental milestones.[2]

However, a static (cerebral palsy like) presentation with atypical neurological features and systemic manifestations also must be a situation for directed investigation for neurometabolic disorder.[3]

Presentation will depend on the area of neuraxis involvement **(Table 4.1)**.

Dementia like presentation (psychomotor retardation) seen when there is diffuse affection and restricted affection produces progressive neurological deficit like progressive ataxic syndrome (e.g. spinocerebellar ataxia), paraplegia (e.g. hereditary spastic paraplegia), or peripheral neuropathy (e.g. hereditary motor sensory neuropathy).

CLINICAL CLUES OF NEURODEGENERATIVE DISORDERS

Following are some of the clinical clues:[4,5]
- Gradually progressive
- Symmetrical affection
- No signs of increased intracranial pressure
- No inflammatory response (no fever)
- Positive family history or consanguinity
- Recurrent coma and vomiting
- Recurrent ataxia or spasticity
- Mental retardation without congenital anomalies
- Associated somatic manifestations.

So after a thorough clinical examination specific neuroimaging and biochemical/molecular tests can be utilized for the diagnosis of neurodegenerative disorders.

Even though inherited metabolic disorders are rare causes of neurologic disease, they should always be considered because many are treatable currently.[6-8]

The characteristics of treatable metabolic disorders are:
- Abrupt onset, episodic relapses and nonspecific clinical/physical features.
- Many are identified through newborn screening programs and thus paves the way for preventive/therapeutic strategies.

Table 4.1 Clinical differentiation of neurodegenerative disorders

Acute encephalopathy (Due to accumulation of small molecules)
- Symptoms
  - Recurrent vomiting, poor feeding, lethargy, dehydration
  - Seizures, coma
- Rapidly progressive course or episodic
- No other specific signs; so investigations only differentiate them

Chronic encephalopathy (Due to accumulation of large molecules)
- Late infancy, children, adolescents
- *Symptoms*: Depends on gray matter (GM) or white matter (WM) involvement
  - *Gray matter symptoms:*
    - Cortical gray matter:
      a. Dementia
      b. Seizures
      c. Fundus showing cherry red spot or retinitis pigmentosa
      d. Affection of other organ systems
    - Deep gray matter:
      a. Dystonia
      b. Choreoathetosis
  - *White matter symptoms:*
    - Spasticity
    - Ataxia
    - Fundus showing optic atrophy
- Gradually progressive
- Specific symptoms and signs may help in clinical differentiation
- Treatable conditions are less

INHERITANCE

Generally, neuromuscular diseases (NMDs) are inherited in an *autosomal recessive* manner. Knowing just the exceptions will help one in remembering the inheritance pattern.
- Exceptions of carbohydrate metabolism—with X-linked recessive (XLR) inheritance—Liver phosphorylase kinase deficiency, Phosphoglycerate kinase deficiency
- Exceptions of lipidoses—XLR; Fabry's disease
- Exceptions of protein metabolic disorders—XLR; Lesch-Nyhan syndrome
- Exceptions of mucopolysaccharidoses (MPS)—XLR; Hunter's syndrome
- Exceptions of urea cycle disorder—XLR; OTC deficiency (ornithine transcarbamylase deficiency).

Autosomal dominant: For example, acute intermittent porphyria, familial hypercholesterolemia.

Progressive neurological manifestation can occur as complications of neurocutaneous syndromes which are *autosomal dominantly* inherited. Exceptions to that general rule are incontinentia pigmentii (X-linked dominant) and Sturge-Weber syndrome (sporadic occurrence).

Approach to a child with acute encephalopathy (small molecule disorders):
- The small molecule disorders are caused by defects in pathways of intermediary metabolism either due to an enzyme deficiency or a cofactor defect (compared to the organelle disorders exemplified by lysosomal storage diseases or peroxisomal disorders). Mainly they are due to defects in amino acid metabolism: organic acidemias (OAs), aminoacidopathies, and urea cycle defects.
- A neonate affected with an OA is usually well at birth and for the first few days of life. The usual clinical presentation is that of toxic encephalopathy and includes vomiting, poor feeding, neurologic symptoms such as seizures and abnormal tone, and lethargy progressing to coma. Outcome is enhanced by diagnosis and treatment in the first ten days of life. In the older child or adolescent, variant forms of the OAs can present as loss of intellectual function, ataxia or other focal neurologic signs, Reye syndrome, recurrent ketoacidosis, or psychiatric symptoms.
- In the setting of an acute encephalopathy, intractable seizures or seizures occurring in sibships, consider an NMD in parallel with more common disorders, especially if fever is not a major symptom.
- Serum and urine metabolic screening **(Table 4.2)** will detect many small molecule disorders. This includes serum ammonia and blood gas analysis for acidosis as the first step. Other associated findings, such as respiratory alkalosis or hypoglycemia with or without ketosis, can narrow the diagnostic possibilities further. Specific diagnosis is possible by doing serum aminogram (for aminoacidopathies) and plasma acyl carnitine and urine organic acids (for organic acidurias).

Approach to Neurodegenerative Disorders

Table 4.2 Screening tests in acute encephalopathy and the usefulness

Urine/serum	Conditions identified
Serum ammonia	Urea cycle disorders (UCDs)[9]
Ammonia and arterial blood gas	Organic aciduria
Serum aminogram	Aminoaciduria, urea cycle disorders, organic aciduria
Urine organic acids	Organic aciduria, aminoacidurias
Plasma acylcarnitine	Organic acidurias

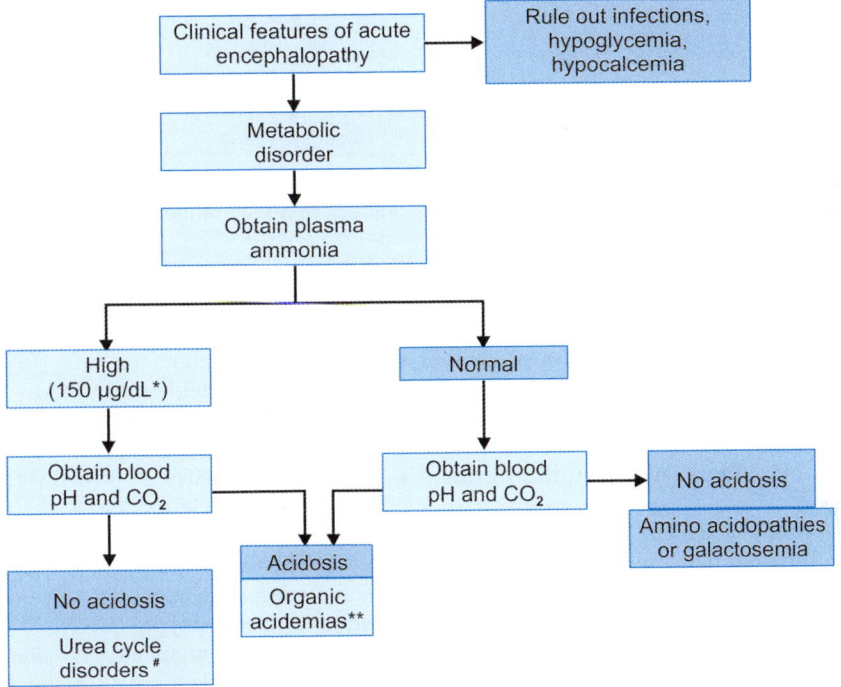

Flow chart 4.1 Stepwise approach for a baby with acute encephalopthy (small molecule disorders)

* 150 µg/dL in neonates, 70 µg/dL in infants to age one month, 35–50 µg/dL in older children and adults
**Organic acidemias can be differentiated by looking for presence of ketosis
\# See text for steps

- If *ketosis is present* with abnormal urine odor consider maple syrup urine disease (MSUD) and without urine odor—methyl malonic acidemia and propionic acidemia (with *neutropenia*)
- With ketosis and skin manifestations like alopecia—multiple carboxylase deficiency
- If *ketosis is not present* with sweaty feet odor—Isovaleric acidemia.
- Organic acidemias without ketosis are glutaric acidemia and Acyl-CoA dehydrogenase deficiency

Following is a step wise approach for a baby presenting with *acute encephalopathy* (**Flow charts 4.1 and 4.2**).

Urea cycle disorders (UCDs) can be differentiated by serum amino acid estimation:

- *Increased arginine* level means arginase deficiency which can be confirmed by red cell enzyme assay
- *Increased citrulline* level means ASS or ASL (elevated arginosuccinate level) deficiency

Flow chart 4.2 Stepwise approach for a baby with acute encephalopathy (when lactic acidosis is detected)

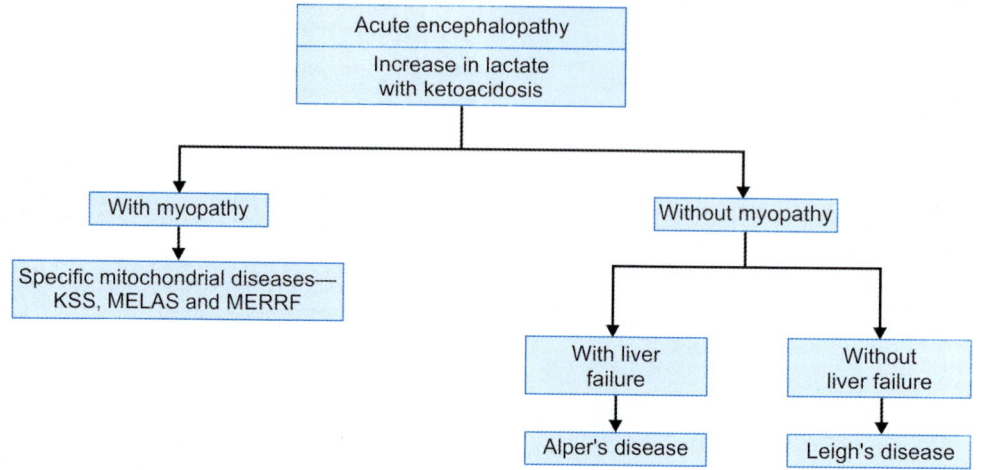

Abbreviations: KSS, Kearns-Sayre syndrome; MELAS, mitochondrial encephalomyopathy, lactic acidosis, and stroke-like episodes; and MERRF, myoclonic epilepsy with ragged-red fibers

which can be confirmed by fibroblast enzyme assay.
- In ASL deficiency elevated arginosuccinate level is seen
- *Low citrulline or arginine* level seen in ornithine transcarbamylase (OTC) or CPS I deficiency; which can be differentiated by urinary orotic aciduria.
  - Orotic aciduria is seen in OTC deficiency
- Final confirmation of acute encephalopathy is possible by
  - Detection of organic acid, aminoacid, and sulfites in urine
  - Detection of specific enzyme deficiency or DNA analysis in WBC and fibroblasts
  - *Clinical distinction* between various diseases coming under each category is not possible
  - Histologic evaluation of affected tissues such as skin, liver, brain, heart, kidney, and skeletal muscle may help but not foolproof.

ORGANIC ACID DISORDERS

The "organic acidemia" or "organic aciduria" (OA) are disorders characterized by the urinary excretion of non-amino organic acids in urine. The majority are caused by abnormal amino acid catabolism of branched-chain amino acids or lysine.

They include:
- Maple syrup urine disease (MSUD)
- Propionic acidemia
- Methylmalonic acidemia (MMA)
- Methylmalonic aciduria-homocystinuria
- Isovaleric acidemia
- Biotin-unresponsive 3-methylcrotonyl-CoA carboxylase deficiency
- 3-hydroxy-3-methylglutaryl-CoA (HMG-CoA) lyase deficiency
- Ketothiolase deficiency
- Glutaric acidemia type I (GA I).

Outcome is enhanced by diagnosis and treatment in the first ten days of life. In the older child or adolescent, OAs can present as loss of intellectual function, ataxia, Reye syndrome, recurrent ketoacidosis, or psychiatric symptoms.

Organic acidurias (OAs) is diagnosed first by urine organic acid analysis using gas chromatography with mass spectrometry (GC/MS). Depending on the specific disorder, plasma amino acid analysis using a quantitative method such as column chromatography, high-performance liquid chromatography (HPLC), or GC/MS can also be helpful. A plasma or serum acylcarnitine profile can also provide a rapid clue to the diagnosis. Finally confirmatory testing involves assay of the activity of the deficient enzyme in lymphocytes or

Approach to Neurodegenerative Disorders

cultured fibroblasts and/or molecular genetic testing.

MRI findings in the Organic Acidurias:

- Distinctive basal ganglia lesions with macrocephaly in glutaric acidemia type I (GA I), Also has wide Sylvian fissure (bat-wing appearance) and nontraumatic subdural hematoma **(Figs 4.1A to E)**
- White matter changes in Maple syrup urine disease **(Figs 4.2A to C)**
- Abnormalities of the globus pallidus in methylmalonic acidemia **(Fig. 4.3)**.

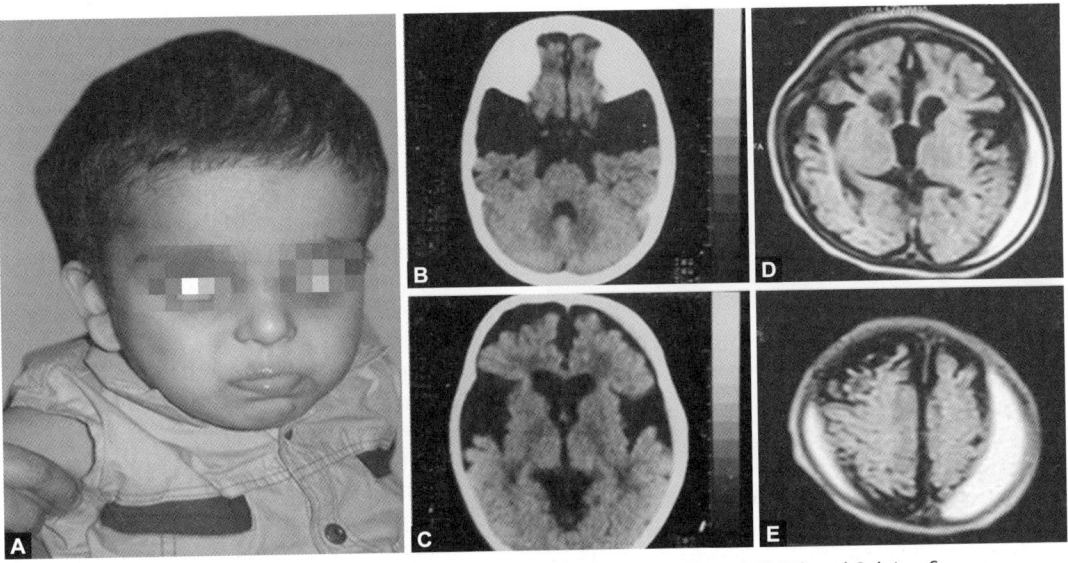

Figures 4.1A to E *Glutaric acidemia type I:* (A) Macrocephaly; (B and C) Dilated Sylvian fissure (Bat-wing appearance); (D and E) Nontraumatic subdural hematoma *(For color version, see Plate 2)*

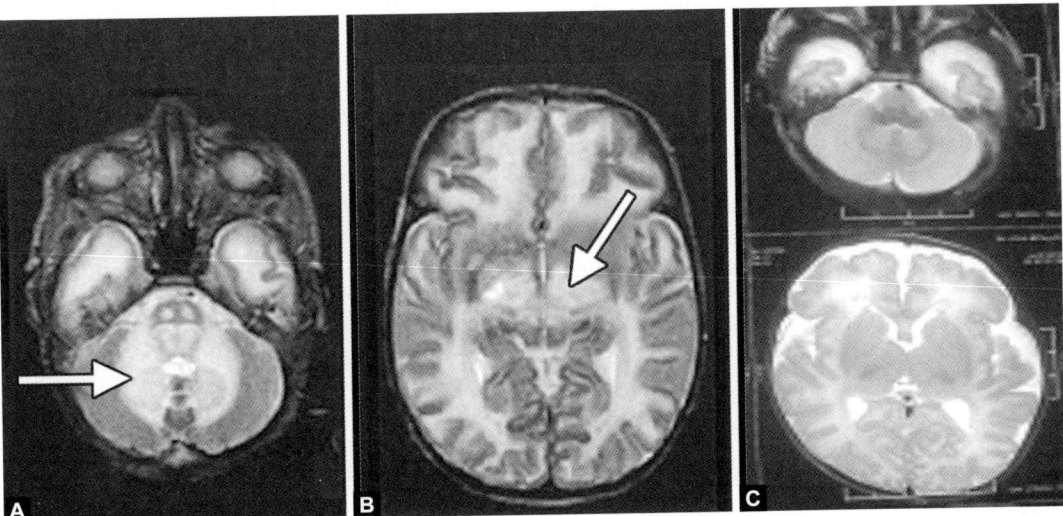

Figures 4.2A to C MRI in MSUD; T2 prolongation seen in already myelinated brain areas: (A) Hyperintensity in posterior brainstem tracts and the central cerebellar white matter; (B) Basal ganglia and ventrolateral thalamic nuclei; (C) Normal T2 images to show normal MRI of same age

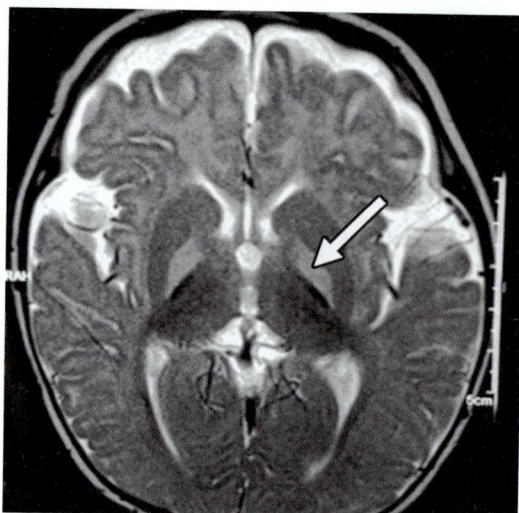

Figure 4.3 Bilateral pallidal hyperintensity in methylmalonic aciduria (arrow)

UREA CYCLE DEFECTS[10]

Severe deficiency of any of the first four enzymes (CPS1, OTC, ASL, ASS-carbamoyl phosphate synthetase I, ornithine transcarbamylase, arginosuccinate lyase; arginosuccinate synthetase) in the urea cycle or the cofactor producer (NAGS—N-acetyl glutamate synthetase) results in the accumulation of ammonia and other precursor metabolites during the first few days of life. Infants are normal at birth but rapidly develop cerebral edema manifested by lethargy, anorexia, hyper- or hypoventilation, hypothermia, seizures, abnormal posturing, and coma. In milder (or partial) deficiencies of the above enzymes and in arginase (ARG) deficiency, symptoms may be triggered by illness or stress at almost any time of life. In these hyperammonia and clinical symptoms are often subtle and the first recognized clinical episode may not occur for months or decades. In ARG deficiency progressive spastic quadriplegia and mental retardation may even mimic cerebral palsy.[11,12]

Traditionally the outcome of newborns with UCDs was considered poor. However, with institution of early treatment with recent protocols, recent data from the NIH-sponsored longitudinal study show IQ measures within a less severe range.

Approach to a Child with Chronic Encephalopathy

Developmental neurological history supplemented with family history will definitely give the diagnostic clues. There will be a decline in the neurological function and the disease keeps worsening as time goes on. But the single most important clue is regression of developmental milestones.

Stepwise Approach to Neurodegenerative Disorders

Step I: Is it a progressive or static disorder?
- *Clues to suspect static encephalopathy:*
  - *History*: High-risk factors, e.g. prematurity, asphyxia, birth trauma
  - *Constellation of signs*: Group of congenital stigmata
    - Suggest malformation of brain
  - *Degenerative diseases mistakenly diagnosed as static encephalopathy*
  - Degenerative diseases with slow evolution may mimic static encephalopathy in infancy
    - For example, progressive disorder that may mimic a "diplegic cerebral palsy"—Arginase deficiency and metachromatic leukodystrophy
    - Dystonia/choreoathetotic cerebral palsy like presentation—Glutaric aciduria type 1 and Lesch-Nyhan syndrome
    - Mixed pyramidal and extrapyramidal cerebral palsy—Pelizaeus-Merzbacher disease
- *Clues to suspect progressive disorder*
  - Positive family history
  - Parental consanguinity
  - Affection of CNS with PNS
  - Presence of neurocutaneous stigmata
  - Dysmorphic features
  - Unusual smell to urine and skin
  - Skeletal abnormalities
- *Somatic involvement (Hepatosplenomegaly and dysostosis multiplex)*:
  - Pitfalls in diagnosing degenerative diseases:
    - Child with hypertonia may turn over early with subsequent delay in milestones
    - Extrapyramidal movements like dystonia may appear late in static encephalopathy.

Approach to Neurodegenerative Disorders

Step II: Find out site/sites of affection:
- The involvement can be either central or peripheral or a combination of central and peripheral nervous system
- By noting selectivity of regression site can be identified.
  - Global deterioration (Regression of motor, social, adaptive and language, milestones) or cognitive regression (dementia dominant) is suggestive of a central disorder
  - Regression only in motor function can be either due to a UMN or LMN lesion
    - *UMN lesion (hyper- or hypotonia with hyper-reflexia)*—Spinal cord lesion (e.g. hereditary spastic paraplegia)
    - *LMN* lesion (Hypotonia with absent reflexes), e.g. Anterior horn cell disease (e.g. SMA); Muscle disease (e.g. Pompe disease); Polyneuropathy (+/- Sensory, e.g. Hereditary motor sensory neuropathy)
  - In both pure central and peripheral disorders, try to find out gray or white matter involvement.

Step III: Always rule out treatable conditions:
- Inflammatory conditions—presence of fever
- Tumors—associated with increased intracranial pressure
- Vascular—lesion has an arterial territory involvement
- Endocrinological conditions, e.g. Hypothyroidism developing myopathy
- Recurrent seizures—progressive encephalopathy

General Examination

It is an important prerequisite for a better diagnosis as external systemic findings will give away the diagnosis. Following are some of the examples:
- Skin/neurocutaneous lesions **(Figs 4.4 and 4.5)**
- Dysmorphic features **(Fig. 4.6)**
- Hair abnormalities
- Micro- or macrocephaly
- Examination of eye
- Hepatosplenomegaly
- Skeletal change (dysostosis multiplex **Figs 4.7A to C)**.

Developmental history and assessment for delay or regression, detailed neurological

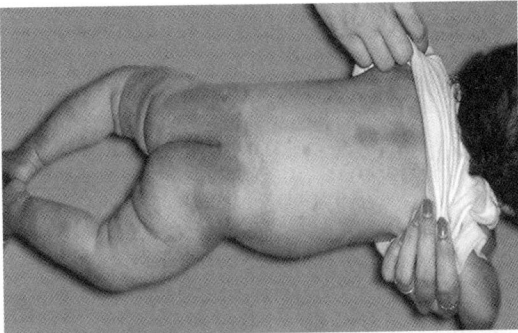

Figure 4.4 Extensive and persistent Mongolian blue spots may be an indicator of gray matter disorders like GM1 gangliosidosis or mucopolysaccharidosis
(For color version, see Plate 2)

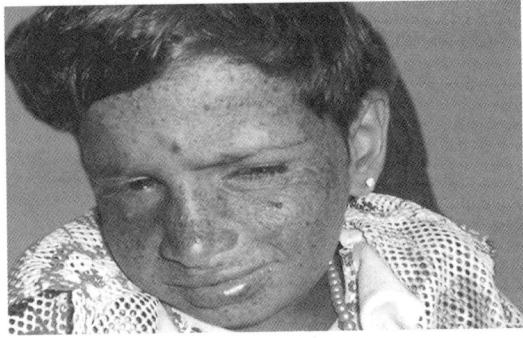

Figure 4.5 A subtle skin change to severe photodermatitis can be seen in xeroderma pigmentosa. This child had severe mental retardation (*DeSanctis-Cacchione syndrome*) *(For color version, see Plate 2)*

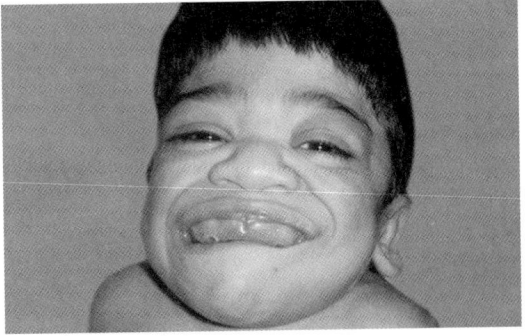

Figure 4.6 Role of facies
- High forehead, puffy eyelids, epicanthal folds
- Flat nasal bridge, anteverted nares, long philtrum
- Gingival hypertrophy, macroglossia—diagnostic of mucolipidosis type 1 (sialidosis I)
(For color version, see Plate 3)

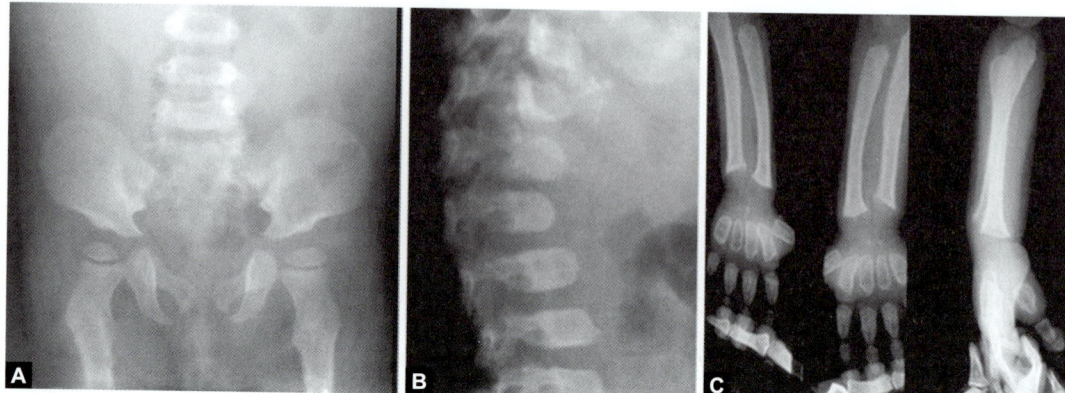

Figures 4.7A to C Disostosis multiplex in gray matter disorders and mucopolysaccharidosis: (A) Round iliac wing, inferiorly tapered ilia; (B) Beaked vertebra; (C) Bullet-shaped phalanges

examination including the motor system and looking for unusual posturing or involuntary movements will further categorize these disorders.

Formulating the Diagnosis

Nonprogressive Central Motor Disorder (Cerebral Palsy)

Features are in history. Positive risk factors in antenatal, natal, postnatal and behavioral soft signs that include colicky behavior, feeding problems and irregular sleep patterns. Physical examination may not yield specific findings. So look for associated findings that may help in rehabilitation.

Neurodevelopmental examination shows delayed milestones or disordered sequence of motor milestones and abnormalities of tone (either hypotonia or poor control of head or a stiffness and rigidity).

In reflex behavior, a combination of delay in disappearance of primitive reflexes and delay in appearance of postural reflexes or incomplete expression is also a powerful predictor of cerebral palsy. Diagnosis of specific type of CP can be done by 1–2 years.

Progressive Central Disorder

When there is delay or regression in development, the pregnancy and birth history is normal with positive family history and consanguinity, progressive central disorder must be thought of.

Progressive disorders can be clinically grouped as gray or white matter disease.

Approach to these disorders are given in the **Flow charts 4.3 to 4.7**.

Among them, a progressive lipidosis may be considered when there are positive eye grounds and hepatosplenomegaly. A Hurler phenotype should be considered in a situation where dysmorphic features combined with dysostosis multiplex are seen.

Nonspecific progressive disorders or gray or white matter should be considered where the history is normally in association with marked subsequent developmental delay. Pelizaeus-Merzbacher disease may masquerade as cerebral palsy. The give away clue is peculiar rhythmic eye movements.

White matter disorders can be differentiated by the imaging finding **(Figs 4.8 and 4.9)**.[13]

Since the demonstration of the DOPA sensitive dystonia (Segawa syndrome), L-dopa has been tried in some of the cases of congenital cerebral palsy where choreoathetotic rigidity is seen. A marked improvement suggests the possibility of Dopa responsive dystonia.[14]

Peripheral Progressive Disorder

Myasthenia gravis and congenital myasthenia, muscular dystrophy and a spectrum of intrinsic muscle disease along with spinal muscular atrophy are considered in this group. Congenital myotonic dystrophy is to be considered in children thought

Approach to Neurodegenerative Disorders

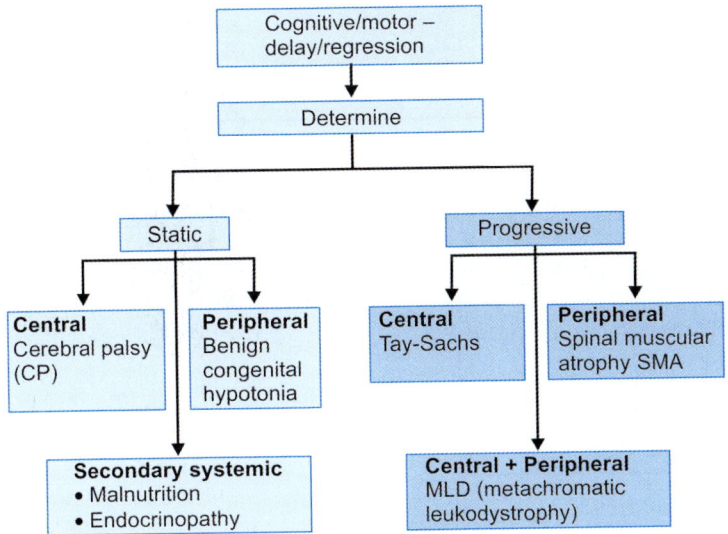

Flow chart 4.3 Chronic encephalopathy—general approach

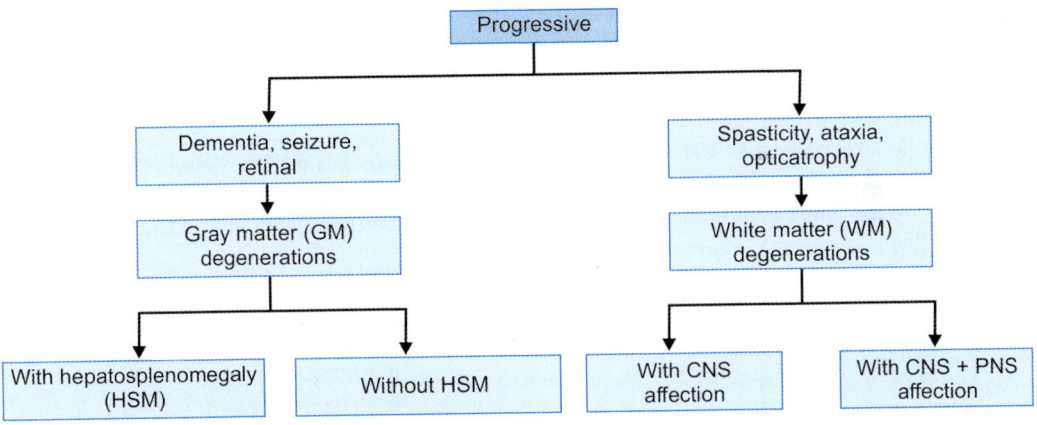

Flow chart 4.4 Chronic encephalopathy—an approach to progressive disorders

to be having cerebral palsy. A maternal myotonia and myopathic facies with history of fetal wastage are the diagnostic clues.

Pure neuromuscular disease in this group are Pompes' disease, Refsum disease, etc.

Other Presentations

Psychomotor retardation with connective tissue involvement homocystinuria.

Investigations

A careful history and physical examination can help more than all the investigations put together.[15,16]

Exercise prudence in the investigations. Some children need little or no testing as part of evaluation for motor delay; others may require an extensive search.

Karyotyping, electroencephalogram, brain electrical activity mapping, brain imaging studies

Flow chart 4.5 Chronic encephalopathy—approach to gray matter disorders-I

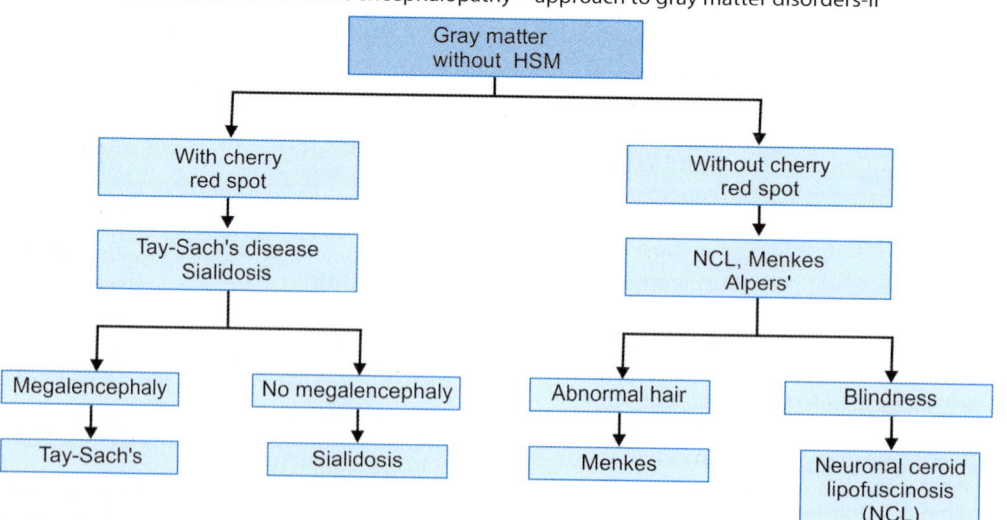

Abbreviations: MPS, mucopolysaccharidosis, HSM, hepatosplenomegaly

Flow chart 4.6 Chronic encephalopathy—approach to gray matter disorders-II

Abbreviations: HSM, hepatosplenomegaly; NCL, neuronal ceroid lipofuscinosis

Approach to Neurodegenerative Disorders

Flow chart 4.7 Chronic encephalopathy—approach to white matter disorders

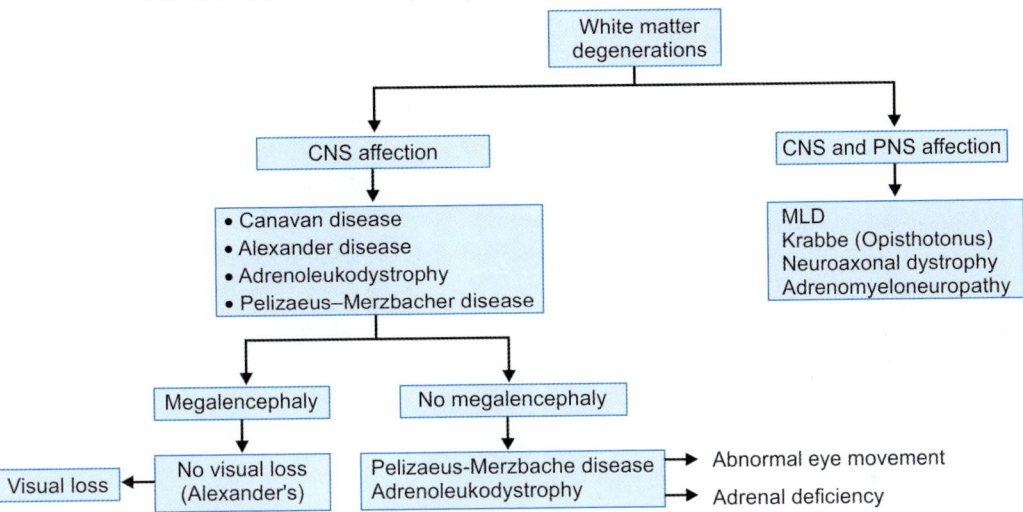

(computed tomography, magnetic resonance imaging and positron emission tomography) and metabolic screening may be utilized in appropriate situations.

Following are some points in deciding on the investigations:

- Although brain imaging may not be required routinely, in the following situations it will be of help: an unexpected change in behavior, head circumference, motor status, cognitive abilities, neurologic examination, or seizure frequency.
- Based on the extremely low prevalence of inborn errors, metabolic screening does not need to be a routine part of an evaluation. If there is a history if intermittent episodes of vomiting and lethargy, failure to thrive, progressive loss of skilled or a plateau in milestone acquisition, an unusual body odor, or a suggestive family history, metabolic screening studies should be performed.
- In peripheral (motor unit) disorders, muscle enzyme studies, electromyography and nerve conduction studies and muscle or nerve biopsy will help in differentiating muscle, nerve, anterior horn cell and for myoneural junction disease neostigmine test.

Diagnostic (molecular) testing: When a pattern of disease and its tissue localization are identified other laboratory testing can be employed to make a specific diagnosis, and direct treatment.

Tissue characterization test are:
- Muscle biopsy
- *Histochemistry*: Diagnosis by specific morpholgic features
  Mitochondrial disease
- *Immunohistochemistry*: Absent or reduced staining for specific protein
  Emery-Dreifuss muscular dystrophy
  Duchenne muscular dystrophy
- *Biochemistry*: Absent or reduced enzyme function
  Myophosphorylase deficiency
- Nerve biopsy
  Vasculitis metachromatic leukodystrophy
- *Antibodies in serum or CSF*: It may define specific immune neuromuscular disorders.

Genetic testing: Defines specific hereditary disorders.
- Usually with symmetric weakness if facilities are available
- Hexosaminidase A (multisystem disorder)
- Spinal muscular atrophy [survival motor neuron (SMN)] deletion
- Bulbo-spinal muscular atrophy (Androgen receptor triplet repeat)
- The age of onset of symptoms is often a helpful guide in deciding which progressive degenerative disorders should be considered.

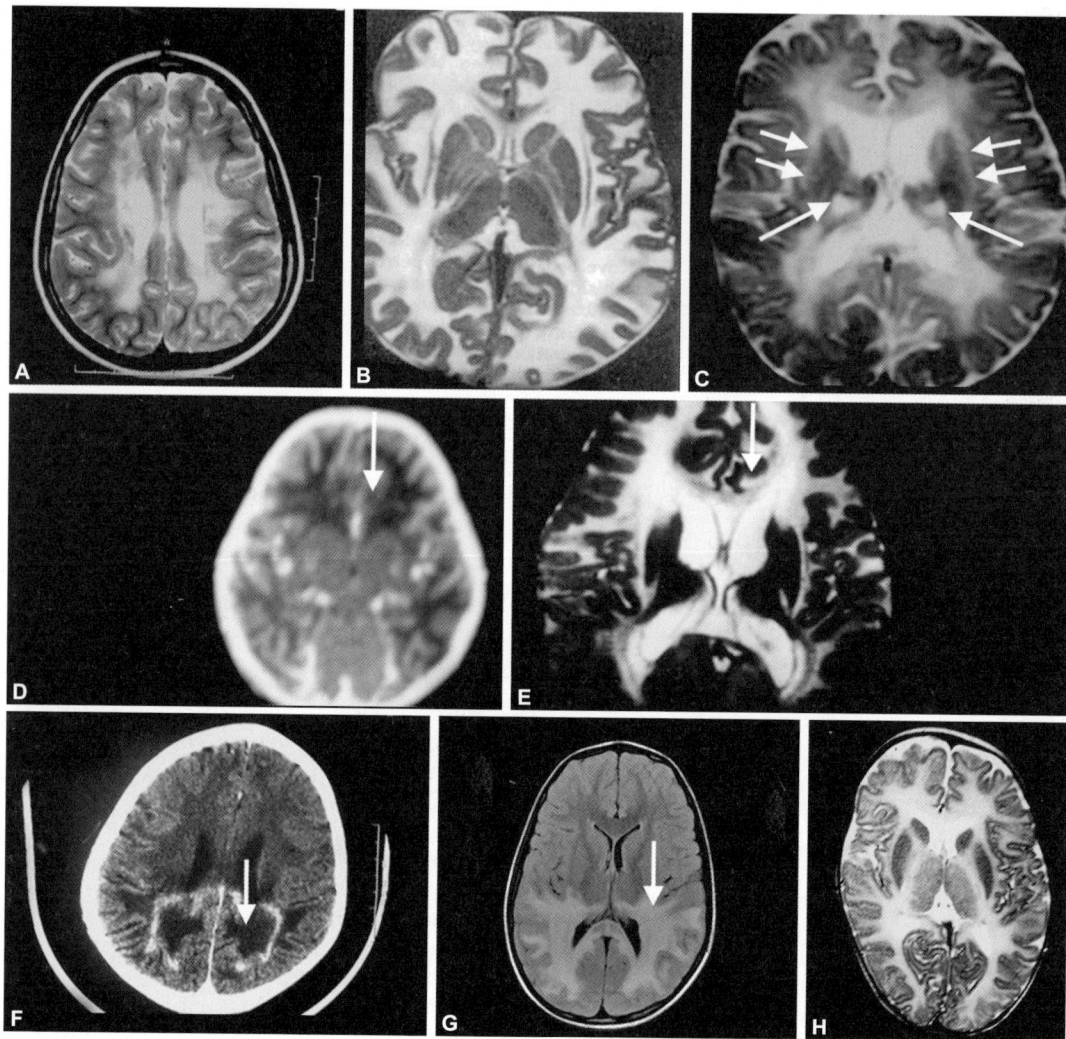

Figures 4.8A to H Imaging in white matter disorders: (A) MLD-symmetric demyelination that spares the subcortical U fibers; (B) Canavan disease—Symmetric demyelination that involves subcortical U fibers; (C) Krabbe disease white matter dysmyelination with high-density basal ganglia; (D and E) Alexander disease; (D) CT scan-frontal hypodensity; (E) MRI—Frontal white matter most involved; (F and G) Adrenoleukodystrophy; Occipital white matter most involved (also callosal splenium) (F) CT scan—Garlanding appearance; (G) MRI hyperintensity posterior brain region; (H) Pelizaeus-Merzbacher disease—extensive dysmyelination including white matter of basal ganglia and thalami showing tigroid appearance

Approach to Neurodegenerative Disorders

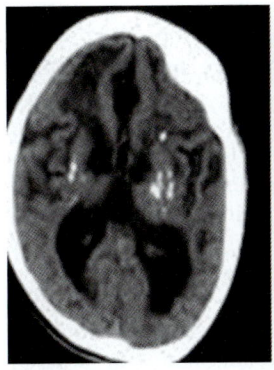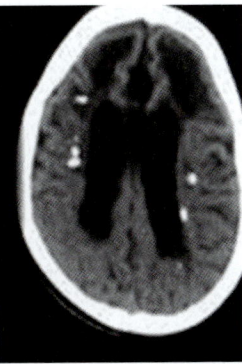

Figure 4.9 Aicardi–Goutières syndrome. See the calcification and the white matter hypodensity and the microcephaly

Specific Diagnostic Entities

Following syndromic groups with characteristic findings will help in identification of other diseases.

Myoclonus Ataxia Dementia Syndrome

- Lafora body disease   Onset in adolescent
- NCL   Retinal degeneration
- MERRF   Ragged red fiber
- Late Gaucher's   Slow saccades
- Sialidosis   Cherry red spot

Progressive Extrapyramidal Symptoms Syndromes (With Mineral Deposits)

- (*Copper*) Wilson Kayser-Fleischer (KF) ring[17]
- (*Iron*) Hallervorden-Spatz—Similar to Wilson, myoclonus, MRI "eye of tiger"
- (*Calcium*) Fahr's syndrome (Familial Basal ganglia calcification syndrome)—Dystonia
- (*Uric acid*) Lesch-Nyhan syndrome—Self mutilation
- Chédiak-Higashi—Mainly neuropathy
- Juvenile Parkinson disease—Parkinson feature, L DOPA response
- Segawa syndrome—Diurnal fluctuation, L DOPA response
- Dystonia musculorum deformans—starting as action dystonia of lower limb
- Juvenile dystonic lipidosis—sea blue histiocytes.

Intermittent Ataxic Syndrome

- Hartnup disease—skin manifestation
- Urea cycle disorders—vomiting
- Pyruvate decarboxylase and dehydrogenase deficiency—alopecia, lactic acidosis
- Intermittent MSUD—acute decompensation during times of physiological stress; ketoacidosis and elevated branched-chain amino acids (BCAAs) level.

Metabolic Causes of Stroke Like Presentations

- MELAS syndrome—nonarterial territory; posterior brain area
- 5,10-methylenetetrahydrofolate reductase deficiency—recurrent venous thromboembolism and have a significant family history of venous thromboembolism. High homocysteine levels
- Fabry's disease—later development of chronic kidney disease or ventricular hypertrophy
- Ethylmalonic-adipic aciduria
- Ornithine transcarbamylase deficiency
- Chédiak-Higashi syndrome
- Homocystinuria.

All needs suspicion and specific metabolic evaluation for the diagnosis.

Treatment

Treatable Small Molecule Disorders:[19]

- *Urea cycle disorders:* CPS (carbamoyl phosphate synthetase I), OTC (ornithine transcarbamylase) ASL (argininosuccinate lyase); ASS, (argininosuccinate synthetase) deficiency Presenting as acute encephalopathy with hyperammonemia.

  Acute phase (hyperammonemic crisis), treat with intravenous arginine and Ammonul (sodium phenylacetate/sodium benzoate), and may require dialysis to reduce ammonia. Long-term management includes high-carbohydrate, low-protein diet; arginine administration to enhance citrulline excretion and nitrogen scavenging with sodium phenylacetate and/or sodium benzoate.

- *Arginase deficiency*: Presenting as progressive spastic quadriplegia and mental retardation;

Treatment includes diet of essential amino acids excluding arginine, and a low-protein diet.

Other Metabolic Disorders

- The acute effects of MSUD require aggressive supportive measures including intravenous fluid hydration and dextrose administration, and branched chain amino acid—free parenteral nutrition solutions

    Maintenance treatment with branched chain amino acid—free formulas, low-protein diet, and avoidance of fasting. Thiamine supplementation is beneficial in some cases.

    Relapses can occur in the setting of illness or increased protein intake.

    Although individuals with less typical presentations generally have some residual enzyme function, their overall prognosis may be poor if their disorder is unrecognized.
- Pyruvate dehydrogenase complex deficiency; pyruvate carboxylase deficiency

    Biotin supplementation (cofactor for PC enzyme), citrate and aspartic acid supplementation as Krebs cycle intermediates

    Treatment of persistent acidosis with chronic bicarbonate therapy

    Avoidance of ketogenic diet and fasting.
- There is currently no known treatment or cure for most (or perhaps all) causes of children with chronic degenerations. But all options are not that gloomy. ERT (enzyme replacement therapy/stem-cell therapies) successful in animal models are now under development for patients with various neurometabolic disorders and some are already available. Example for Fabry, Gaucher, Hunter and Hurler syndrome. Megavitamin therapy with biotin for biotinidase deficiency, thiamin for Leigh's syndrome and riboflavin for glutaric aciduria are some of the established treatment strategies.

    Physical, occupational, and speech therapies are often recommended and used, with very good results. Hypotonic/hypertonic, infant may need extra stimulation. Toddlers and children with speech difficulties may benefit greatly by using sign language within the family until speech has become intelligible by the family.

Prognosis

The outcome in any particular case depends largely on the nature of the underlying disease. Typically the hypotonia does not get much worse, and sometimes improves. Usually, life expectancy is not seriously threatened in peripheral/central nonprogressive disorders. As of today in progressive disorders nothing much can be offered. Recently a few cases with dysmyelinative features trial of steroids have yielded unexpected and dramatic positive outcome. So we recommend a course of steroid in children with MRI/CT evidence of dysmyelination. Similarly in children with CP, no response with physiotherapy warrants a trial of levodopa since some of these cases may be dopa responsive dystonia.

REFERENCES

1. Jaeger C, Glaab E, et al. The mouse brain metabolome region-specific signatures and response to excitotoxic neuronal injury. Am J Pathol. 2015;185:1699e1712.
2. G Pierre. Neurodegenerative disorders and metabolic disease. Arch Dis Child. 2013;98: 618-24.
3. Minassian BA. The progressive myoclonus epilepsies. Prog Brain Res. 2014;213:113-22.
4. Kwon JM, D'Aco KE. Clinical neurogenetics—neurologic presentations of metabolic disorders. Neurol Clin. 2013;31:1031-50.
5. Sultan T, Qureshi AA, Rehman Mu, Khan MM. The spectrum of neurodegeneration in children. J Coll Physicians Surg Pak. 2006;16(11):721-4.
6. Hoffman GF, Nyhan WL, Zschocke J. Inherited metabolic diseases. Philadelphia: Lippincott Williams and Wilkins; 2002.
7. Lyon G, Kolodny EH, Pastores GM. Neurology of hereditary metabolic disease of children. 3rd edn. McGraw-Hill Professional, 2006.
8. William L Nyhan, Bruce A Barshop, Pinar T Ozand. Atlas of metabolic diseases, 2nd edn. A Hodder Arnold Publication, 2005.
9. Lanpher BC, Gropman A, Chapman KA, Lichter-Konecki U. Urea cycle disorders overview. GeneReviews® [Internet] *http://www.ncbi.nlm.nih.gov/books/NBK1217*.
10. Nassogne MC, Heron B, Touati G, et al. Urea cycle defects: management and outcome. J Inherit Metab Dis. 2005;28:407-14.

11. Pierre G. Neurodegenerative disorders and metabolic disease. Arch Dis Child. 2013;98:618-24.
12. Fernandes J, Saudubray JM, Van den Berghe G, et al. Inborn metabolic diseases: diagnosis and treatment. 4th, rev edn. Springer; 2006.
13. Gropman A. Brain imaging in urea cycle disorders. Mol Genet Metab. 2010;100(Suppl 1):S20-30.
14. Brusilow SW. Urea cycle disorders: clinical paradigm of hyperammonemic encephalopathy. Prog Liver Dis. 1995;13:293-309.
15. Daroff RB, Fenichel GM, Jankovic J, Mazziotta JC. Bradley's. Neurology in Clinical Practice, 6th edn. Saunders; 2012.pp.69-78.
16. Barkovich AJ, Moore KR, Grant E, Jones BV, G Vezina G, Koch BL, Raybaud C, Blaser S, Hedlund GL, et al. In: Diagnostic imaging: pediatric neuroradiology: Amirsys-Elsevier Salt Lake City, Utah; 2007.pp.1-124.
17. Bandmann O, Weiss KH, Kaler SG. Wilson's disease and other neurological copper disorders. Lancet Neurol. 2015;14(1):103-13.
18. Gouider-Khouja N, Kraoua I, Benrhouma H, Fraj N, Rouissi A. Movement disorders in neurometabolic diseases. Eur J Paediatr Neurol. 2010;14(4):304-7.

CHAPTER 5

Neural Tube Defects: Prevalence, Predisposing Factors and Prevention

TM Ananda Kesavan, Ciju Ravindranath

INTRODUCTION

Neural tube defects (NTDs) accounts for the largest proportion of congenital anomalies of central nervous system. It results from the incomplete closure of neural tube between the 3rd and 4th week of *in utero* development. NTD assume significance by virtue of morbidity, mortality, health care expenditure, and human suffering. In this chapter we will discuss about 3Ps of NTDs.

PREVALENCE

The incidence of NTDs shows a wide variation; by race, ethnicity, nutritional status, geographic location, and socioeconomic conditions.[1] The highest incidence of NTD has been reported from Ireland and Wales (6.38–10.92 per 1000 births), whereas its incidence in other European countries has only been 0.1–0,6 per 1000 births.[2] The prevalence of NTD in the US and worldwide is about 1 per 1000.[2] Other parts of the world with high prevalence of NTD are northern India,[3] northern China, Egypt and Lebanon.[4]

The incidence of NTDs ranges from 0.5 to 11/1000 births in different regions of India.[5] In general the prevalence in northern states, namely, Punjab, Haryana, Delhi, Rajasthan, Uttar Pradesh and Bihar has been much higher (3.9-9.0/1000) compared to eastern, western and southern parts of the country (0.5-2.64/1000). One exception to this statement, is the reported high incidence of NTD from Davangere, Karnataka.[6,7] The true incidence of NTDs is difficult to access, as some affected pregnancies end up in spontaneous abortions, or may be medically terminated.

EMBRYOLOGY

Neural tube formation (neurulation) is a highly intricate biological process controlled by a number of genes, growth factors, adhesion molecules and receptors.[8] In the 3rd week of embryonic development, invagination of the neural groove is completed, and the neural tube is formed, by separation from the overlying surface ectoderm. usually, the rostral end of the neural tube closes on the 23rd day and the caudal neuropore closes by a process of secondary neurulation by the 27th day of development. Failure to do so results in NTDs.

CLASSIFICATION

Neural tube defects (NTDs) can be classified based on:
- Embryological considerations
- Presence or absence of exposed neural tissue
- Open or closed types
- Affected parts of the CNS:
  - Cranial
  - Spinal types

Open NTDs frequently involve the entire CNS (e.g. associated hydrocephalus, Chiari II malformation) and are due to failure of primary neurulation. Exposure is associated with cerebrospinal fluid (CSF) leakage.

Closed NTDs, resulting from a defect in secondary neurulation are localized and confined to the spine (brain rarely affected). Neural tissue is not exposed as the defect is fully epithelialized, although the skin covering the defect may be dysplastic. Cranial presentations include anencephaly, encephalocele (meningocele or meningomyelocele), craniorachischisis totalis, congenital dermal sinus. Spinal presentations include spina bifida aperta (cystica) and myelomeningocele.

PREDISPOSING FACTORS

- *Environmental factors*: The variation in incidence in different geographical area may be due to genetic and environmental factors. In a study from Haryana, India, a high incidence of NTDs was reported following dengue fever.[9] A presentation of a "flu" or "cold" syndrome or a febrile illness in the first trimester has been associated with a two- to three-fold increase in risk for NTDs.[10]
- *Genetic factors*: Polymorphism of genes involved in folic acid metabolism (MTHFR C677T polymorphism): NTD are related to genes encoding proteins that are directly or indirectly connected with folic acid and methionine metabolism; a significantly higher number of female fetuses are afflicted with NTD compared to male fetuses. A significantly higher incidence of consanguinity has been noticed among the parents of NTD-afflicted babies; parents who have had an affected pregnancy would be at an increased risk of recurrence, that is, a three to fivefold higher risk than the general population. A common mutation in the 5, 10-methylenetetrahydrofolate reductase (*MTHFR*) gene, which is a risk factor for NTD, has been identified. The risk of recurrence of NTDs after one affected pregnancy is 2–3% and may approach 10% with two previous abnormal pregnancies.[1]
- *Folic acid deficiency in mother*: Up to 70% increased incidence is seen in offspring of mothers with FA deficiency.[11]
- *Exposure to drugs*:
  – *Antiepileptics drugs (AED)*: AED crosses placenta, alter folate metabolism, and decrease the plasma folate or red-cell folate concentration. The suggested mechanisms of AED include: liver enzyme induction by AED, the impairment of folate absorption, competitive interaction between folate coenzymes and drugs, and an increased demand for folate as a coenzyme for antiepileptic hydroxylation.[12]
  The prevalence of malformations is increased with the number of drugs administered; the rate of malformation was 7.8% for one AED, 9.6% for two AED, 11.5% for three AED, 13.5% for four AED, and 15.4% for five AED.
  According to recent data, Valproate is found to be more teratogenic than carbamazepine, and a combination of valproate and lamotrigine is chiefly teratogenic. The Japanese government has banned the prescription of both trimethadione and valproate to pregnant women and has cautioned that primidone should be prescribed only when its usefulness exceeds the risk of harm to the mother and fetus.
  – *Other drugs*: A variety of drugs are known to interfere with folate metabolism and prevent the absorption of folic acid. These drugs comprise of sulfamethoxazole-trimethoprim, methotrexate, aspirin, sulfadoxine-pyrimethamine, sulfasalazine, azathioprine, antacids and rifampicin.[3] A high dietary intake of preformed vitamin A appeared to be teratogenic, thus required to be completely avoided.[13]
- *Zinc deficiency*: Inadequate zinc intake is associated with NTDs in both animals and humans. The essentiality of zinc in neural tube formation is further supported by the observation that women with acrodermatitis enteropathica, a disorder of impaired zinc absorption from the intestine, are at high-risk for babies with NTDs.[14]
- *Maternal hyperthermia*: Heat exposure in general has been associated with an increased risk for NTDs. The use of Hot-tub in the first trimester was associated with a threefold

increase in the risk. Any combination of hot-tub use and febrile illness was associated with a six-fold increase in the risk.[15]
- *Maternal diabetes*: The mothers with insulin-dependent diabetes mellitus reported an incidence of 15.5 infants.[16]
- *Obesity*: Maternal obesity and elevated body mass index have been consistently associated with an increased risk for NTDs. Body mass index >29 doubles the risk.[17]
- *Age*: Risk tends to be elevated in mothers of extremes of age; younger or older. Studies have shown both a "modest risk in mothers of parity more than two" and an increased risk in primiparous mothers.[18] Twin pregnancies may be associated with a higher risk for NTDs.[19] Prevalence of anencephaly in twins at birth was 0.99 per 1,000, significantly higher than the birth prevalence of anencephaly in singletons.[20]
- *Cigarette smoking*: During the first and early second trimester; serum folate concentration levels are found to be significantly lower in smokers, compared nonsmokers.[19]

PREVENTION

Therapeutic options are limited. Therefore, high priorities are given for preventive strategies.

Primary Prevention

Primary prevention implies the prevention of the birth of a child with NTD, prior to its occurrence in any family. Primary prevention aims at targeting preventive measures to concerned maternal population or to high-risk individuals who can be identified by suitable screening methods.

The approaches are:
- Maternal serum alpha-fetoprotein (msAFP): Screening, to identify the presence of open NTD in the 16th–18th week of gestation.[21] In presence of open NTD, much higher amounts of AFP ooze into amniotic fluid and consequently to maternal serum. Thus, the level of msAFP is significantly higher if the fetus *in utero* carries an open NTD. At cut-off value of greater than 2.5 XMOM (Multiple of Median), more than 90% cases of anencephaly and 80% of spina bifida cystica may be detected by msAFP measurement.[11] The test has decreased specificity however, is not very high since it may be elevated in several other fetal disorders as well.[22]
- *Other tests*: The utility of combining serum uE3 measurement along with msAFP has been proposed.[23] The diagnosis of NTD can be confirmed by high-resolution fetal ultrasonography and/or amniotic fluid acetylcholine-esterase estimation, both of which are capable of making a correct diagnosis of NTD, in great majority of cases.
- *Periconceptional folic acid supplementation*: It has been proposed that supplementation of folic acid 0.4 mg/day to all women in the reproductive age group reduces the incidence of NTDs.[24] The double blind randomized trial of Medical Research Council, Great Britain has shown that supplementation of 4 mg folic acid per day, for at least one month prior to conception to three months postconception reduces the risk of recurrence of NTD by 70%.[25] The timing of folic acid supplementation for prevention of NTD is very critical, since neural tube in humans closes between days 17 and 30 post-ovulation, which corresponds to day 2 and 15 post-LMP. The mechanism of action of folic acid in preventing the occurrence of NTD has been a subject of speculation. Many of these women were found to have higher levels of serum homocysteine (and methionine), indicating a metabolic block in the folic acid pathway.
- *Identification of genes predisposing to NTD*: The common sporadic type of isolated NTD is considered to be a polygenic multifactorial disorder. The role of genes in causation of NTD is supported by higher risk of recurrence in first degree relatives compared to general population. The observation that periconceptional folic acid supplementation can prevent recurrence and even the first occurrence of NTD has led to investigation of the role of genes involved in folic acid metabolism. It has been reported that C to T mutation at nucleotide 677 in the *MTHFR* gene is 1.7–1.9 (95% CI 1.1–3.1) times more prevalent in mothers, fathers and fetuses affected with NTD compared to the general population.[26] While in isolated families *Pax 3* as well as Paxl have been implicated in NTD.

Secondary Prevention and Genetic Counseling

The prevention of recurrence of the condition after the birth of one affected child is known as secondary prevention. The risk of recurrence of NTD after birth of one affected child is 3–5%, which is 10 times higher than that of general population.[27] It increases to 10% after birth of two affected children and to 25% after three such births.

Periconceptional folic acid supplementation and antenatal diagnosis can prevent the birth of NTD child in the subsequent pregnancy. It is, therefore, important that all women who have given birth to a child with NTD, is requested to be discharged with folic acid supplementation and is referred for genetic counseling prior to conception of the next child. The affected child is expected to be examined by a geneticist to make a correct diagnosis of the disorder since there are several monogenic syndromes and chromosomal disorders which are associated with NTD. These syndromes carry different risks of recurrences and may not be preventable by folic acid supplementation. In case of stillbirths and neonatal deaths, where obtaining immediate genetic advice is impossible, it is important to take a photograph, a whole body radiograph and to carry out chromosomal study and autopsy, if feasible, of the affected child.

SUMMARY

Our ultimate objective is to reduce the genetic burden and to achieve the desired reproductive goal of the couple without undue harm to mother and fetus. It is the responsibility of physicians to communicate the risk of the occurrence and reoccurrence of the disease with discussing the various reproductive options. The couples need to bed informed about the availability, utility, limitations and safety of various tests and procedures for carrier screening and antenatal diagnosis. For prevention of genetic disorders, it is important to start preconception clinics where individuals with high-risk predisposing factors of having a child with genetic disease could be screened and those who are found to be at risk are counselled and managed.

REFERENCES

1. Chen CP. Syndromes, disorders and maternal risk factors associated with neural tube defects. Taiwan J Obstet Gynecol. 2008;47:267-75.
2. Lemire RJ. Neural tube defects. JAMA. 1988;259: 558-62.
3. Verma IC. High incidence of neural tube defects in North India. Lancet. 1978;i: 879.
4. Moore CA, Li S, Li Z, Hong SX, Gu HQ, Berry RJ, et al. Elevated rates of severe neural tube defects in high-prevalence areas in northern China. Am J Med Gen. 1997;73:113-8.
5. Sharma AK, Upreti M, Kamboj M, Mehra P, Das K, Mishra A, et al. Incidence of neural tube defects in Lucknow over a 10-year period from 1982-1991. Indian J Med Res. 1994;99:223-6.
6. Kulkarni ML, Mathew MA, Ramehandran B. High incidence of neural tube defects in South India. Lancet. 1987;i:260.
7. Kulkarni ML, Mathew MA, Reddy V. The range of neural tube defects in southern India. Arch Dis Child. 1989;64:201-4.
8. Padmanabhan R. Etiology, pathogenesis and prevention of neural tube effects. Congenit Anom (Kyoto). 2006;42:55-67.
9. Sharma JB, Gulati N. Potential relationship between dengue fever and neural tube defects in a Northern District of India. Int J Obstet Gynaecol. 1992;39:291-5.
10. Lynberg MC, Khoury MJ, Lu X, Cocian T. Maternal flu, fever, and the risk of neural tube defects: a population-based case-control study. Am J Epidemiol. 1994;140: 244-55.
11. Hernandez-Diaz S, Werler MM, Walker AM, Mitchell AA. Folic acid antagonists during pregnancy and the risk of birth defects. N Engl J Med. 2000;343:1608-14.
12. Kaneko S, Battino D, Andermann E, et al. Congenital malformations due to antiepileptic drugs. Epilepsy Res. 1999;33:145-58.
13. Rothman KJ, Moore LL, Singer MR, Nguyen U-SDT, Mannino S, Milunsky A. Teratogenicity of high vitamin A intake. N Engl J Med. 1995; 333:1369-73.
14. Tamura T, Goldenberg R. Zinc nutriture and pregnancy outcome. Nutr Res. 1996;16:139-81.
15. Graham JM Jr, Edwards MJ, Edwards MJ. Teratogen update: Gestational effects of maternal hyperthermia due to febrile illness and resultant patterns of defects in humans. Teratology. 1998;58:209-18.

16. Becerra JE, Khoury MJ, Cordero JF, Erickson JD. Diabetic mellitus during pregnancy and the risks for specific birth defects: A population-based case-control study. Pediatrics. 1990;85:1-9.
17. Shaw GM, Velie EM, Schaffer D. Risk of neural tube defect-affected pregnancies among obese women. JAMA. 1996;275:1093-6.
18. Elwood JM, Little J, Elwood JH. Epidemiology and control of neural tube defects. New York: Oxford University Press, 1992.
19. Tuthill DP, Stewart JH, Coles EC, Andrews J, Cartridge PHT. Maternal cigarette smoking and pregnancy outcome. Paediatr Perinat Epidemiol. 1999;3:245-53.
20. Windham GC, Bjerkedal T. Malformations in twins and their siblings, Norway, 1967-79. Acta Genet Med Gemellol (Roma). 1984;33:87-95
21. UK Collaborative Study on Alpha-fetoprotein in Relation to Neural Tube Defects. Maternal scrum alpha-fetoprotein measurement in antenatal screening for anencephaly and spina bifida in early pregnancy. Lancet. 1977;i:1323-32.
22. Adams MJ, Windham GC, Greenberg, JF Clayton-Hopkins JA, Reimer CB, Oakley GP. Clinical interpretation of maternal alphafetoprotein concentrations. Am J Obstet Gynecol. 1984;148:241-54.
23. Yaron Y, Hamby DD, O'Brian JE, Critchfield G, Lcon J, Ayoub M, et al. Combination of maternal scrum alpha-fetoprotein (MSAFP) an low estriol is highly predictive of anencephaly. Amer J Med Genet. 1998;75:297-9.
24. Centers for Disease Control: Recommendations for the use of folic acid to reduce the number of cases of spina bifida and other neural tube defects. JAMA. 1993;269:1233-8.
25. MRC Vitamin Study Research Group. Prevention of neural tube defects: Results of the Medical Research Council Vitamin Study. Lancet. 1991; 338:131-7.
26. Van Der Put NM, Eskes TK, Blom HJ. Is the common 677---@T mutation in the methylene tetrahydrofolate reductase gene a risk factor for neural tube defects? A meta-analysis. QJM. 1997;90:111-5.
27. Tolmie J. Neural tube defects and other congenital malformations of the central nervous system. In: Rirnoin DL, Connor JM, Pyeritz RE (Eds). Principles and Practice of Medical Genetics, 3rd edition. New York, Churchill Livingstone; 1996. pp. 2145-76.

CHAPTER 6

Cerebral Palsy

PA Mohammed Kunju

INTRODUCTION

Cerebral palsy (CP) is a group of permanent disorders of movement and posture causing activity limitation which are attributed to nonprogressive disturbances that occur in the developing fetal or infant brain.[1,2]

Following aspects are to be considered—*Nonprogressive central motor deficit due to disorders affecting developing brain.*
- *"Nonprogressive"*—to be differentiated from progressive disorders like metabolic or progressive genetic disorders by loss of acquired milestones or occurrence of systemic manifestations.
- *"Central"*—to be differentiated from peripheral nervous system disorders by presence of upper motor neuron (UMN) signs and cognitive dysfunctions.
- *Motor deficit*—dominant motor and less mental and sensory disturbances. All disturbances of motor system can be present in varying degree. Weakness, tone changes (hypotonia, spasticity, rigidity), incoordination, and abnormal movements.
- *Due to disorders affecting developing brain*—i.e. it can occur due to problems from first trimester to 2 years; and not a problem of mature brain.

Incidence: 1–2/1000.

ETIOLOGY

- Congenital malformations of brain[3]
- Perinatal hypoxia
- Birth trauma
- Acid base imbalance
- Indirect hyperbilirubinemia
- Metabolic disturbances
- Intrauterine growth restriction (IUGR)
- Infections
- Low birth weight (LBW) babies.

CLASSIFICATION

Cerebral palsy may be classified according to the pattern of neurologic involvement, neuropathology, and etiology.
- Physiological
  – Pyramidal (spastic)
    - Diplegic
    - Hemiplegic
    - Quadriplegic
  – Extrapyramidal
    - Athetoid, dystonic
    - Cerebellar (ataxic)
  – Mixed
    - Ataxic diplegic
    - Dystonia + choreoathetoid + spastic CP

- Etiological
  - Prenatal (For example: infections, metabolic, anoxia, genetic)
  - Perinatal (anoxia)
  - Postnatal (toxin, trauma)
- Functional
  - Class I: No limits of activity
  - Class II: Mild → moderate
  - Class III: Moderate → severe
  - Class IV: No useful physical activity.

TERMINOLOGIES USED IN TOPOGRAPHIC DEFINITION OF CEREBRAL PALSY[4]

- *Diplegia*: When the legs are more affected than arms. Approximately 80% of preterm infants who manifest motor abnormalities have spastic diplegia (**Figs 6.1A to C**).
- *Quadriplegia*: Weakness of all four extremities along with weakness of trunk, neck and face.
- *Hemiplegia*: Weakness of upper and lower limb on one side of the body; upper limbs will be more affected than legs (**Figs 6.2A and B**).
- *Double hemiplegia*: Weakness of all four extremities, arms are more affected than legs.
- *Triplegia*: Weakness of both lower extremity and one upper extremity.
- *Monoplegia*: Weakness of a single extremity. It is a very rare condition.

Diplegic Cerebral Palsy

- Bilateral spasticity of legs
- Classical form of CP in preterm
- First indication when an affected infant begins to crawl. Uses the arms normally, tends to drag leg (commando crawl).

On Examination

- Increased tendon jerks + increased plantar + ankle clonus
- Scissoring and spasm of extensors and group of muscles
- When grown up, walks on tiptoes with lower limb internally rotated at hip and all of lower limb in semiflexion
- Severe spastic diplegia → disuse atrophy and impaired growth of lower extremities
- Most common neuropathologic finding → periventricular leukomalacia
  Water shed area in preterm is periventricular → decreased white matter between vascular territories
  Close → Lower limb (LL) → Upper limb (UL) → Facial fibers
- Visual disturbances, strabismus (+)
- If mental retardation (MR) + epilepsy + spastic diplegia = cortex
- In term, water shed area → parasagittal cortex between the vascular territories of anterior,

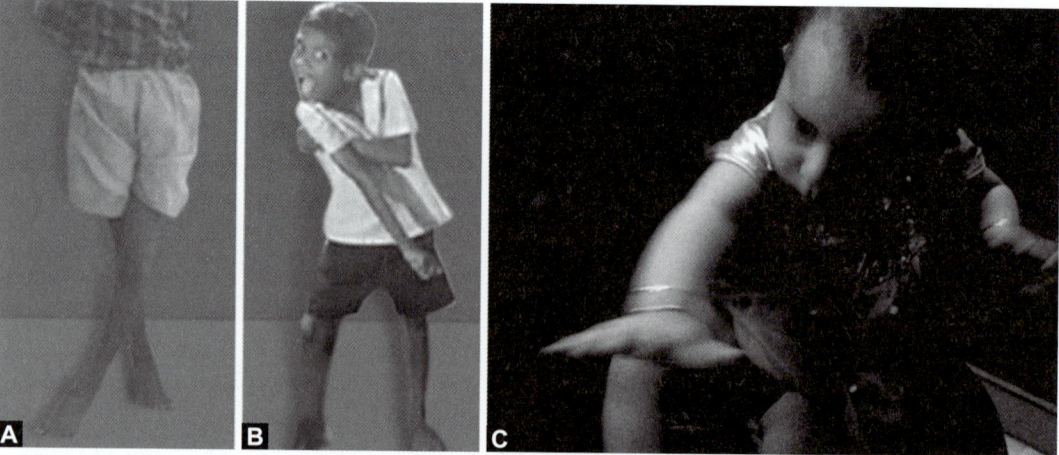

Figures 6.1A to C Types of cerebral palsy: (A) Diplegic CP—notice the scissoring; (B) Choreoathetotic CP—notice the twisted posturing; finger posturing; (C) Ataxic CP—early evidence of incoordinated approach
(For color version, see Plate 3)

Cerebral Palsy

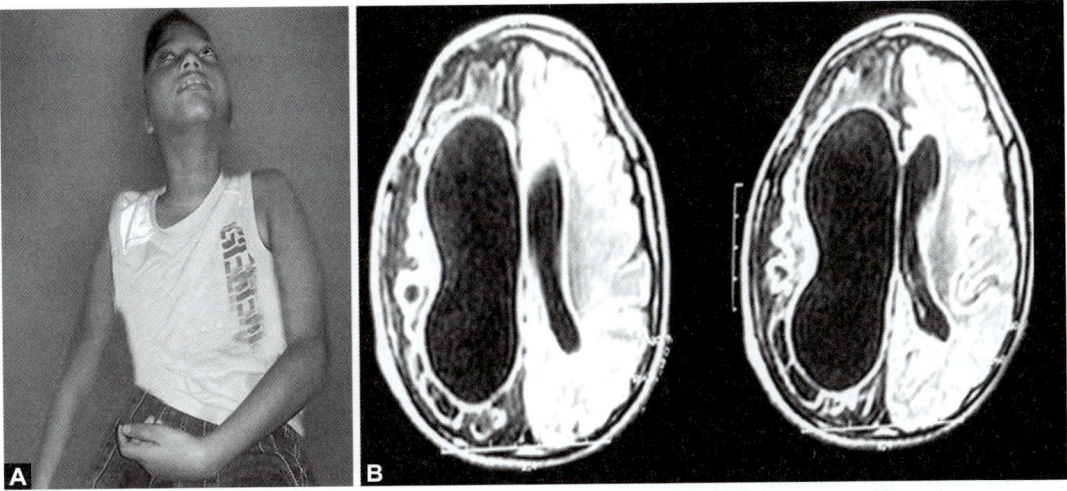

Figures 6.2A and B (A) Left hemiplegic CP; (B) MRI—notice the right hemispheric atrophy; dilated right lateral ventricle cystic changes in the atrophied brain *(For color version, see Plate 4)*

middle and posterior cerebral arteries. As severe hypoxia → cortex → quadriplegia (hip shoulder weakness).

Spastic Quadriplegic Cerebral palsy

- Severe form of CP because of marked motor impairment of all extremities and high association with mental retardation and seizures
- Result of bilateral cortical involvement by multifocal cortical necrosis
- UMN type of spasticity in all 4 limbs with pseudo-bulbar palsy (PB), severe mental retardation and epilepsy
- PB palsy → difficulty in swallowing nasal regurgitation and increased gag reflex. PB palsy result loss of bilateral UMN connections to the lower cranial nerve nuclei and hence exaggerated gag reflex.

On Examination

- Increased tone and spasticity in all extremities, brisk reflex and extensor plantar
- Associated with develop disabilities like speech, visual abnormality

- Other cranial nerve nuclei, sub cortical nuclei and other specific areas destroyed
- Various cranial nerve palsies and extra pyramidal symptoms may be associated with quadriplegic CP.

Spastic Hemiplegic Cerebral Palsy

- Vascular occlusion
- Decreased spontaneous movements on affected side
- Unilateral cortical thumb
- Hand preference at early age
- Arm involved > leg and difficulty in hand manipulation by 1 year
- Walking delayed until 18–24 m
- Extremities show growth arrest, especially hands and thumbnail—if contralateral parietal lobe is abnormal
- Spasticity more in the ankle → equinovarus deform, walks on tip toes.

On Examination

- Ankle clonus (+), increased plantar, DTR increased
- Weakness of hand and foot dorsiflexors.

Computed Tomography/Magnetic Resonance Imaging

- Atrophic cerebral hemisphere with dilated lateral ventricles contralateral to the side of affected extremity (Dyke Davidoff Mason syndrome)
- If middle cerebral artery territory undergoes infarction with residual cystic change
- Porencephalic cyst in some part of parietal lobe.

Dystonic and Choreoathetoid Cerebral Palsy

(Extrapyramidal CP).

Hallmarks

- Defective coordination of movements. Defective regulation of muscle tone. These cause inability to execute the intended movements.
- Muscle tone at rest normal or even reduced, but on attempted movements there is dystonic posturing and unintended involuntary movements in many muscle groups → execution of parallel movements impossible.
- No gross mental retardation, but child can perform only like a retarded child due to the above handicap.

Causes

Hyperbilirubinemia and hypoxia:
- Dysmyelination in place of gray matter of the basal ganglia (the appearance is described as *status marmoratus* = Marbled appearance) Kernicterus → Athetoid tetrad = Choreo athetosis, high tone deafness, enamel hypoplasia, upgaze palsy.
- Bilirubin interferes with O_2 utilization of specific cerebral tissues → damage.

Cerebellar (Ataxic) Cerebral Palsy

Pure case is rare. Ataxia manifest in the 2nd year of life
- Before 2nd year child floppy
- Pyramidal tract signs +/–
- Cerebellar signs → Titubation, truncal ataxia, gait ataxia, hypotonia
- Look for congenital cerebellar malformations.

Mixed Cerebral Palsy (Ataxia + Diplegia)

- Corticocerebellar fibers pass around the periventricular area (+LL fibers)
- In hydrocephalus → or on the fibers → presents with mixed CP.

Hypotonic (Atonic) Cerebral Palsy

- Despite pyramidal involvement → child is atonic
- Tendon reflexes—Brisk
- Extensor plantar
- Severe mental retardation
- Delayed CNS maturation.

Associated Features

- *Eyes*: Squint, gaze palsy, cataract, coloboma, refractory error.
- *Ears*: Partial/complete loss of hearing.
- *Speech*: Aphasia, dysarthria.
- *Sensory defects*: Astereognosis.
- *Seizures*: Generalized, focal tonic.
- *Intelligence*: 50% will have severe mental retardation, inadequate thermoregulation.

Diagnosis

- If a child with LBW, perinatal insult has increased tone, feeding difficulty, neurological and behavioral abnormality, abnormal posture, involuntary movements
- Perinatal history
- Neurological and developmental examination
- EEG
- Assessment of language and learning disability
- Psychometric and sensory evaluation
- Asymmetric tonic neck reflex persists >6 months → CP.

Common Pathologies Occurring in Perinatal Asphyxia Resulting in CP[4,5]

- Parasagittal cerebral injury of term babies leading to a hip shoulder type of weakness resulting in quadriplegia
- Periventricular leukomalacia in preterm babies resulting in diplegia (Figs 6.3A and B)
- Focal and multifocal brain necrosis with cognitive defects and seizures

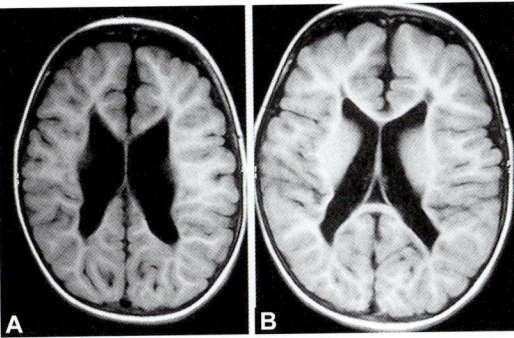

Figures 6.3A and B Periventricular leukomalacia: (A) Dilatation of the lateral ventricle by the loss of Periventricular white matter; (B) Squared posterior horn

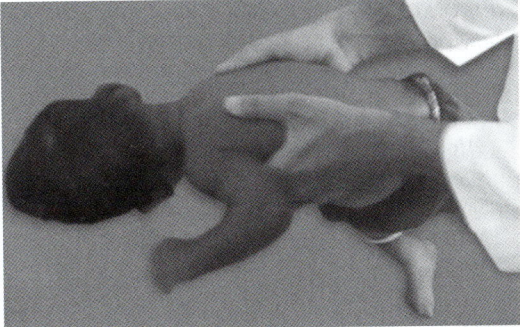

Figure 6.4 An early sign of cerebral palsy. On ventral suspension abnormal head and shoulder retraction; stiff extension of lower limbs *(For color version, see Plate 4)*

- Selective neuronal necrosis producing varying degrees of spastic cerebral palsy, or spastic hemiparesis
- Status marmoratus (marbled basal ganglia and thalami) with resultant extrapyramidal cerebral palsy
- Diffuse neuronal injury producing mixed or severe forms.

Clues Towards Early Diagnosis of Cerebral Palsy

A newborn with high risk factors and following:
- *Abnormal behavior*: Colicky behavior; excessive docility or irritability, poor eye contact, irregular sleep pattern, feeding problem (failure to establish breastfeeding and failure to thrive).
- *Oromotor problems*: Frequent vomiting, poor sucking, tongue retraction, grimacing, difficulty in chewing and swallowing.
- *Poor mobility*: Poor head control, abnormal tone, hand preference before 2 years of age, abnormal crawl, abnormal posturing **(Fig. 6.4)**.
- Persistent fisting (cortical thumb >50% of time before 2 months of age and at any time after 2 months **(Fig. 6.5)**.
- *Delayed milestones*: Social smile not attained by 3 months, inability to sit without support by 8 months.
- Persistence of neonatal reflexes (For example, ATNR—asymmetric tonic neck reflex) or late or non-appearance of infantile reflexes (For example, Landau reflex).

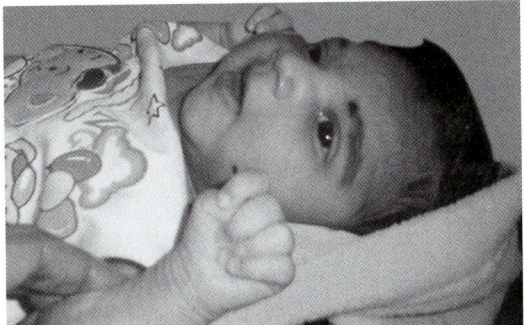

Figure 6.5 Persistent fisting *(For color version, see Plate 4)*

Utilization of a simple *developmental observation card* with following items will help in identification and early intervention:
- Social smile by 2 months completed
- Head steadiness by 4 months completed
- Sitting without support by 8 months completed
- Standing without support by 12 months completed.

Make sure that "baby sees, hears and listens".

Differential Diagnosis

- Neurodegenerative disorders
  - Progressive, familial, consanguinity, vomiting, seizures, failure to thrive (FTT). *Apparent regression in static encephalopathy* may be noticed due to new onset seizures, new onset movement disorders (usually during second year), increasing spasticity, progressive hydrocephalus

enlarging porencephalic cyst and parental misperception of attained milestones
- Hydrocepahlus with subdural effusion
  - Head large, fontanel bulge, sutures separate
- Brain tumor or intracranial space occupying lesions (ICSOL)
  - Progressive, increased ICT
- Muscle disorders—Congenital myopathy, myotonic dystrophy mimic CP EMG and biopsy diagnostic
- Ataxia telangiectasia.

Prevention of Cerebral Palsy[6]

- Prevention of maternal infection
- Prevention of fetal/perinatal insults
- Early diagnosis, adequate management plans can reduce the residual neurological and psychological emotional handicaps for the child and family.

Early Intervention Measures for Cerebral Palsy

In early intervention programs, the primary care giver (either a pediatrician or a developmental therapist) works to create a developmental setting in which the key to child's improvement is by mother-child participation.

The basis of early intervention is that there are critical periods of development and if interventions happens before that, delay and disabilities can be minimized. This focuses on mobility, manipulation, and communication.

So anticipate CP in high risk babies including preterm and use early screening for motor milestone delay and tone change by Amiel Tison angles.

Regular passive exercises can be done at home by the parents as per the assessment.

By utilizing the head steadiness, sitting, standing and walking developmental observation, manipulative techniques can be utilized for facilitating achievement of each milestone. Multilevel and repeat sensory inputs and appropriate experiences in early life will contribute to information gains and achievement in various developmental spheres. The components of early intervention depend on the primary impairment and can be tailored as per the needs.

Management of Established Cerebral Palsy[7-9]

- Holistic—involve the family
- Physiotherapy
- Occupational therapy
- Symptomatic treatment
  - Seizures—anticonvulsants
  - Behavioral disturbance—tranquilizers
  - Improving muscle function—muscle retardation
    - Dantrolene Na—relax of skeletal muscles, 1 mg/kg BD (gradually increased)
    - Local phenol blocks
  - Prevent contractures—plastic orthoses
  - Spasticity—Diazepam, nitrazepam, baclofan, dantrolene sodium.

Physiotherapy

- Mother must do it at home
- Prevention of contractures
- Avoid/make use of abnormal patent reflexes
- Reflex stimulation of muscles
- Training in motor activities
- Feeding—Tongue thrust: Mass movements precipitated by stimuli—avoid such stimuli
  - In severe quadriplegia—NG feeding.

Drooling

- Anticholinergics—(atropine)
- Surgical transposition of salivary ducts
- Hyperactivity- Methylphenidate
- Education- If IQ good → (N) schooling
- Special education centers.

Orthopedic and Neurosurgical Measures

- Arthrodesis of wrist, ankle, etc.
- Muscle lengthening
- Surgical transfer of tendons
- Peripheral nerve section
- Selective motor fasciculotomy

Cerebral Palsy

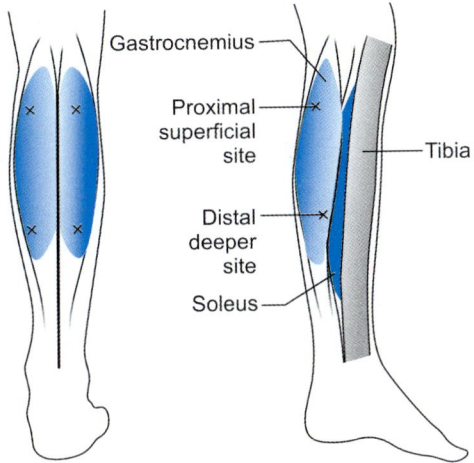

Figure 6.6 Sites of calf muscle botulinum toxin injection for tendo achilles spasm

- Spinal stimulation with surgical implants of electrodes
- Porencephalic cyst—neurosurgical, placement of shunt.

Spasticity

- Diazepam, nitrazepam, baclofen, dantrolene sodium
- Local vibration/application of ice
- Some for dystonia—trihexyphenidyl
- For athetosis—levo-dihydroxyphenylalanine (L-DOPA)
- Neuromuscular blocks[10-12]
  - Local anesthetics
  - Phenol
- Botulinum toxin injections—Multilevel injection after assessing spasticity and deciding point of injection sites of giving injection gastrosoleus for tendoachillis spasm is given in **Figure 6.6**.

Independence

- Wheel chairs, sitting type of toilet, pressing type of buttons
- Mode of communication (sound a bell- indicate toilet needs)
- Spastic societies
  - Guide the parents.

REFERENCES

1. Mutch L, Alberman E, Hagberg B, Kodama K, Perat MV. Cerebral palsy epidemiology: where are we now and where are we going? Dev Med Child Neurol. 1992;34(6):547-51.
2. Bax M, Goldstein M, Rosenbaum P, Leviton A, Paneth N, Dan B, et al. Proposed definition and classification of cerebral palsy, April 2005. Dev Med Child Neurol. 2005;47(8):571-6.
3. Shevell MI, Bodensteiner JB. Cerebral palsy: defining the problem. Semin Pediatr Neurol. 2004;11(1):2-4.
4. Russman BS, Ashwal S. Evaluation of the child with cerebral palsy. Semin Pediatr Neurol. 2004; 11(1):47-57.
5. Volpe JJ. Neurology of the Newborn. 4th edition. Philadelphia, PA: WB Saunders; 2001. pp. 45-99.
6. Nelson KB. Can we prevent cerebral palsy? N Engl J Med. 2003;349(18):1765-9. Capute AJ, Accardo PJ (Eds). Developmental Disabilities in Infancy and Childhood, 2nd edition. Baltimore, Md: Brookes Publishing; 2001. Vol 2.
7. Vincer MJ, Allen AC, Joseph KS, Stinson DA, Scott H, Wood E. Increasing prevalence of cerebral palsy among very preterm infants: a population-based study. Pediatrics. 2006; 118(6):e1621-6.
8. Delgado MR, Hirtz D, Aisen M, et al. Practice parameter: pharmacologic treatment of spasticity in children and adolescents with cerebral palsy (an evidence-based review): report of the Quality Standards Subcommittee of the American Academy of Neurology and the Practice Committee of the Child Neurology Society. Neurology. 2010;74(4):336-43.
9. Edwards P, Sakzewski L, Copeland L, Gascoigne-Pees L, McLennan K, Thorley M, et al. Safety of Botulinum Toxin Type A for Children With Nonambulatory Cerebral Palsy. Pediatrics. 2015;136 (5):895-904.
10. Dai AI, Wasay M, Awan S. Botulinum toxin type A with oral baclofen versus oral tizanidine: a nonrandomized pilot comparison in patients with cerebral palsy and spastic equinus foot deformity. J Child Neurol. 2008;23(12):1464-6.
11. Rahmati H, Martens H, Aamo OM, Stavdahl O, Stoen R, Adde L. Frequency-based features for early cerebral palsy prediction. Conf Proc IEEE Eng Med Biol Soc. 2015;2015:5187-90. doi: 10.1109/EMBC.2015.7319560.
12. Kedem P, Scher DM. Evaluation and management of crouch gait. Curr Opin Pediatr. 2016;28(1):55-9.

CHAPTER 7

Neuronal Migration Disorders

TM Ananda Kesavan

INTRODUCTION

Anomalies of the central nervous system are common. As many as 2000 congenital brain malformations have been described. Incidence of cerebral congenital malformations is in 1% of live birth. 75% of fetal deaths have cerebral malformation and one third of all major anomalies involve the central nervous system.

Neuronal migration disorder (NMD) is a group of brain malformations resulting from interference in normal neuronal migration at the time of brain development (8–20 weeks of gestation). The migrating neurons fail to reach their intended destination in the cortex and normal neurons lie in abnormal locations.[1]

Normal development of the brain will have the following stages in sequence:
- Induction
- Neural tube formation
- Regionalization and specification
- Proliferation
- Neuronal migration
- Connection, selection and apoptosis.

Neuronal migration is very important stage in brain development.[2] Cerebral gyri and sulci are formed due to migration of the neuron. If there were no gyri and sulci, the brain will be so large that a normal delivery would not be possible!

Layers of cortex are (outside to inner):
- Molecular layer
- Outer granular layer
- Pyramid layer
- Inner granular layer
- Ganglionic layer and
- Polymorphic layer.

Neuronal migration takes place in the 7th week of intrauterine life by mitotic activity in the sub-ependymal layer (germinal matrix). Cells migrate from this germinal matrix to form the cortical plate. Migration begins first centrifugally and then radially.[1]

MECHANISM OF NEURONAL MIGRATION

Much is now known about the mechanics of how neurons move from their birthplace to their final destination. Depending on the area of the developing nervous system in which they originate, migrating neurons follow one of the two strategies. Neural crest cells are largely guided along distinct migratory pathways by specialized adhesion molecules in the extracellular matrix or by molecules on the surfaces of cells in the embryonic periphery.[3] At different developmental stages, similar molecules are probably used to guide axonal outgrowth. In contrast, neurons in many regions, including the cerebral cortex, cerebellum, hippocampus, and spinal cord, are guided to their final destinations by crawling along a particular type of glial cell, called radial glia, which acts as a cellular guide (**Fig. 7.1**). Specialized molecules (integrin) help to find the correct path. Once

Neuronal Migration Disorders

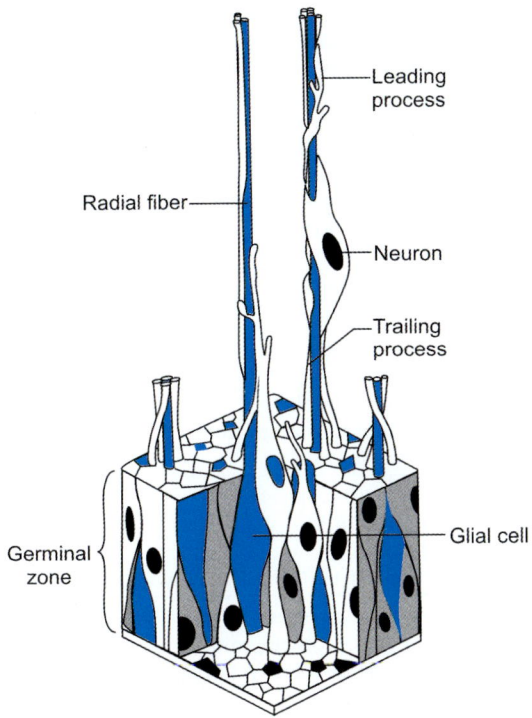

Figure 7.1 Role of radial glial cells in neuronal migration. A migrating neuron is ascending on the radial fiber

neurons reached the correct location, it will detach from the radial glia by the stop signal given by REELIN. There are several ways they can do this, e.g. by radial migration or tangential migration.[4]

RADIAL MIGRATION

Neuronal precursor cells proliferate in the ventricular zone of the developing neocortex. The first postmitotic cells to migrate form the pre-plate which are destined to become Cajal-Retzius cells and sub plate neurons. These cells do so by somal translocation. Neurons migrating with this mode of locomotion are bipolar and attach the leading edge of the process to the pia. The somal is then transported to the pial surface by nucleokinesis, a process by which a microtubule "cage" around the nucleus elongates and contracts in association with the centrosome to guide the nucleus to its final destination. Radial glia, whose fibers serve as a scaffolding for migrating cells, can itself divide or translocate to the cortical plate and differentiate in to astrocytes or neurons.[5]

Subsequent waves of neurons split the preplate by migrating along radial glial fibers to form the cortical plate.[6] Each wave of migrating cells travel past their predecessors forming layers in an inside-out manner, meaning that the youngest neurons are the closest to the surface. The first neuron migrates to form the interior brain structure (layer 1). The neurons which form the deepest layer (layer VI) migrate early. It is followed by formation of layer 5 to 2. This is called *"inside out theory"*. It is estimated that glial guided migration represents 90% of migrating neurons in human.[5]

TANGENTIAL MIGRATION

Most interneurons migrate tangentially through multiple modes of migration to reach their appropriate location in the cortex. An example of tangential migration is the movement of inter neurons from the ganglionic eminence to the cerebral cortex.

OTHER MODES OF MIGRATION

There is also a method of neuronal migration called multipolar migration. This is seen in multipolar cells, which are abundantly present in the cortical intermediate zone.

Major pathways of neuronal migration are: Migration via the corpus pontobulbar, migration via the corpus ganglio thalamic, cerebellar migration, migration to the cerebral cortex from periventricular germinal matrix.

NEUROTROPHIC HYPOTHESIS

According to the neurotrophic hypothesis, advanced by Victor Hamburger and Rita Levi-Montalcini, neurons compete for limiting amounts of survival factors produced by target structures. These factors are called neurotrophic factors. The first neurotrophic factor to be purified was nerve growth factor.[7]

ETIOLOGY

The majority of neuronal migration disorders are thought to have a genetic cause.[8] The widespread abnormal expression of defective genes leads to the global nature of the disorders, contrary to acquired developmental brain insults, which lead to more localized defects. Several genes have been implicated in causing the various disorders. The most well characterized genes include DCX on the X chromosome, responsible for double cortex syndrome.[9] Some other identified genes are given in **Table 7.1**.

DCX, LIS 1, and filamin 1 are genes responsible for controlling the mechanics of cell movement during neuronal migration.

Any antenatal insult before 20th intrauterine life may lead to development of neuronal migration disorder.[10] Many conditions are associated with NMD **(Table 7.2)**.

CLINICAL FEATURES

Jaw et al. described from 36 patients the various clinical features of NMD. They are in order of frequency: Seizure—64%, delayed development-42%, mental retardation—25%, motor deficit-42% and others–dysmorphic features, poor schooling.[2,10] Some of them may be normal also. Clinical features also depends on the associated conditions **(Table 7.2)**.

Common migration disorders are: lissencephaly, schizencephaly, heterotopia, and cortical dysplasia.

Lissencephaly

The word Lissos (Gk) means—smooth. It is the most common migration disorder. It occurs due to insult to fetal brain occur during 8-14 weeks gestation. Characteristic feature is paucity of gyral and sulcal formation. In lissencephaly, cortex shows 4 layers

Table 7.1 Neuronal migration disorder and the associated genes

Migration disorder	Chromosome	Gene
Schizencephaly	–	EMX2
Lissencephaly	17p13.3	LIS 1
Periventricular heterotopia	Xq28	XIS3, Filamin 1
Cobble stone lissencephaly	9q31-33	Fukutin
Band heterotopia	Xq22.3-q24	Double cortin

Table 7.2 Conditions are associated with neuronal migration disorder

- *Metabolic disorders*
  - Zellweger syndrome
  - Neonatal adrenoleukodystrophy
  - Glutaric aciduria Type-II
  - Nonketotic hyperglycinemias
  - Pyruvate dehydrogenase deficiency
  - Kinky Menkes disease
  - GM2 gangliosidosis
- *Brain anomaly*
  - Hydrancephaly
  - Porencephaly
  - Cerebellar hypoplasia
  - Agenesis of corpus callosum
  - Holoprosencephaly
- *Chromosomal anomalies*
  - Trisomy 13,18, 21
  - Deletion 4p
  - Deletion 17p13 (Miller-Dieker syndromes)
- *Neuromuscular diseases*
  - Walker-Warburg syndrome
  - Fukuyama muscular dystrophy
  - Myotonic dystrophy
  - Anterior horn arthrogryposis
- *Neurocutaneous syndromes*
  - Incontinentia pigmenti
  - Neurofibromatosis
  - Hypomelanosis of Ito
  - Epidermal nevus syndrome
  - Tuberous sclerosis
- *Multiple congenital anomalies/syndromes*
  - Smith-Lemli-Opitz syndrome
  - Potter syndrome
  - Cornelia de Lange syndrome
  - Meckel-Gruber syndrome
  - Orofacial digital syndrome
  - Coffin-Siris syndrome
  - Aicardi syndrome
  - Joubert syndrome
  - Hemimegalencephaly
  - Thanatophoric dysplasia
  - Dandy-Walker syndrome
- *Maternal infection*
  - CMV, Rubella, toxoplasmosis
- *Intoxication*
  - Alcohol-CO, Isoretinoic acid
  - Methyl mercury
- *Ionizing radiation*

(layer III and IV missing). It is associated with deletion and mutation in LIS1 on 17p.

Clinical features of lissencephaly: Intractable seizures, mental retardation, microcephaly, delayed development. Lissencephaly broadly divided in 2 types.

Type I is classical Agyria—pachygyria spectrum. It is classically seen in Miller-Dieker syndrome (microcephaly, long upper lip, narrow temples, anteverted nares, wide spaced eyes, etc.) and lissencephaly with cerebellar hypoplasia.

Type II lissencephaly has disorganized cluster of neurons with haphazard orientation and no definitive layer or pattern (cobblestone lissencephaly) associated with Walker-Warburg syndrome, muscle-eye disease and Fukuyama congenital muscular dystrophy.

MRI in lissencephaly is very characteristic. It shows smooth brain with thick, broad cortex **(Fig. 7.2)**. Shallow vertically oriented sylvian fissures giving an overall figure of eight (8) appearance in axial imaging.

Schizencephaly

Gray matter-lined clefts extend from subarachnoid space to lateral ventricle (Schiz *Greek*-Cleft). It is caused by defect in neuronal migration in fourth month of gestation. Two types are described. Close lip schizencephaly where no connection of the cleft to the ventricle and present with hemiparesis or motor delay. In minor deformity, child may asymptomatic.[8]

Open lip schizencephaly where clefts are filled with CSF. It may be unilateral or bilateral and common clinical features are: hemiplegia, epilepsy, mental retardation **(Fig. 7.3)**. 80–90% is associated with absent septum pellucidum.

MRI shows clefts that may be open and filled with CSF or closed with the sides of cleft touching and lined by dysplastic cortex.

Heterotopia

It is another form of NMD in which there is focal collection of ectopic neurons in cerebral hemispheres.[11] *Three types of heterotopias are:*
1. *Subependymal*: Nodules develop from sub ependymal region to ventricular system.
2. *Focal*: Gray matter (mass lesion) in deep subcortical white matter.
3. Diffuse underlying band of gray matter and white matter in band manner—band heterotopias or double cortex syndrome **(Fig. 7.4)**. It is commonly associated with corpus callosum agenesis also.

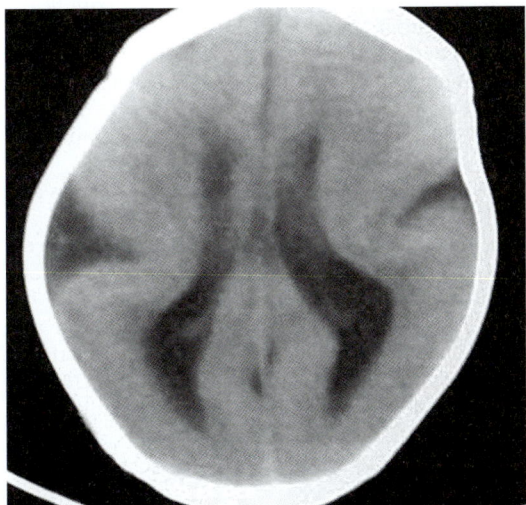

Figure 7.2 MRI in lissencephaly. Smooth brain with diminished white matter, Figure of 8 appearance and shallow vertically oriented Sylvian fissure

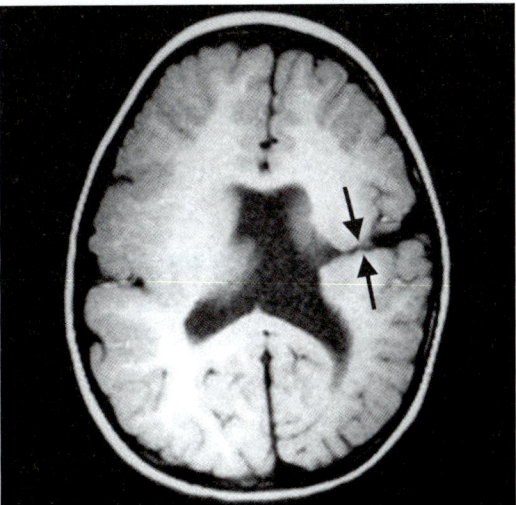

Figure 7.3 Open lip schizencephaly. Gray matter lined clefts extend from subarachnoid space to lateral ventricle

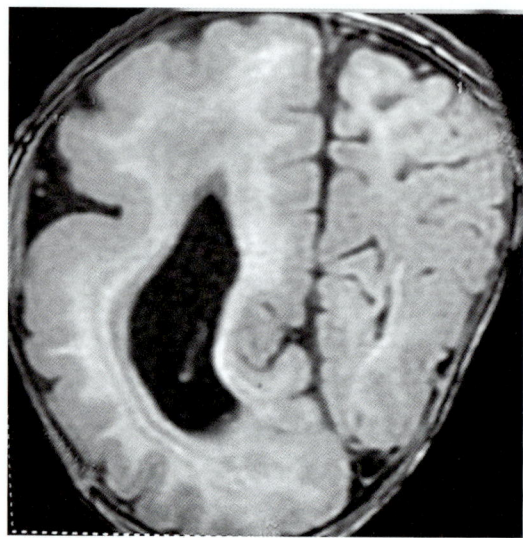

Figure 7.4 Abnormal gray-white matter differentiation with neuronal heterotopia, thickened cortex and broad gyres. Also note the associated hemimegalencephaly enlarged right cerebrum, ventricular asymmetry and subdural hygroma

Cortical Dysplasia

Disorder in which developing neurons complete the initial phase of neuronal migration, i.e. to the cortex, but fail to organize themselves in a six layered cortical pattern.[12]

Different types are:
- *Focal*: Irregular inner and outer surface of sulci and gyri.
- *Diffuse*: Bilateral involvement.
- *Bilateral perisylvian syndrome*: Insular, opercular and perisylvian dysplasia and underdeveloped Sylvian fissures.

Treatment of Neuronal Migration Disorders

No definite treatment. Only symptomatic and supportive treatment for seizures and physiotherapy are available. Surgical intervention are tried with variable results in localized form of NMD.

Prevention

Antenatal diagnosis is possible nowadays. Genetic testing is available for patients with lissencephaly to identify whether the DCX or LIS 1 gene is defective. Knowledge of the genes affected enables counseling and family planning.

REFERENCES

1. Guerrini R, Parrini E. Neuronal migration disorders. Neurobiol Dis. 2010;38:154-66.
2. Sarnat HB. In: Child neurology, 6th edn., Menkes JH, Sarnat HB (Eds). Lippincott; 2010. pp.186-98.
3. Crino PB. mTOR: A pathogenic signaling pathway in developmental brain malformations. Trends Mol Med. 2011;17:734-42.
4. Curran TD, Arecangelo G. Role of reelin in the control brain development. Brain Res Rev. 1998;26:285-94.
5. Dodd J, Schuchardt A. Axon guidance: a compelling case for repelling growth cones. Cell. 1995;81:471-4.
6. Barkovich AJ, Kuzniecki RI, Jackson GD, et al. A developmental and genetic classification for malformations of cortical evelopment. Neurology. 2005;65:1873-87.
7. Guerini R, Dobyns WB, Barkovich AJ. Abnormal development of the human cerebral cortex: genetics, functional consequences and treatment options. Trends Neurosci. 2008;31:154-62.
8. Faina GT, Cardini FA, D'Incerti L. Familial schizencephaly associated with EMX2 mutation. Neurology. 1997;48:1403-6.
9. Mc Ginnis W, Krumlauf R. Homebox genes and axial patterning. Cell. 1992;68:283-302.
10. Guerrini R, Dobyns WB. Malformations of cortical development: clinical features and genetic causes. Lancet Neurol. 2014;13(7):710-26.
11. Leventer RJ, Jansen A, Pilz DT. Clinical and imaging heterogeneity of polymicrogyria: a study of 328 patients. Brain. 2010;133:1415-27.
12. Gaitanis JN, Donahue J. Focal cortical dysplasia. Pediatr Neurol. 2013;49(2):79-87.

CHAPTER 8

Acute Disseminated Encephalomyelitis

Ciju Ravindranath

Acute disseminated encephalomyelitis (ADEM) is an immune-mediated inflammatory disorder of the central nervous system (CNS) with acute or subacute polyfocal onset, which predominantly affects the white matter of the brain and spinal cord. ADEM typically starts with an abrupt onset of neurological symptoms and signs within days to weeks after a viral infection or immunization. It is also known as *postinfectious, parainfectious, postexanthematous,* or *postvaccinal* encephalomyelitis.[1,2]

DEFINITIONS

Acute Disseminated Encephalomyelitis (Monophasic)

A first clinical event with a polysymptomatic encephalopathy, with acute or subacute onset, showing focal or multifocal hyper intense lesions predominantly affecting the CNS white matter. Typically, the subcortical white matter is affected; sometimes additional gray matter lesions are also seen.[3]

If a relapse takes place within 4 weeks of tapering steroid treatment or within the first 3 months from the initial event, this early relapse is considered temporally related to the same acute monophasic condition.

Recurrent ADEM

New demyelinating event fulfilling diagnostic criteria for ADEM, occurring at least 3 months after the initial ADEM event and at least 4 weeks after completing steroid therapy, showing the same clinical presentation and affecting the same areas on MRI as the initial ADEM episode.

Multiphasic ADEM

Refers to one or more ADEM relapses, including encephalopathy and multifocal deficits, but involving new areas of the CNS on MRI and neurological examination.

Epidemiology

The ADEM can occur at any age, but it is more common in pediatric patients than in adults. Peak incidence in children of 3–10 years of age.[4] No gender predominance is seen in ADEM. Viral illnesses and immunizations are the most common antecedent events.

CAUSES OF ACUTE DISSEMINATED ENCEPHALOMYELITIS

Viral Infections

- Measles, *Varicella zoster virus*, Rubella, Mumps
- Influenza A and B, Hepatitis A, Hepatitis C
- Epstein-Barr virus, Human immunodeficiency virus, Herpes simplex virus
- Dengue virus, Coronavirus.

Nonviral Infections

- Group A β-hemolytic streptococci, *Legionella pneumophila*

- Salmonella typhi, Leptospirosis
- *Plasmodium falciparum*, Mycoplasma pneumoniae
- *Rickettsia rickettsii, Borrelia burgdorferi*.

Postvaccinal ADEM

- Rabies vaccine made in brain or spinal cord preparations
- Measles, Japanese encephalitis virus
- Oral poliovirus, Tetanus toxoid
- Influenza, Hepatitis B recombinant vaccine.

PATHOGENESIS

Immune activation is a major contributor to the pathogenesis, initial events induced by the infectious agent might be more subtle and alternative nonimmune mechanisms are likely to contribute.

Immune-mediated Mechanisms

Molecular mimicry is one of the proposed mechanisms by which pathogens might lead to autoimmune responses.

Nonimmune Mechanisms

Myelin damage by viral products has been proposed.

ADEM is typically described as demyelination with relative preservation of axons, histologically characterized by perivenular infiltrates of T-cells and macrophages. It is associated with the human leukocyte antigen (HLA) class II alleles.

CLINICAL PRESENTATION

The diagnosis requires encephalopathy to be present, which may include behavioral change or alteration in consciousness. ADEM classically described as monophasic disorder.

Symptoms

- Motor weakness
- Fever
- Seizures
- Headache/vomiting/Malaise, Myalgia
- Visual problems
- Aphasia
- Psychiatric symptoms
- Behavioral changes.

Signs

- Altered sensorium.
- *Pyramidal signs:* Unilateral or bilateral long tract signs, acute hemiparesis and ataxia, DTR is brisk, normal or diminished with extensor plantar response.
- Cranial nerve palsy
- Meningeal signs
- Spinal cord involvement
- Extrapyramidal signs
- Cerebellar sign

Involvement of peripheral nervous system is rare in childhood ADEM but more common in adult patients, usually in the form of acute polyradiculoneuropathy. Optic neuritis is typically bilateral in ADEM.

Acute Hemorrhagic Leukoencephalitis

Acute hemorrhagic leukoencephalitis (AHL), acute hemorrhagic encephalomyelitis (AHEM) and acute necrotizing hemorrhagic leukoencephalitis (ANHLE) of Weston Hurst are rapidly progressive, and frequently fulminant inflammatory hemorrhagic demyelination of CNS white matter. Death from brain edema is common within 1 week of onset of the encephalopathy unless treated aggressively.

Differential Diagnosis

The differential diagnosis of ADEM can be narrowed by careful history, appropriate lab evaluations and MRI.[5] The principle disease in differential diagnosis being multiple sclerosis and acute bacterial or viral encephalitis **(Table 8.1)**.

INVESTIGATION

Blood and CSF Features

Patients with ADEM frequently have raised inflammatory markers (white cell count and erythrocyte sedimentation rate (ESR)) and lymphopenia.

CSF more commonly shows an increased protein and lymphocytosis in ADEM.

Acute Disseminated Encephalomyelitis

Table 8.1 Clinical and MRI features that may distinguish ADEM from first attack of multiple sclerosis[6]

	ADEM	MS
Age	<10 year	>10 year
Stupor/coma	+	–
Fever/vomiting	+	–
Family history	No	20%
Sensory complaints	+	+
Optic neuritis	Bilateral	Unilateral
Manifestations	Polysymptomatic	Monosymptomatic
MRI imaging	*Widespread lesions*: Basal ganglia, thalamus, cortical gray-white junction	*Isolated lesions*: Periventricular white matter, corpus callosum
CSF	Pleocytosis (lymphocytosis)	Oligoclonal bands
Response to steroids	+	+
Follow-up	No new lesions	New lesions
Female: Male	Almost equal	2:1 strong female preponderance
Recurrence	Chiefly monophasic, recovery 1–6 months. Self-limiting disease even in absence of therapy	Recurrent relapsing remitting disease course

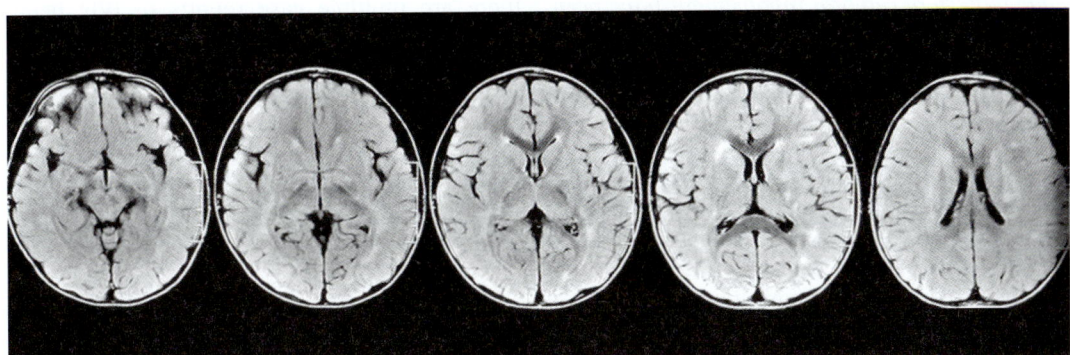

Figure 8.1 Patchy confluent hyperintense signals on FLAIR image noted in the subcortical white matter of both temporoparietal lobes, pons, medulla, bilateral basal ganglia, corona radiata, periventricular white matter, bilateral thalamic and both internal capsules

Intrathecal synthesis of Oligoclonal bands (oligoclonal IgG in CSF but not in serum) which occur in 0–29% of ADEM patients.

Stools to be sent as a part of acute flaccid paralysis (AFP) surveillance.

Neuroimaging

Magnetic resonance imaging abnormalities are most frequently identified on T2-weighted and fluid-attenuated inversion recovery (FLAIR) sequences as patchy, poorly marginated areas of increased signal intensity. Lesions in ADEM are typically large, multiple, and asymmetric. They typically involve the subcortical and central white matter and cortical gray-white junction of both cerebral hemispheres, cerebellum, brainstem, and spinal cord.

MRI lesions were classified according to system described by Tenebaum et al. (**Figs 8.1 and 8.2**).

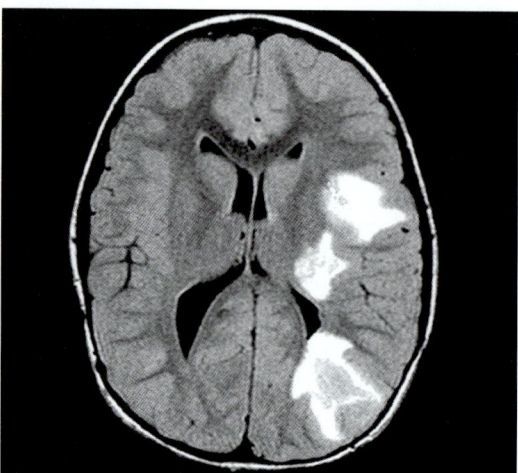

Figure 8.2 T2 FLAIR shows areas of demyelination and edema in deep subcortical and periventricular white matter as well as the basal ganglia and thalamus on the left side

Four pattern of cerebral involvement have been proposed.
1. ADEM with small lesions (less than 5 mm).
2. ADEM with large, confluent, or tumefactive lesions, with frequent extensive perilesional edema and mass effect.
3. ADEM with additional symmetric bithalamic involvement
4. Acute hemorrhagic encephalomyelitis (AHEM), when some evidence of hemorrhage can be identified in the large demyelinating lesions.

The MRI pattern does not appear to correlate with any particular outcome or disability. Since most lesions tend to resolve on follow-up imaging studies.

The typical spinal cord lesion is large and swollen, showing variable enhancement, and predominantly affects the thoracic region.

Advanced Neuroimaging Techniques

- *MR spectroscopy in acute stage*: Low levels of N-acetylaspartate (NAA) and elevated lactate levels within regions of prolonged T2-MRI signal, without increase in choline.
- Positron emission tomography (PET) scanning to show decreased cerebral metabolism.
- Single-photon emission computed tomography (SPECT) using 99m Tc-HMPAO shown areas of hypoperfusion that are more extensive than the MRI lesions.

TREATMENT AND MANAGEMENT

Steroids

High dose intravenous steroids are commonly employed, typically methylprednisolone 20–30 mg/kg/day for 5 days with maximum dose of 1 g/day. An oral prednisone taper over 1 month may prevent relapse. There is increased risk of relapse has been reported with steroid taper of 3 weeks or less.[7]

Adverse effects of long-term steroids include gastritis, hyperglycemia, hypokalemia, high blood pressure, facial flushing, and mood disorders.

Immunoglobulin

There are multiple case reports of IVIg being used successfully alone or in combination with corticosteroids in both pediatric and adult cases of ADEM, but there have been no studies which have directly compared IVIg with steroids, plasmapheresis, or other immunomodulatory treatments. In some cases, IVIg was administered after failed IV pulse steroid therapy or in cases of recurrent demyelination.

Plasma Exchange

The use of plasma exchange in ADEM has been reported in only a small number of cases, typically severe cases when steroid treatment has failed.

Other Therapies

There have been no published reports of interferon—alpha or glatiramer acetate used in the acute stage of ADEM although there are anecdotal descriptions of interferon-beta use for episodes of recurrent demyelination consistent with multiphasic ADEM. There are no published reports of cyclophosphamide, azathioprine, or other cytostatic drug use in pediatric ADEM.

OUTCOME AND PROGNOSIS

Untreated ADEM

The natural history of ADEM in most children is gradual improvement over several weeks, with 50–70% of patients experiencing full recovery. Limited data exist about the natural history of ADEM in the post-MRI era. There is considerable diversity with respect to antecedent infections, clinical presentation, and neuroimaging findings, further complicating outcomes analysis.

Treated ADEM

Over half the patients treated had a good recovery with minimal or no deficit. The most common problems seen following ADEM were focal motor deficits ranging from mild clumsiness and ataxia to hemiparesis or blindness. Behavioral and cognitive problems were identified in 6–50% of children, but are likely under reported in some series.[8] Less frequent late effects included development of seizures following ADEM resolution.

REFERENCES

1. Singhi PD, Ray M. Acute disseminated encephalomyelitis in North Indian children: clinical profile and follow-up.
2. Garg RK. Acute disseminated encephalomyelitis. Postgrad Med J. 2003;79:11-7.
3. Tenembaum S, et al. Acute disseminated encephalomyelitis; Silvia for the international pediatric MS study group. Neurology. 2007; 68(Suppl 2):S23–S36.
4. Noorbakhsh F. Acute disseminated encephalomyelitis: clinical and pathogenesis features. Neurol Clin. 2008;26:759-80.
5. Dale RC, et al. ADEM, MDEM and MS in children. Brain. 2000;123:2407-22.
6. Ketelslegers IA, Neuteboom RF. A comparison of MRI criteria for diagnosing pediatric ADEM and MS. Neurology. 2010;74:1412–5.
7. Bunyan RF. Acute demyelinating disorders: emergencies and management. Neurol Clin. 2012;30:285-307.
8. Dundar NO, et al. Relapsing acute disseminated encephalomyelitis in children: further evaluation of the diagnosis. J Child Neurol. 2010;25:1491.

CHAPTER 9

Guillain-Barré Syndrome

Shaji Abraham

INTRODUCTION

Guillain-Barré syndrome (GBS) is an acute inflammatory polyneuropathy commonly characterized by a rapidly progressive, essentially symmetric, flaccid weakness and areflexia. Sensory, autonomic, and cranial nerve involvement may also be seen. With the eradication of poliomyelitis, GBS is the most common cause of acute flaccid paralysis in children.

Guillain-Barré syndrome was first described by Jean Baptiste Landry, A French Physician in 1916, Georges Guillain, Jean Alexandre Barré, and André Strohl provided the first comprehensive description including clinicopathological features and CSF findings. GBS is a syndrome that encompasses different specific disorders, including the demyelinating form—acute inflammatory demyelinating polyneuropathy (AIDP), and axonal form, acute motor axonal neuropathy (AMAN), other forms like Miller Fisher syndrome.

EPIDEMIOLOGY

Annual incidence of GBS range from 0.5 to 1.5 cases per 100,000 populations in individuals younger than 18 years. About two third of children with GBS have an antecedent infection usually within 4 weeks prior to the onset of neurologic symptoms. The common preceding infection is respiratory (50–70%) followed by gastrointestinal (7–14%). The common pathogenic organisms are, Epstein-Barr virus, cytomegalovirus, varicella, and other herpes viruses, enteroviruses, hepatitis A and B, *Mycoplasma pneumoniae*, and *Campylobacter jejuni*; which is perhaps the most common with organism associated with GBS. An Indian case-control study reported that 27.7% of childhood GBS cases were associated with *C. jejuni* infection. Males appear to be at greater risk for GBS than females.

PATHOGENESIS

The GBS is an autoimmune-mediated disease triggered by with environmental factors. Demyelinating and axonal forms of GBS have both been described. In the demyelinating form, segmental demyelination of peripheral nerves is thought to be immune mediated and both humoral and cell-mediated immune mechanisms have been implicated. These pathogens are believed to activate $CD4^+$ helper-inducer T cells, which are particularly important mediators of disease. A variety of specific endogenous antigens, including myelin protein P-2, gangliosides GQ1b, GM1, and GT1a, may be involved in this response. Resemblance of the triggering pathogens to antigens on peripheral nerves (i.e. molecular mimicry) leads to an exaggerated autoimmune response initiated by T-lymphocytes and macrophages. Strong evidence now exists that axonal subtypes of Guillain–Barré syndrome, acute motor axonal neuropathy (AMAN), and acute motor and sensory axonal neuropathy (AMSAN), are caused by antibodies to gangliosides on the axolemma that target macrophages to invade the axon at the node of Ranvier.

CLINICAL FEATURES

Children with Guillain-Barré syndrome usually presents with acute onset of paresthesia/pain followed by progressive limb weakness. Pain and gait difficulty is also a common mode of presentation in children. The disease progresses rapidly and about 50% of patients reach the peak by 2 weeks and more than 90% by 4 weeks. Back, buttock or leg pain, which is presumed to result from nerve root and peripheral nerve inflammation, is the initial manifestation in as many as 50% of children. In small children GBS can present with pain and decreased movement or refusal to weight-bear. Neurological examination is characterized by relatively symmetrical weakness involving the proximal and distal muscles with hyporeflexia/areflexia in the classic form. Although GBS is essentially a motor neuropathy, sensory symptoms in the form of paresthesias and pain are common, but objective sensory losses are usually minimal. Cranial nerve involvement is common, facial nerve involvement (often bilateral) in 50–70% cases followed by bulbar muscles. Diaphragmatic weakness due to phrenic nerve involvement is also common. Approximately one third of hospitalized GBS patients require mechanical ventilation due to respiratory muscle oropharyngeal weakness. Tachycardia is common however, more serious autonomic nervous system dysfunction may occur, including life-threatening arrhythmias, hypotension, hypertension, and gastrointestinal dysmotility.

Clinical Variants of GBS

The clinical variants of GBS are characterized based on the types of nerve fiber involvement (motor, sensory, cranial and autonomic), or predominant mode of fiber injury (demyelinating versus saxonal). The common clinical variants are:
- *Acute inflammatory demyelinating polyradiculoneuropathy (AIDP)*: Most common form of GBS presents with predominantly symmetrical motor weakness with areflexia, bilateral facial and pharyngeal, occasional sensory, and autonomic disturbance. It is characterized by an immune-mediated attack on myelin with infiltration of lymphocytes and macrophages with segmental stripping of myelin.
- *Acute motor axonal neuropathy (AMAN)*: Most commonly seen in China and Japan (50–60% of cases), as opposed to Western countries (10–20% of cases). In this form, axonal degeneration occurs by immune attack within 1–2 weeks after infections. *C. jejuni* is the most common preceding infection, antiganglioside antibodies are usually found in this type. Electrophysiology shows reduction in muscle action potentials with relatively preserved motor nerve conduction velocity and normal sensory nerve action potentials and F waves.
- *Acute motor and sensory axonal neuropathy (AMSAN)*: This type is rare and resembles AMAN except sensory nerves are also affected. This type is associated with a severe course and poor prognosis.
- *Miller-Fisher syndrome*: Characterized by triad of ophthalmoplegia, ataxia, and areflexia. The characteristic autoantibodies are against gangliosides GQ1b. GQ1b plays a key role in the pathogenesis of MFS.
- *Pharyngio-cervical-brachial syndrome*: Presents with neck, arm and oropharyngeal muscle weakness and upper limb areflexia. Up to 40% have anti-GQ1b antibodies, and other antibodies include anti-GT1a.
- *Sensory variant*: Presents with acute sensory ataxia. Some patients have antibodies to GD1b and Gq1b gangliosides.
- *Acute pandysautonomia*: Presents with orthostatic hypotension, gastroparesis, constipation, urinary disturbance and pupillary abnormalities.

DIAGNOSIS

Diagnosis of GBS is essentially clinical, based on the history and characteristic neurologic examination findings. Electrophysiological tests (NCV, EMG), blood investigations and lumbar puncture (LP- CSF) studies helps in confirming the diagnosis and to exclude other possible causes **(Tables 9.1 and 9.2)**.

Electrodiagnostic Studies

Eectrodiagnsotic studies (nerve conduction studies and electromyogram) are helpful in confirming the diagnosis and to differentiate between axonal and demyelinating forms. Early findings include prolonged F wave latencies, absent H reflex and the pattern of a normal sural but abnormal median sensory response.

The cardinal features of demyelination are:
- Prolonged distal motor latency
- Slowed motor conduction velocity
- Prolonged F wave latencies
- Partial motor conduction block and/or abnormal temporal dispersion.

The findings evolve over a period of one to weeks. Axonal forms shows reduction in compound muscle action potential (CMAP) or absent CMAP in severe case.

The CSF findings in GBS includes; albuminocytological dissociation—an elevated protein with less than 10 white cells. Half of the cases of GBS may have a normal CSF protein in the first week, by 2nd week 90% cases shows elevated protein. Pleocytosis of 10–20 cells/mm^3 may be seen in approximately 5% cases. If more than 50 cells/mm^3 one should consider other causes like early HIV infection, CMV polyradiculitis, sarcoidosis, etc.

MANAGEMENT

Children with GBS who are symptomatic but are able to walk unaided and who are stable can be managed conservatively. However, they should be observed for progression of the disease, especially if they are still within the first week of the onset of the disease. Blood pressure and heart rate fluctuations, clinical signs of respiratory failure should be carefully and meticulously monitored. Clinical signs of paralytic ileus should be observed. If any of these signs are detected they should be immediately shifted to specialized centers for further management.

Management of Respiratory Failure and General Supportive Care

Despite advances in respiratory management and immunotherapy, mortality from GBS is as high as 20% for ventilated patients. Mechanical ventilation is usually required for one-third of the patients. Involvement of the neck muscles (particularly neck flexion) and weakness of infraspinatus correlate best with phrenic nerve involvement and diaphragmatic paralysis. Weakness of laryngeal and pharyngeal muscles as well as limited tongue movement suggests impaired ability to manage secretions and protect the airway. The patient should be asked or observed to cough, as weakness of intercostal muscles can significantly impair this important reflex, which expels secretions and prevents lung collapse. Patients who are unable to converse in full sentences or count to 20 in a single breath likely have respiratory compromise. Other signs of respiratory distress are restlessness, tachycardia, tachypnea, excessive sweating, and use accessory muscles of respiration, asynchronous movements of chest and abdomen. In cooperative children older than 5 years, serial monitoring of respiratory function using a spirometer is a valuable tool for detecting respiratory distress. A vital capacity <20 mL/kg, maximal inspiratory pressures <30 mm

Table 9.1 Diagnostic criteria for Guillain-Barré syndrome

Required	Supportive	Exclusionary
Progressive weakness of more than one limb. Hyporeflexia or areflexia	Progression less than 4 weeks Symmetric weakness Sensory symptoms or signs Cranial nerve involvement, Especially facial N Autonomic dysfunction CSF protein elevation CSF cell count < 10/mm^3 Electrophysiologic features of demyelination.	Other causes excluded (toxins, botulism, porphyria, diphtheria)

Table 9.2 Differential diagnosis of Guillain-Barré syndrome

Diseases	Points to differentiate from GBS
Acute transverse myelitis • Paraparesis or quadriparesis • Spinal shock may lead to areflexia	• No facial or bulbar weakness • May have sensory level • Extensor plantar response • CSF pleocytosis
Poliomyelitis, West Nile virus, and other viruses infection • Rapid onset of weakness appearing after a viral prodrome • May have respiratory impairment	• Asymmetric patchy weakness • Reflexes preserved in unaffected limbs and lost only in very weak muscles. No sensory loss CSF pleocytosis
Botulism • Diffuse symmetric weakness with frequent respiratory impairment • Hyporeflexia may be present	• Ptosis, abnormal pupils, and neck weakness common in early disease. Descending paralysis • No sensory loss • Normal CSF • Abnormal repetitive nerve stimulation
Myasthenia gravis • Diffuse, symmetric weakness with frequent respiratory impairment	• Slower onset • Preserved reflexes • Ptosis, ophthalmoplegia, neck and bulbar weakness disproportionate to limb weakness • No sensory loss • Normal CSF • Acetylcholine receptor/muscle specific kinase antibodies in most patients • Abnormal repetitive nerve stimulation
Acute toxic neuropathies (thallium, arsenic, lead) • Generalized weakness with loss of reflexes	• Usually slower onset (weeks) • Distal >proximal weakness • Cranial nerves preserved • Prominent nausea, vomiting, and abdominal pain • Rash (thallium, arsenic) • Mee's line (lead, arsenic)
Hypokalemic periodic paralysis • Acute symmetric flaccid weakness • Hyporeflexia may be present	• Predominant proximal muscle weakness • No cranial nerve involvement • Diminished reflexes only in severely affected muscles.

H_2O, maximal expiratory pressure <40 cm H_2O predicts imminent respiratory failure. In general it takes 2–6 weeks to wean out of ventilatory support. Tracheostomy may be performed 2 weeks following intubation and should be based on status of individuals. If pulmonary function is improving, it may be preferable to wait one more week to attempt at weaning from ventilator.

Good supportive therapy is vital in GBS which includes:
- Prevention of complications of immobility (aspiration, constipation, pressure sores, contractures)
- Pain management
- Management of autonomic instability
- Management of gastroparesis, ileus and urinary retention
- Proper nutritional care, as inadequate calorie and protein intake can cause accelerated muscle catabolism
- Proper limb positioning, posture, orthotics, strengthening exercise, chest physiotherapy.

IMMUNOTHERAPY

Both plasma exchange (PE) and intravenous immunoglobulin (IVIg) are effective immunotherapies for adult and pediatric patients with GBS if given during the first few weeks of disease. IVIg has been shown to be safe and effective in the treatment of pediatric GBS. Although only one prospective, randomized treatment trial in childhood GBS has been published, multiple studies have shown that IVIg seems helpful in reducing the severity of the disease as well as duration of hospitalization and duration and need for mechanical ventilation. The proposed mechanism of action include neutralization of circulating myelin antibodies through anti-idiotypic antibodies; down-regulation of proinflammatory cytokines, including interferon-gamma; blockade of Fc-receptors on macrophages; suppression of inducer T and B cells and augmentation of suppressor T cell. Several regimens have been used. Most commonly used regimen includes 0.4 g/kg of IVIg daily for five days. Some authors use 2 g/kg of IVIg given as a single dose or 1 g/kg/day over 2 days in children who are showing rapid signs of deterioration. Although, in a small, randomized trial, the outcomes between the 2 treatment regimens were equivalent, treatment-related fluctuation (deterioration after receiving IVIg) occurred more often in children who received the 2-day course of IVIg.

Mild reactions of IVIg includes, headache, nausea, chills and myalgia. Moderate and rare reactions includes chemical meningitis, neutropenia, maculopapular skin rashes. Rare and serious adverse reactions include anaphylaxis and pulmonary embolism. In patients with renal dysfunction the rate of infusion should be decreased to half of the normal infusion rate.

PLASMAPHERESIS

Plasmapheresis directly removes humoral factors, such as autoantibodies, immune complexes, complements, cytokines, and other nonspecific inflammatory mediators. Studies in children using both historical and case controls indicate that patients treated with PE fared significantly better in the following outcome measures: Time to recover walking without aid, percentage of patients requiring artificial ventilation, duration of ventilation, full muscle strength recovery after 1 year. The availability of plasmapheresis is generally limited to major referral centers and requires equipment and trained personnel. PE is usually administered as one plasma volume, 50 mL/kg, on 5 separate sessions on alternate days. PE requires placing and maintenance of a central catheter. Significant adverse events of PE include pneumothorax, hypotension, sepsis, pneumonia, abnormal clotting, and hypocalcemia. Plasmapheresis is limited to larger children; in most institutions, children less than and weighing less 10–15 kg may not be considered for plasma exchange therapy. The advantage of IVIg over PE is that it can be given to smaller children and can be administered via peripheral IV line at ward level hospital settings.

CORTICOSTEROIDS

In a Cochrane systematic review of 6 trials with 587 patients it has been shown that corticosteroid therapy is ineffective for treating GBS.

MILLER FISHER SYNDROME

No randomized controlled trials (RCTs) have studied the effect of PE or IVIg in patients with Miller Fisher syndrome (MFS). Observational studies have suggested that the final outcome in patients with MFS is generally good. In a large uncontrolled observational study, IVIg slightly hastened the amelioration of ophthalmoplegia and ataxia. However, in view of good natural recovery, patients with mild or uncomplicated MFS may perhaps be treated conservatively.

TREATMENT OF PATIENTS WHO DETERIORATE IN SPITE OF THERAPY

Some patients with GBS continue to deteriorate after PE or a standard course of IVIg. In these cases, the best treatment options are not available. The combination of PE followed by IVIg is no better than PE or IVIg alone. PE after IVIg is also not advised, because PE would probably wash out the IVIg previously administered. A study in a small series of patients investigated the effect of a second course of IVIg in severe unresponsive patients with GBS. This uncontrolled study suggested that a repeated course of IVIg could be effective. About 5–10% of patients with GBS deteriorate after initial improvement or stabilization following IVIg treatment. Although no RCTs have assessed the effect of a repeated IVIg dose in this condition, it is common practice to give a second IVIg course. These patients are thought to have a prolonged immune response that causes persistent nerve damage that needs treatment for a longer period of time. A longer interval between onset and treatment and longer time to nadir may be associated with a greater chance of relapse.

VACCINATION AND GBS

The association of vaccination and GBS is controversial. There was an increased incidence of GBS within 6 weeks of administration of influenza vaccine in 1992 to 1993 and 1993 to 1994 seasons in US. The estimated risk was excess of one GBS cases per million vaccinations. Hepatitis vaccine is also associated with a slight increased risk of GBS. H1N1 immunization is associated with an excess GBS risk of 0.8 cases per million vaccinations. Immunizations are not recommended during the acute phase and should be avoided for one year after onset. If GBS occurs within 6 weeks after a specific immunization, it is better, the vaccine should be avoided in the future.

PROGNOSIS

The long-term prognosis of GBS is good in children even for patients who are severely affected. Death is uncommon when good supportive care is available. About 80% of patients are able to walk independently 6 months after onset of illness. Full recovery within 3–12 months is experienced by 90–95% of pediatric patients with GBS. Between 5% and 10% of individuals have significant permanent disability. Overall mortality rate in childhood GBS is estimated to be less than 5%. Deaths are usually caused by respiratory failure, often in association with cardiac arrhythmias and dysautonomia.

SUMMARY

The GBS is a monophasic immune-mediated neuropathy characterized by acute onset of predominantly motor weakness and is a common cause of acute flaccid paralysis and neuromuscular respiratory failure in children. The diagnosis is essentially clinical, supported by electrophysiological studies and CSF analysis. Electrodiagnostic tests aids in the diagnosis. Both PE and IVIg are equally effective. However in children; IVIg may be preferred because of its low side-effect profile and ease of administration.

BIBLIOGRAPHY

1. Asbury AK, Cornblath DR. Assessment of diagnostic criteria for Guillain-Barré syndrome. Ann Neurol. 1990;27(Suppl):S21-4.
2. Baranwal AK, Ravi RN, Singh R. E*xchange transfusion:* a low-cost alternative for severe childhood Guillain-Barré syndrome. J Child Neurol. 2006;21(11):960-5.
3. Farcas P, Avnun L, Frisher S, et al. Efficacy of repeated intravenous immunoglobulin in severe unresponsive Guillain-Barré syndrome. Lancet. 1997;350:1747.
4. Hughes RA, Cornblath DR. Guillain–Barré syndrome. Lancet. 2005;36(9497):1653-66.
5. Hughes RA, Swan AV, van Koningsveld R, et al. Corticosteroids for Guillain-Barré syndrome. Cochrane Database Syst Rev. 2006;2:CD001446.
6. Kalita J, Misra UK, Das M. Neurophysiological criteria in the diagnosis of different clinical types of Guillain–Barré syndrome. J Neurol Neurosurg Psychiatry. 2008;79:289-93.
7. Kalra V, Chaudhry R, Dua T, Dhawan B, Sahu JK, Mridula B. Association of Campylobacter jejuni infection with childhood Guillain-Barré syndrome: a case-control study. J Child Neurol. 2009;24(6):664-8.
8. Kalra V, Sankhyan N, Sharma S, Gulati S, Choudhry R, Dhawan B. Outcome in childhood Guillain-Barré syndrome. Indian J Pediatr. 2009;76(8):795-9.
9. Korinthenberg R, Schessl J, Kirschner J, et al. Intravenously administered immunoglobulin in the treatment of childhood Guillain-Barré syndrome: a randomized trial. Pediatrics. 2005;116(1):8-14.
10. Lee JH, Sung IY, Rew IS. Clinical presentation and prognosis of childhood Guillain-Barré syndrome. J Paediatr Child Health. 2008;44: 449-54.
11. McKhann GM, Cornblath DR, Griffin JW, Ho TW, Li CY, Jiang Z, et al. Acute motor axonal neuropathy: A frequent cause of acute flaccid paralysis in China. Ann Neurol. 1993;33:333-42.

12. Meché FG, Meulstee J, van Doorn PA. Risk factors for treatment related clinical fluctuations in Guillain-Barré syndrome. Dutch Guillain-Barré Study Group. J Neurol Neurosurg Psychiatry. 1998;64:242-4.
13. Meena AK, Khadilkar SV, Murthy J. Treatment guidelines for Guillain-Barré syndrome. Ann Indian Acad Neurol. 2011;14:73-81.
14. Paul BS, Bhatia R, Prasad K, Padma MV, Tripathi M, Singh MB. Clinical predictors of mechanical ventilation in Guillain-Barré syndrome. Neurol India. 2012;60:150-3.
15. Sarada C, Tharakan JK, Nair M. Guillain-Barré syndrome: A prospective clinical study in 25 children and comparison with adults. Ann Trop Paediatr. 1994;14:281-6.

CHAPTER 10

Autoimmune Encephalitis in Children

V Viswanathan

INTRODUCTION

More children are being diagnosed/detected with this condition over the last few years ever since some of the tests for certain antibodies became freely available in India. Although in the past, one may have considered this diagnosis in some children. While lack of testing facilities made it impossible for us to identify this condition. It is true that the word autoimmune encephalitis includes few different conditions and not just a single entity. What is generally accepted is that the body's immune mechanisms get triggered due to certain factors and this in turn attacks the brain in the same person resulting in the clinical features of the disease.

Some of the common types of autoimmune encephalitis recognized are N-methyl-D-aspartate (NMDA) receptor-associated encephalitis, Rasmussen's encephalitis, Voltage-gated potassium channel complex antibody associated encephalitis, Hashimoto's encephalopathy and acute disseminated encephalomyelitis.

ACUTE DISSEMINATED ENCEPHALOMYELITIS

This accounts for about 10% of all encephalitis seen in children. Most of these children have a history of preceding viral infections or immunization. The latent period can be from a few days to a few weeks. There has been large number of viruses associated with this condition including measles, mumps, rubella, varicella zoster, Epstein–Barr virus, Cytomegalovirus, herpes simplex virus, hepatitis A, influenza and entero-viruses.[1] The association between inflammatory reaction following vaccination has been temporal and direct connection between a vaccine and an immune attack has not been established. Post vaccinal acute disseminated encephalomyelitis (ADEM) has been associated with immunization for rabies, hepatitis B, influenza, Japanese B encephalitis, diphtheria/pertussis/tetanus, measles, mumps, rubella, *Pneumococcus*, polio, smallpox and varicella.[2]

The classical picture is that of patchy demyelination seen in the brain in these children associated with neurological signs/symptoms. Initial symptoms can be quite subtle with fever, headache, nausea, vomiting, neck stiffness followed by progressive depression in the level of consciousness. The rapidity of deterioration can be quite variable with progression over hours in some to a few days. There may be progressive drowsiness to coma, weakness on one side of the body, clumsiness, deterioration in vision, seizures, etc. In some children, there may be predominant involvement of the spinal cord with weakness in one or both legs and there may be associated dysfunction of the bowel and bladder depending on the level of the lesion in the spinal cord. One needs to have a high index of suspicion to do the appropriate tests to make an early diagnosis and treat appropriately.

Magnetic resonance imaging (MRI) brain scan as in **(Fig. 10.1)** below shows patchy areas of demyelination. CSF examination may reveal increase in protein and cell counts and this is helpful in suggesting an inflammatory picture. The role of antibiotics and acyclovir in this condition is questionable but in most centers this is usually started along with IV methyl prednisolone (steroids) until the results of the CSF cultures and viral studies are available. Rarely IVIg is considered if there is poor response to steroids. Most children appear to show good response to treatment with steroids and show good recovery and are not left with any residual neurological signs. The duration of IV steroids followed by oral steroids is usually a clinical decision made by the attending neurologist but in general 5 days of IV methyl prednisolone followed by tapering course of oral steroids over 3–4 weeks is given.

It is rare for ADEM to recur in children but if it does so then a consideration multiple sclerosis needs to be entertained. Periodic evaluation with MRI for these children with ADEM is generally not required, although it is usual for doctors to perform at least one repeat MRI brain to see whether the lesions seen previously have resolved a few weeks later. However, whenever there are even early symptoms or signs suggestive of possible recurrence a repeat MRI is mandatory as recurrences do occur and needs to be carefully identified early and treated.

N-METHYL D-ASPARTATE RECEPTOR-ASSOCIATED ENCEPHALITIS

This is an acute form of encephalitis which is potentially lethal but has a high probability of recovery. NMDA stands for N-methyl D-aspartate.[3] The autoimmune reaction in this condition is primarily against the NR 1 subunit of the NMDA receptor. The condition is associated with tumors in particular teratomas of the ovaries.[4] In many cases no tumor may be identified. A multicenter, population-based prospective study of causes of encephalitis in adults and children in the UK showed that 4% of patients had anti-NMDAR encephalitis; the disorder was the second most common immune-mediated cause, after acute disseminated encephalomyelitis and before all antibody-associated encephalitis, including encephalitis attributed to voltage-gated potassium channels.[5] In yet another series, they found that 80% of the sufferers are usually females.[6] The age range was said to be between 20 months and 84 years with mean age of presentation around 18.5 years.[7,8]

The prodromal symptoms may include flu-like illness with upper respiratory infection, headaches, etc. These symptoms could precede the illness by quite a few weeks. Behavior changes are quite common in children including agitation, violent behaviors, memory deficits, impaired cognition, making rhythmic movements of the lips, mouth and some pedalling movements of the legs or hand movements resembling playing the piano, etc. and speech problems including aphasia and mutism. As the symptoms are predominantly psychiatric in nature many of these children come to neurologists late. As the disease progresses, autonomic dysfunction, hypoventilation, cerebellar ataxia, hemiparesis, progressive drowsiness and gradual

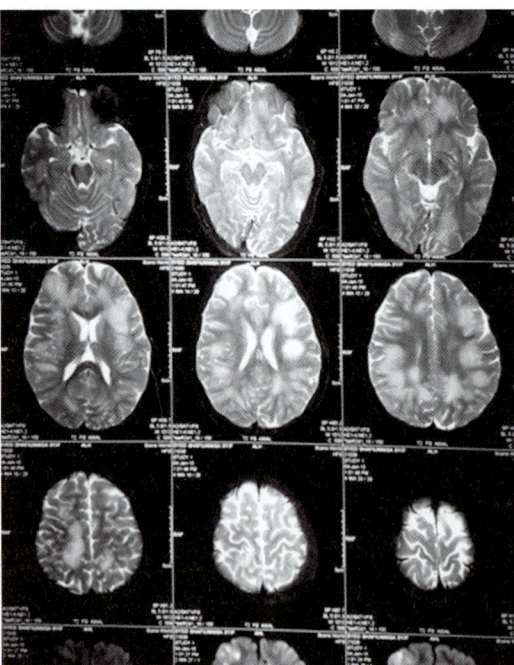

Figure 10.1 Patchy demyelination in the brain for this child who presented in coma
Courtesy: CHILDS Trust Medical Research Foundation and Apollo Hospitals, Chennai

onset of coma are not unusual. Many times these children need to be admitted to the intensive care units to stabilize their breathing, blood pressure and heart rate.

The seizures in this condition are difficult to control and require multiple anticonvulsant medications or an infusion of benzodiazepines.[9]

Investigations apart from the routine tests show high levels of serum and CSF antibodies to NMDA receptor. The serum levels are usually almost 10 times higher than the CSF antibody levels. Abdominal ultrasound/CT abdomen may reveal the ovarian tumor which may require removal **(Fig. 10.2)**. MRI brain scan may reveal hyperintense signals over the hippocampus of the temporal lobes as in **Figure 10.3**.

"One-third of patients presenting with acute noninfective encephalitis would be positive for NMDAreceptor antibodies with the remaining two-thirds with clinically suspected autoimmune encephalitis being antibody-negative."[10] The important consideration is on the diagnostic method and the reliability of the tests for autoimmunity.[11] There is no data on this aspect. Based on literature search, there is no report confirming the reliability and acceptability of the test kit.

Apart from the regular supportive measures in the intensive care these children respond well to a course of steroids/IVIg apart from the removal of the tumor if identified as in this girl. If there is history of seizures, anticonvulsant medications may be required. Some children may benefit from haloperidol if there are lot of choreoathetoid movements. The recovery is usually gradual, may take a few weeks or months. Plasmapheresis, Rituximab and cyclophosphamide have been tried in a few difficult cases.[12]

RASMUSSEN'S ENCEPHALITIS

This is a rare form of chronic focal encephalitis that occurs predominantly in children. This rare disorder is characterized by focal seizures, hemiparesis, loss of motor skills, speech, vision and dementia in most cases.

As in the other forms of autoimmune encephalitis this is also preceded a few weeks to months by a prodromal phase of flue like illness. The characteristic symptom of this condition is

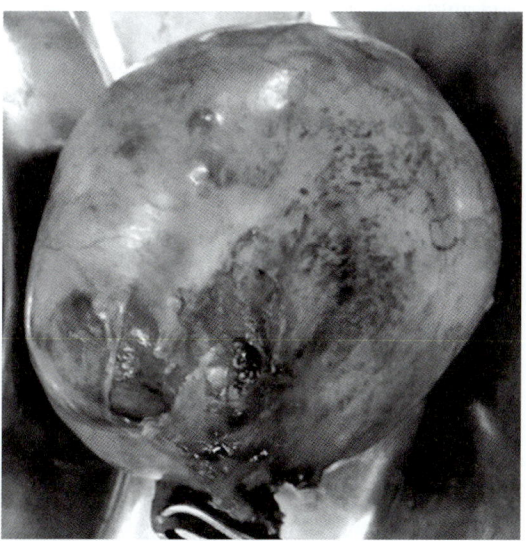

Figure 10.2 Ovarian tumor removed from a girl presented with encephalitis
Courtesy: CHILDS Trust Medical Research Foundation and Apollo Hospitals, Chennai
(For color version, see Plate 4)

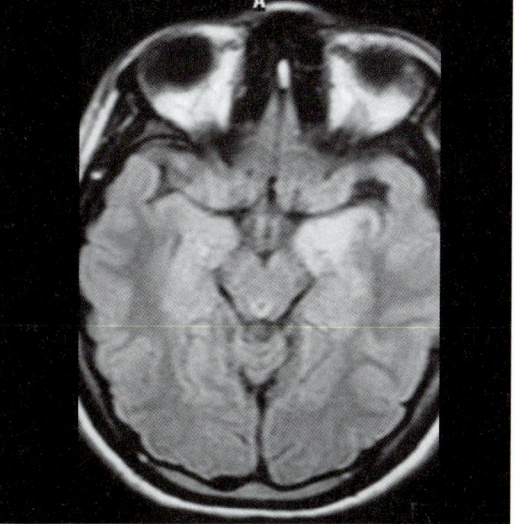

Figure 10.3 MRI brain scan showing hyperintense signals over the hippocampus
Courtesy: CHILDS Trust Medical Research Foundation and Apollo Hospitals, Chennai

focal seizures and progressive weakness of one side of the body. This is usually accompanied by progressive loss of vision on one side along with loss of cognitive abilities including learning, memory, language and speech. The seizures are usually very difficult to control and many evolve into epilepsia partialis continua. In the long-term, most patients are left with epilepsy, weakness/paralysis of one side of the body, cognitive problems, learning difficulties, etc. but the severity of the disability varies from child to child. In most cases, CT/MRI brain shows significant atrophy on one side of the brain and EEG shows focal spikes/slow waves on that side.

Initially, this disease was thought to be due to viral infection but the evidence for this is inconclusive.[13] There was also a suggestion that anti-GluR3 antibodies were important in causing the disease.[14] This has been refuted more recently and new antibodies to the NMDA type glutamate receptor subunit Glu Repsilon 2 in a subset of patients has been described.[15]

As in the other forms of autoimmune disorders steroids may be used. In some children, IV immunoglobulins may be of value. Anticonvulsant medications will be needed and the seizures may be quite difficult to control. Most of these children are left with hemiparesis, severe cognitive and speech difficulties, refractory seizures, feeding and swallowing difficulties necessitating prolonged/frequent hospitalization and multidisciplinary rehabilitation including physiotherapy, speech therapy, dietary advice, etc.

HASHIMOTO'S ENCEPHALITIS

This is a rare form of autoimmune encephalitis associated with Hashimoto's thyroiditis. Occurs primarily in adults around 40 years of age and rare in children.[16] A relapsing form of encephalopathy associated with antithyroid antibodies.[17] The onset of symptoms tends to be gradual over 1–7 days. Symptoms may include personality changes, aggression, coma, seizures, tremors, sleep abnormalities. MRI brain may show features suggestive of encephalopathy and single photon emission computed tomography (SPECT) may be more helpful and show focal/global hypoperfusion. This condition is quite difficult to differentiate from other autoimmune encephalitis like the NMDA receptor encephalitis. Like any autoimmune disorder they also respond to steroids/IVIg although no clear randomized controlled trials are there to say which is better.[18]

VOLTAGE-GATED POTASSIUM CHANNEL ANTIBODY LIMBIC ENCEPHALITIS

A form of autoimmune encephalitis that is more common in adults than children but being more and more recognized in children of late.[19] Common presentation is with amnesia, seizures, psychiatric manifestations including aggression and sleep difficulties. The typical pattern of seizures described in this condition is faciobrachial dystonic type of seizures usually involving only one side of the body. The seizures are usually difficult to control. Hyponatremia is a regular feature in this condition. Diagnosis is usually made by the high levels of VGKCC complex-associated LG1 antibodies which are more frequent than CASPR2 antibodies.[20] MRI brain shows high signal in the Hippocampus. CSF analysis is usually normal. There is good response to steroids, IVIg or plasma exchange.

SUMMARY

Autoimmune encephalitis is of very many types although the most common among them is acute disseminated encephalomyelitis. The next common is NMDA receptor encephalitis and all other disorders described above are rare in children in particular. The difficulty is in differentiating the various types of disorders as the clinical manifestation are similar. Although we are better over the recent past in making a diagnosis as compared to the past there has been very little progress in the form of treatment and we are left with immunomodulation using steroids or IVIg or other immunosuppressive medications, such as rituximab and cyclophosphamide. More research is needed into these disorders.

REFERENCES

1. Dale RC. Acute disseminated encephalomyelitis. Semin Pediatr Infect Dis. 2003;14(2):90-5.

2. Huynh W, Cordato DJ, Kehdi E, et al. Post-vaccination encephalomyelitis: literature review and illustrative case. J Clin Neurosci. 2008;15(12):1315-22.
3. Mohammad SS, Sinclair K, Pillai S, Merheb V, Aumann TD, Gill D, et al. Herpes simplex encephalitis relapse with chorea is associated with autoantibodies to N-Methyl-D-aspartate receptor or dopamine-2 receptor. Mov Disord. 2014;29:117-22.
4. Irani SR, Bera K, Waters P, Zuliani L, Maxwell S, Zandi MS, et al. Brain. 2010;133(6):1655-67.
5. Granerod J, Ambrose HE, Davies NW, et al. Causes of encephalitis and differences in their clinical presentations in England: a multicenter, population-based prospective study. Lancet Infect Dis. 2010.
6. Dalmau J, Lancaster E, Martinez-Hemandez E, Rosenfield MR, Rossi, Peng X, et al. Anti-NMDA receptor encephalitis: case series and analysis of the effects of antibodies. Lancet Neurol. 2008;7:1091-8.
7. Gable MS, Gavali S, Radner A, et al. Anti-NMDA receptor encephalitis: report of ten cases and comparison with viral encephalitis. Eur J Clin Microbiol Infect Dis. 2009;28:1427-9.
8. Wong-Kisiel LC, Ji T, Renaud DL, et al. Response to immunotherapy in a 20-month-old boy with anti-NMDA receptor encephalitis. Neurology. 2010;74:1550-1.
9. Maramalttom BV, Philip C, Sundaram PS. Idiopathic anti-NMDA receptor encephalitis in a young Indian girl. Neurol India. 2010;58:671-2.
10. Cyril AC, Nair SS, Mathai A, Kannoth S, Thomas SV. Autoimmune encephalitis: Clinical diagnosis versus antibody confirmation. Ann Indian Acad Neurol. 2015;18:408-11.
11. Probst C, Saschenbrecker S, Stoecker W, Komorowski L. Antineuronal autoantibodies: Current diagnostic challenges. Mult Scler Relat Disord. 2014;3:303-20.
12. Titulaer MJ, McCracken L, Gabilondo I, et al. Treatment and prognostic factors for long-term outcome in patients with anti-NMDA receptor encephalitis: An observational cohort study *The Lancet Neurology*. 2013;12(2):157-65.
13. Bien CG, et al. Pathogenesis, diagnosis and treatment of Rasmussen encephalitis: a European consensus statement. Brain. 2005;128 (Pt 3):454-71.
14. Rogers SW, Andrews PI, Gahring LC, et al. Autoantibodies to glutamate receptor GluR3 in Rasmussen's encephalitis. Science. 1994;265 (5172):648.
15. Takahashi Y, Mori H, Mishina M, et al. Autoantibodies and cell-mediated autoimmunity to NMDA-type GluRepsilon2 in patients with Rasmussen's encephalitis (RE) and chronic progressive epilepsia partialis continua. Epilepsia. 2005;46(Suppl 5):152-8.
16. Brain L, Jellinek EH, Ball K. Hashimoto's disease and encephalopathy. Lancet. 1966;2(7462):512-4.
17. Yoneda M, Fujii A, Ito A, Yokoyama H, Nakagawa H, Kuriyama M. High prevalence of serum autoantibodies against the amino terminal of alpha-enolase in Hashimoto's encephalopathy. Journal of Neuroimmunology. 2007;185(1-2):195-200.
18. Flanagan EP, McKeon A, Lennon VA, et al. Autoimmune dementia: clinical course and predictors of immunotherapy response. Mayo Clinic Proceedings. 2010;85(10):881-97.
19. Cakmakli HF, Oguz KK, Haliloglu G, et al. Limbic encephalitis in a 9-year-old child due to voltage-gated potassium channel antibody (VGKC-Ab) (IAP 043). Eur J Paediatr Neurol. 2007;11:97-8.
20. Vincent A, Bien CG, Irani SR, Waters P. Autoantibodies associated with diseases of the central nervous system: New developments and future challenges. Lancet Neurol. 2011;10:759-72.

CHAPTER 11

Tuberculous Meningitis in India

Jitendra Kumar Sahu, Sumeet R Dhawan

'When the family doctor has good reason to suspect the diagnosis, he should send the child to hospital without delay....so...may have the great advantage of early treatment'

Illingworth RS 1950[1]

INTRODUCTION

India has the highest of incidence of tuberculosis, accounting for almost 20% of all new cases globally—an estimated 2.25 million cases annually.[2] Central nervous system (CNS) tuberculosis encompasses tubercular meningitis (TBM), TBM with miliary tuberculosis, space occupying lesions like tuberculomas, tuberculous encephalopathy, tubercular vasculopathy and tuberculous abscesses. TBM is a severe form of tuberculosis and remains an important cause of hospitalization, death, and permanent neurological disability in India. Indian scientists have made immense contribution to the understanding of pathogenesis, pathology, diagnosis, management and prognosis of the condition. Children with HIV are five times more likely to have CNS TB and infants are 40 times more likely to develop CNS TB compared to older children.[3]

PATHOGENESIS

Predisposing factors for all kind of tuberculosis are similar and include poverty, immunodeficiency, overcrowding and malnourished state. The pathogenesis is unexplained and based on autopsy series by Rich and McCordock in early part of 20th century. CNS TB is caused by hematogenous dissemination of *Mycobacterium* from primary complex in lungs to the meninges causing inflammation and tubercles. These subpial tubercles known as Rich's foci rupture in the subarachnoid space causing meningitis.[4]

The likelihood of development of TBM and primary bacteremia is dependent on immune status and age of child. Infants are at maximum risk and are more likely to develop TBM compared to older children who may have disease localized to lungs. In the series by Rich, it was suggested that miliary TB and CNS TB constitute separate entities. Some cases of miliary TB and disseminated TB without CNS involvement have been described suggesting that miliary TB may not a prerequisite for CNS TB. Immunosuppressed children like HIV positive, children on prolonged corticosteroids therapy like nephrotic syndrome and systemic arthritis, children on cancer chemotherapy and immunomodulators like cyclophosphamide, infliximab and cyclosporine are at maximum risk. In a small frequency of patients, hematogenous seeding may involve choroid plexus and ventricular wall. Rarely focus from vertebra and middle ear may involve meninges and cause TBM.

PATHOLOGY

In all cases of TBM, meninges as well as brain are involved. From this perspective TBM is meningoencephalitis rather than pure meningitis. In almost all cases, blood vessels are pathologically involved though clinical manifestations of vasculitis are present in less than 50% of cases.

Meningeal involvement is mainly basal and consists of serofibrinous exudates, large areas of caseous necrosis, lymphocytes, plasma cells with infrequent epitheloid cells and giant cells. Dense basal meningitis also involves optic chiasma and optic sheath causing vision loss. These exudates may extend down to spinal cord causing spinal meningitis, arachnoiditis and radiculomyelopathy. Brain parenchyma manifests border zone inflammation, hydrocephalus, and in some cases, infarction or tuberculoma.

Pathologically, blood vessels of all types (arteries, veins, capillaries) and size (small, medium, large) are involved. Findings described include periarteritis, medial fibrinoid necrosis, vessel wall granuloma, panarteritis, thrombosis and luminal occlusion.

DIAGNOSIS OF TUBERCULAR MENINGITIS

Tubercular meningitis poses a diagnostic challenge. Various diagnostic issues have been discussed in detail in first author's published article.[5] Early diagnosis is difficult as the initial symptoms are minimal, nonspecific and commonly treated as upper respiratory tract infection, viral infection, enteric fever and pyrexia of unknown origin. A high degree of suspicion is needed for early diagnosis. The most important clue to presence of TBM is the 'persistence' of symptoms. Persistence of symptoms is often missed due to frequent change of medical practitioners. The early diagnosis of TBM is the most desirable and of paramount importance but difficult due to non-specific presenting clinical features of the disease, poor sensitivity of conventional bacteriology, misinterpretation of investigations, and incompletely assessed alternative diagnostic methods.

An important clinical clue to early diagnosis of TBM is evaluation of TBM in all meningitis of more than 5 days duration.[6] Differentiation of pyogenic meningitis can be difficult in early disease with minimal meningeal involvement. Diagnosis requires combination of clinical features, cerebrospinal fluid examination, neuroradiology and features of extracranial tuberculosis. Several clinical algorithms have been developed and reported for diagnosis of TBM but none has been accepted universally. Therefore, a consensus case definition for diagnosis of TBM is recently developed for use in research.[7]

Clinical Diagnosis

The clinical presentation of TBM is variable **(Table 11.1)**. In adults, the characteristic clinical features consist of fever, headache, vomiting and in some cases neck pain developing gradually over 2–6 weeks, progressing if untreated to altered sensorium with or without motor deficits. In children, apathy, lack of interest in play, irritability, restlessness at night, minor headache, vomiting, loss of appetite and abdominal pain are the usual presenting symptoms. Intermittent low-grade

Table 11.1 Presenting features of tubercular meningitis[14]

Clinical features	Frequency
Symptoms	
Pyrexia	60–95%
Headache	50–80%
Weight loss	60–80%
Seizures-children Adults	50% 5%
Photophobia	5–10%
Signs	
Meningeal signs	40–80%
Alteration in sensorium	30–60%
Cranial nerve palsy Oculomotor Abducens Facial	30–50% 5–15% 30–40% 10–20%
Confusion	10–30%
Hemiparesis	10–20%
Paraparesis	5–10%

fever may be present. It is very unusual but possible for TBM to present acutely; there is more often than not a subacute presentation over a number of weeks or even months.

Seizure and altered sensorium are common symptoms which bring attention to the underlying CNS illness. Intracranial hypertension manifesting as papilloedema in adults and enlargement of head in children and infants can occur in the early stage of illness. Cranial nerve palsies are common and seen in almost half of children. The sixth cranial nerve is most commonly affected. Cranial nerves are involved due to entrapment in basal exudates or due to hydrocephalous. Vision impairment is a devastating complication of TB. It may be due to optic atrophy due to prolonged hydrocephalous, optochiasmatic arachnoiditis, chiasmal tuberculoma, ethambutol toxicity.[3,8] Extrapyramidal movements are common due to basal ganglia stroke due to involvement of thalamoperforating arteries.

In some children the condition called "tuberculous encephalopathy" has been seen. This condition presents with convulsions and coma with little or no meningeal symptoms or signs and characterized by white matter edema, demyelination with little evidence of meningitis. However, this was seen in pre-CT era. Now in an era of advanced neuroimaging this entity is practically non-existent.

Atypical presentations of TBM are not rare and include acute (meningitis like or stroke like) presentations, intracranial hypertension, psychoses, locked in syndrome, sphenoidal fissure syndrome, brainstem syndrome and movement disorders.

Radiological Diagnosis

A computed tomogram in tuberculous meningitis may reveal basal contrast enhancing exudates, hydrocephalus, cerebral infarction, or tuberculoma **(Fig. 11.1)**. Basal contrast enhancing exudates **(Fig. 11.2)** and hydrocephalus are the most common CT features of TBM. Mild meningeal enhancement in absence of basal exudates is a nonspecific finding and can be present in any type of meningitis. A combination of basal exudates, hydrocephalous and tuberculoma is virtually diagnostic of TBM with high sensitivity and

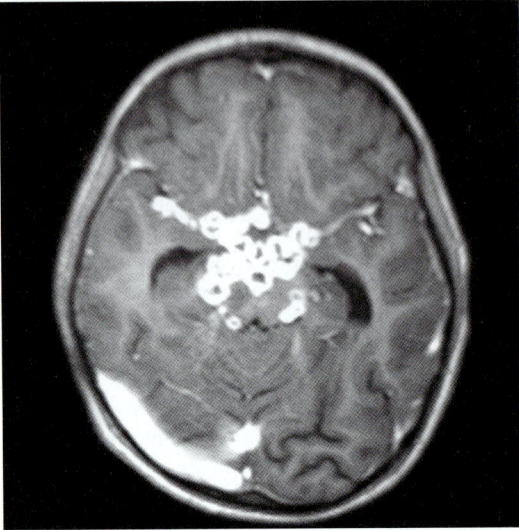

Figure 11.1 Contrast T1 weighted MRI image showing conglomerate subpial tuberculomas

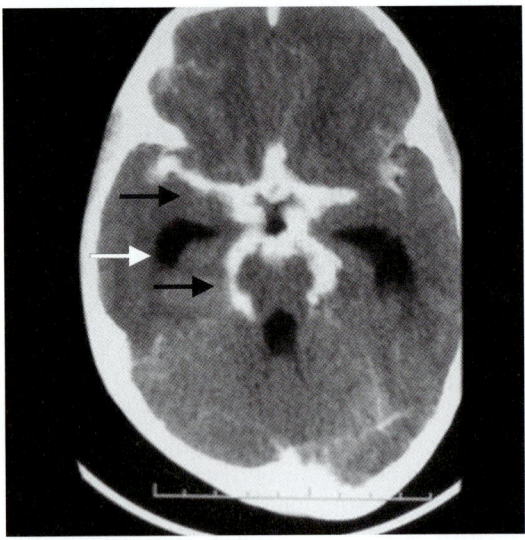

Figure 11.2 Contrast CT scan showing basal exudates (black arrows) and hydrocephalous (white arrow)

specificity. Cerebral infarctions were described in 19–67% and tuberculoma were seen in 10–56% children with TBM in one review.[9] In one series, 80% infarcts were seen in basal ganglia and internal capsule. One third children had bilateral infarcts and half had evidence of hemispheric infarct.[10] Tuberculoma might increase in size or appear fresh during treatment but remain usually asymptomatic. Recently precontrast hyperdensity in the basal cisterns has been described as the most specific sign (sensitivity 46%, specificity 100%, positive predictive value 100%), but needs to be correlated with clinical features.[9] In children with normal initial radiology seen in 5–10% of cases, a repeat scan after 2–4 weeks with persistent abnormal CSF parameters may be new findings.[11] The radiological picture may evolve in the first 2–8 weeks even after starting antitubercular therapy (ATT) with increasing hydrocephalous, increasing exudates, new strokes, increasing size of tuberculomas.

The MRI may show mild features of TBM not seen with CT scan. Mild meningeal enhancement, basal exudates, small tuberculomas, small lacunar infarcts may be frequently missed with CT scan. Cryptococcal meningitis, cytomegalovirus encephalitis, acanthamoeba, brucella meningitis, toxoplasmosis, non-tubercular mycobacterial meningitis, neurosyphilis, sarcoidosis, meningeal spread of malignancies and lymphoma may have similar radiological appearance.

About 50% of patients with tuberculous meningitis may have abnormalities on the chest radiograph including a primary complex, miliary shadowing, parenchymal change, mediastinal glands, and pleural effusion. Although chest CT is more sensitive than conventional X-ray to find out these changes, it is not routinely indicated.

All children with suspected chronic meningitis warrant a contrast CT head scan as initial evaluation. It is not common to see TBM being missed in the developing countries due to use of noncontrast radiology especially CT scan for initial assessment. Though MRI has better anatomical delineation, role of CT scan in delineation of hydrocephalous cannot be undermined and emergency CSF drainage procedure can be lifesaving. Chest radiograph of child and family members should be part of the diagnostic assessment.

A MRI should include T1, T2, FLAIR, T1 contrast, diffusion weighted imaging in axial, coronal and sagittal planes as a minimum mandatory protocol. FLAIR contrast image may help in picking up minimal basal exudates not seen on other MRI sequences. Additionally magnetic resonance spectroscopy and MRI perfusion imaging may help in differentiating tuberculous abscesses from malignant masses. MRI angiography may help in assessment of extent of vasculitis. The role of trained neuroradiologist cannot be undermined in the assessment of complex lesions. HIV positive children have less basal exudates and hydrocephalous.

Microbiological Diagnosis

The diagnosis of TBM is most often presumptive and is based on the dictum: "a subacute or chronic illness with compatible clinical picture and a characteristic cerebrospinal fluid profile is TBM unless proved otherwise". The compatible clinical picture with the diagnosis is described above. Examination of cerebrospinal fluid (CSF) is necessary to diagnose tuberculous meningitis. CSF pressure is usually elevated. Appearance is clear, colorless, and may in some cases form a cobweb. Cobweb formation is not specific and should not be considered diagnostic. It is believed that staining the cobweb may increase the chance of finding acid fast bacilli (AFB), but it has not been systematically studied. The signature CSF picture consists of predominantly lymphocytic pleocytosis (usually 100–500, range 20–1000), moderately low (less than 50% of the plasma concentration) or normal glucose and raised protein concentration (usually 100–500 mg, often 1.0–3.0 g/L). Protein concentrations as high as this are very rare in other bacterial meningitis outside the neonatal period. Very low or absent CSF glucose should raise suspicion of pyogenic meningitis. It is important to mention that absolute glucose values may be normal; it is essential to draw blood sample for plasma glucose estimation to allow proper interpretation of the results. The cellular response in CSF usually shows lymphocytic pleocytosis of less than 500×10^6/L. In the first few weeks of illness the CSF pleocytosis may be predominantly polymorphonuclear cells. Atypical CSF picture includes normocellular CSF, hemorrhagic CSF, or xanthochromic CSF and one resembling pyogenic meningitis.

Definitive diagnosis of TBM requires the detection of the AFB in the CSF, either by Ziehl-

Neelsen (ZN) staining or culture (solid or liquid). Large amount of CSF (>6 mL),[12] frequent CSF examination, centrifugation of CSF and prolonged examination time (>30%) have been shown to increase the sensitivity to 79%. Fluorescent microscopy has helped increasing sensitivity by 10%. Once ATT has started, the bacterial yield by ZN staining and culture drops rapidly. Though culture is gold standard, the antitubercular treatment must be initiated in clinical grounds. However, culture may provide valuable decision on drug susceptibility. Liquid culture like MGIT BACTEC 960 has better sensitivity. However, dedicated certified lab requiring processing AFB culture are scarce and limited to tertiary care hospitals and medical colleges. Additionally, the RNTCP does not process extrapulmonary samples and culture is done in under RNTCP only in suspected drug resistant cases further makes access to AFB cultures more difficult. To overcome strict biosafety precautions to conventional culture, WHO has suggested use of microscopic observed drug susceptibility (MODS assay) which is liquid culture with rapid detection rates and better sensitivity than conventional culture.

Molecular Diagnosis

A meta-analysis on utility of commercial nucleic acid amplification (NAA) assays concluded that commercial NAA assays were 64% sensitive (95% confidence interval 56–72%) and 98% specific (95% CI 96-99%) with positive likelihood ratio of 20.36 (range 11.29–36.73).[13] However, for inhouse PCR compared to commercial PCR, sensitivity and specificity were 73% and 92% respectively. Therefore, a commercial NAA assay on CSF should be performed in all cases of suspected TBM, although a negative test does not exclude TBM. NAA tests may remain positive till one month of initiation of ATT; and so they are more useful than AFB Z-N staining and culture once ATT has been initiated.[11] WHO has advocated use of Xpert MTB/Rif as the first test to be used for diagnosis of TBM. The advantage of this test is that the results are available within 2 hours and provides early timely information on rifampicin resistance based on detection of mutations in rpoB gene. The sensitivity of Xpert MTB/Rif in one recently conducted meta-analysis was 70%.[14,15] WHO has advocated that Xpert MTB/Rif replace the smear examination as first test for CSF analysis in all cases with suspected TBM.[16] A word of caution must be exercised in respect to all PCR based tests (including Xpert MTB/Rif). These tests are 'good rule in' tests but 'not good rule out' tests (negative test result does not exclude disease). Secondly the high cost of Xpert MTB/Rif also needs to be considered until it is freely available under the National Program.

Ancillary Diagnosis

Tuberculin Skin Test (TST) and Interferon-Gamma Release Assays (IGRAs)

The IGRA detect sensitization to *M. tuberculosis* by measuring IFN-γ release in response to *Mycobacterium tuberculosis* antigens. Recent WHO guideline suggested that IGRA is more specific, though evidence is low grade and evidence in high group population like children is scarce. A positive test like Mantoux test indicates only active infection and not disease. Also negative result does not rule out tuberculosis. Also IGRA are costly and results may be indeterminate and nonconclusive. So WHO has suggested that IGRA should not be used for ancillary diagnosis of extrapulmonary tuberculosis.[16]

Cerebrospinal Fluid Adenosine Deaminase Activity (ADA)

The ADA is an enzyme of purine metabolism and is used for diagnosis of extrapulmonary TB like pleural, pericardial and meningeal TB. The test is inexpensive and widely available. In a meta-analysis, the sensitivity and specificity were 79% (range 75–83%) and 91% (range 89–93%) respectively with a positive likelihood ratio of 6.85 (range 4–11). In another study, using a cut-off of 10 U/L, sensitivity and specificity were 92.5% and 97% respectively. However, 21% adults with pyogenic meningitis also had elevated CSF >8 U/L in the same study.[17] So utility of CSF ADA remains limited especially with low sensitivity and false positivity in pyogenic meningitis.

COMPLICATIONS AND SEQUELAE

Motor Deficits

Hemiplegia, paraplegia and tetraplegia have been reported. Rapid or sudden onset of deficits suggests a vascular cause. Paraplegia or tetraplegia is usually a manifestation of myeloradiculopathy due to spinal arachnoiditis. Focal deficits may be present in 50-65% patients. Strokes are often asymptomatic (silent stroke) at admission as most of children have encephalopathy at admission. They are noticed later during the admission stay when the encephalopathy improves. Strokes are due to subcortical (basal ganglia) or cortical involvement. Cortical stroke (hemispheric) is associated with poor outcome.

Symptomatic High Pressure Hydrocephalus

Hydrocephalus is a common feature of TBM. It is usually self-limiting and surpassed by features of meningitis. In some cases, the features of high pressure hydrocephalus (headache, vomiting or papilloedema) are detected when other features of meningitis have subsided/or are subsiding, The hydrocephalus is mostly communicating but in some cases, obstruction at foramen of Monro or at the aqueduct may occur.

Optochiasmatic Arachnoiditis

Dense exudates at the chiasmatic cistern in some cases, give rise to fibrosis and adhesions in the midst of persistent inflammation thus strangulating the optic chiasm or optic nerves. This may lead to bilateral or unilateral primary optic atrophy and visual impairment.

TREATMENT OF TUBERCULAR MENINGITIS

There is currently no general consensus about the form of chemotherapy or optimal duration of treatment of TBM due to lack of solid clinical evidence. Therefore, below is the treatment policy followed in our clinical practice.

Antituberculosis Chemotherapy

The chemotherapy for TBM is divided in 2 phases: Intensive phase and maintenance phase as for pulmonary tuberculosis. The treatment is started as soon as TBM is suspected. This suspicion is based on the characteristic clinical symptoms and CSF cells, protein and sugar profile as described earlier. A combination of isoniazid, rifampicin, pyrazinamide and streptomycin or ethambutol (HRZE or HRZS) given for a period of two months (Intensive phase) followed by isoniazid, rifampicin and pyrazinamide (HRZ) for minimum ten months (maintenance or continuation phase). The dosage of various drugs is listed in **Table 11.2**. Dosages may need to be adjusted according to changes in weight.

Isoniazid is effective in killing rapidly replicating bacilli but is less effective against low replicating organisms. Rifampicin kills both rapidly and low replicating organisms. Pyrazinamide has good blood brain barrier penetration. In patients with over six years of age pyridoxine is routinely given to this combination to reduce the risk of INH neuropathy.

A daily treatment regimen is advised. No controlled trial in CNS TB comparing intermittent verses daily therapy is available. Some physicians believe that in severe infections recognized by deep coma or evidence of miliary disease, five drug regimen may be employed.

Table 11.2 Recommended doses of antitubercular drugs

Drug	National guidelines[28]	WHO[29]
Isoniazid	10 mg/kg	10 (range 10–15 mg/kg)
Rifampicin	10–12 mg/kg	15 mg/kg (range 10–20 mg/kg)
Ethambutol	20–25 mg/kg (max 1500 mg/day)	25 mg/kg (range 15–25 mg/kg)
Pyrazinamide	30–35 mg/kg (max 2000 mg/day)	35 mg/kg (range 30–40 mg/kg)
Streptomycin	15 mg/kg (max 1 g/day)	15–25 mg/kg

Role of Adjunctive Steroids

The majority of sequelae in TBM is due to inflammation of vessels and parenchyma at the base of the brain. Corticosteroids decrease meningeal inflammation and swelling and congestion of meninges thus decreasing cerebral edema and causing symptomatic improvement. It has been postulated that steroids may reduce the organization and fibrosis of basal exudates that is responsible for raised intracranial pressure, periarteritis and hydrocephalous. Theoretical worry regarding use of corticosteroids is that decrease in meningeal inflammation due to steroids may decrease the penetration of antitubercular drugs. In a Cochrane review, corticosteroids reduced risk of death by 22% (range 9–33%). And risk of severe neurological deficits by 18% (range 3–30%).[18] The benefit is more in stage 1 compared to stage 2 and 3. Either dexamethasone or prednisolone can be used. Dexamethasone 0.4–0.5 mg/kg/day or prednisolone 2 mg/kg/day can be used. A maximum dose of 4 weeks followed by tapering over 4 weeks have to be used.

Management of Complications

Hydrocephalus

Hydrocephalus is a main cause of morbidity and mortality in TBM. Grading of TBM hydrocephalous (TBMH) can help in prognosticating and management of children with TBMH. Modified MRC staging and Vellore grading system **(Table 11.3)** can help in grading. The most important step is to define whether is hydrocephalous is communicating or non-communicating. Though CT scan can differentiate these 2 entities reliably in 80% cases, air encephalography is the suggested gold standard for confirmation.[19] Children with noncommunication hydrocephalus need urgent CSF diversion procedure.

The most important is to assess the severity of alteration in GCS. All children with hydrocephalous need to be started on acetazolamide (dose range 30–100 mg/kg/day). Mannitol is used for acute control of cerebral edema if hemodynamic is stable. Furesemide and glycerol can also be used for cerebral edema due to their diuretic effect.

Table 11.3 The modified British Medical Research Council clinical criteria for tuberculous meningitis

Grade I	Alert and orientated without focal neurological deficit
Grade II	Glasgow coma score 14–10 with or without focal neurological deficit or Glasgow coma score 15 with focal neurological deficit
Grade III	Glasgow coma score less than 10 with or without focal neurological deficit

Vellore grading of tuberculous meningitis hydrocephalus[30]

I. Minimal symptoms with no neurological deficit and normal sensorium

II. Normal sensorium with neurological deficit

III. Altered sensorium but easily arousable with or without dense neurological deficit

IV. Deeply comatose, decerebrate or decorticate posturing

The decision for shunt surgery needs to be taken in light of affordability, access to medical care and abnormality in sensorium.

Different centers follow different treatment policy for grade 1 and 2 hydrocephalous. Early shunt in moderate hydrocephalous with grade I and II hydrocephalous have better outcome. However, this option must be exercised with the lifelong risk of shunt *in situ* and shunt block, displacement and infection. Conservative approach with medical therapy for 4 weeks can also be tried. However, this need prolonged monitoring in the hospital and should be considered provided patients have easy access of medical care in case patient deteriorates.

Grade 3 hydrocephalous generally benefit with surgery. The optimal management of grade 4 hydrocephalous is controversial. In MRC stage 3 and Vellore grade 4, the etiology of severely depressed sensorium is multifactorial which including infarcts and encephalitis and VP shunt alone may not lead to improvement in condition. An external ventricular drainage (EVD) may be inserted for 2–5 days and monitored for improvement in sensorium. Ventriculoperitoneal shunt (VP shunt) may be done, if there is improvement in sensorium with EVD.[20]

Indications of VP shunt are:
- Clinical symptoms of raised ICT
- CT scan showing severe hydrocephalous with periventricular ooze
- Evidence of improvement in sensorium after ventricular tap.

Ventricular tap may bed in emergency room for urgent control of life threatening raised pressure if immediate surgery cannot be done. A EVD can be placed for external CSF drainage. Alternatively if prolonged external drainage is needed (high CSF pleocytosis and elevated proteins which increases risk of VP shunt block and infection), Ommaya reservoir can be placed and CSF removed periodically.[20]

Endoscopic third ventriculostomy (ETV) can be used for management of obstructive hydrocephalous as an alternative to VP shunt with success rate of 60-85%.

Parents must be counseled for risk of complications of VP shunt like blockage of ventricular end, shunt migration, subdural hematoma, overdrainage, peritoneal pseudocyst formation, ascites, peritonitis and perforation of bowel.

Intracerebral Tuberculoma

Paradoxical expansion or appearance of tuber culoma, is a well-known complication, can occur during antitubercular treatment. Majority are clinically silent or they may manifest as new focal deficits, vision loss, increase in basal exudates, hydrocephalous, and enlargement of tuberculomas or spinal involvement with bowel bladder symptoms depending upon their size, number, pressure symptoms, peri lesional edema, and location. Corticosteroids may decrease perilesional edema and lead to improvement in pressure symptoms. There is anecdotal evidence of benefit of mycophenolate, cyclophosphamide, thalidomide, pulse methyl prednisolone, interferon-gamma and infliximab. Rarely, tuberculomas may coalesce to form tuberculous abscess which may need surgery.

Hyponatremia

Hyponatremia is common and seen in 50-60% individuals in TBM. It may alteration in sensorium, convulsions and worsening neurological signs in children on treatment for TBM. Sodium and water replacement may be done depending on volume status. Management need to tailored depending on daily weight, flu`id balance, plasma and urine sodium and plasma and urine osmolarity. There is evidence to suggest that syndrome of inappropriate antidiuretic hormone (SIADH) and elevated atrial natriuretic peptide may co-exist and the term 'hyponatremic natriuretic syndrome' is a more suitable term. Fludrocortisone and demeclocycline may be useful treatments.[21]

Hepatic Toxicity

Separate guidelines for ATT induced hepatitis in TBM are lacking. Management principles are similar to pulmonary TB. In asymptomatic individuals, if ALT is elevated to more than 5 times (3 times in symptomatic individuals) the upper normal limit, all hepatotoxic drugs should be stopped (INH, rifampicin and pyrazinamide). All attempts should be made to rule out other causes. The management depends on whether child is in intensive phase or maintenance, severity of hepatitis and severity of disease. In severe disease like miliary tuberculosis and TBM, a regimen comprising ethambutol, streptomycin and fluoroquinolone should be started. Liver function tests should be done twice weekly. When the LFT are normal, isoniazid should be introduced initially at low dose (5 mg/kg) and dose increased after 3 days. Subsequently low dose rifampicin (5 mg/kg) should be introduced and hiked to 12-15 mg/kg over 7 days. Subsequently, gradual reintroduction of pyrazinamide may be done.

Total duration of ATT will depend on the implicated drug. Two months of INH, streptomycin and ethambutol followed by 10 month of ethambutol and isoniazid are to be used if hepatotoxicity is associated with rifampicin. 6-9 months of rifampicin, ethambutol and pyrizinamide is to be used if isoniazid is hepatotoxic. 9 months of isoniazid and rifampicin is to be used if pyrazinamide was not used in intensive phase.[22,23] Pyridoxine should be used in all children receiving isoniazid >10 mg/kg and in all children who are malnorished and HIV positive.

Management of Drug Resistance

Drug resistance (DR) is an increasing problem, particularly in developing countries. Rising prevalence of drug resistant strains threaten to disrupt treatment and control programs. Studies estimate that three percent of all new TB cases in India and roughly 14% of patients undergoing treatment for the disease have developed resistance to drugs. In a recent study, multidrug resistant tuberculosis (resistant to rifampicin and isoniazid) was seen in 5.6%, monoresistance to either of first line ATT was seen in 24% cases. A history of poor compliance to ATT and contact with known resistant tuberculosis may lead to early suspicion on drug resistant TB. Such susceptibility testing should be done in high risk cases with liquid (BACTEC) cultures and gene Xpert. A recent study from Delhi showed that genotype MTBDRplus assay identify resistance to isoniazid and rifampicin. Though the sensitivity was only 55% compared to BACTEC MGIT system, the rapidity of the test result can permit early initiation of second line ATT.[24]

Suspected isoniazid monoresistance should be treated initially with conventional four drug ATT. In cases of low level resistance to isoniazid, children should be treated with 12 months HRZ in maintenance phase (isoniazid, rifampicin, pyrizinamide) In case of high level isoniazid resistance, fluoroquinolone, rifampicin and pyrazinamide is given in maintenance phase ethambutol is given along with these drugs in intensive phase.

Multidrug resistance (resistance to both isoniazid and rifampicin) has a far worse outcome. Treatment for MDR TB with extrapulmonary involvement like TBM is difficult and challenging. Firstly, the isolation of AFB from CSF is rare and so susceptibility is not known. There are no standard guidelines for treatment of MDR TB with TBM. In cases of proven resistance, children must be enrolled in supervised DOTS plus program in which children should be treated with 4 drugs which are susceptible and includes pyrazinamide, fluoroquinolone, ethionamide or prothionamide, and an injectable agent.[22] At our setting, when we suspect drug-resistance, we initiate treatment with a combination of isoniazid, rifampicin, pyrazinamide, ethambutol, streptomycin and fluoroquinolone. Treatment regimen and duration should be guided by expert, individualized according to patient response to treatment and knowledge of prevalence of drug resistance in the practice setting. Isoniazid and rifampicin should not be stopped until resistance is proven.

OUTCOME

Outcome in tuberculous meningitis is strongly associated with the stage of disease at presentation. Disease staging was first proposed by the Medical Research Council in 1948 **(Table 11.3)**.[25] The incidence of residual neurological handicap or death rises steeply where appropriate treatment is not initiated until after the emergence of reduced conscious level and focal neurological signs. Evidence from epidemiological studies found complete recovery was the rule in appropriate treated stage I cases, but was seen in only about 20% in stage III. Severity of coma, hydrocephalous, cranial nerve palsies, brain stem dysfunction, hypertonia and seizures at admission were the important variables predicting adverse outcome.[3,26,27]

KEY MESSAGES

- TBM should be considered as differential diagnosis of meningitis more than five days duration.
- Diagnosis is made by combination of clinical features, CSF, neuroradiology and evidence of extracranial tuberculomas.
- Gene Xpert may be used for rapid diagnosis of TBM.
- Empirically ATT before prior microbiological confirmation may be lifesaving.
- Parents should be counseled that a prolonged duration of ATT with a minimum of 12 months duration of ATT will need to be given.
- All neuroimaging must be carefully preserved to allow comparison from baseline to see for improvement or worsening.
- Parents should be counseled for the worsening of symptoms during therapy.
- Dose of ATT should be adjusted for weight gain.

REFERENCES

1. Illingworth RS. The early diagnosis of tuberculous meningitis. British medical journal. 1950;1(4651):479-81. Epub 1950/02/25.
2. Global Tuberculosis Report. [Internet] 2014 [updated 15 May 2015]; Available from: *http://www.who.int/tb/publications/global_report/gtbr14_executive_summary.pdf?ua=1*.
3. Garg RK. Tuberculous meningitis. Acta Neurol Scand. 2010;122(2):75-90. Epub 2010/01/09.
4. Rich AR, McCordick HA. The pathogenesis of tuberculous meningitis. Bull Johns Hopkins Hospital. 1933;52:5-37.
5. Prasad K, Menon GR. Tuberculous meningitis JAPI. 1997;45:722-29.
6. Thwaites GE, van Toorn R, Schoeman J. Tuberculous meningitis: more questions, still too few answers. Lancet Neurol. 2013;12(10):999-1010. Epub 2013/08/27.
7. Marais S, Thwaites G, Schoeman JF, Torok ME, Misra UK, Prasad K, et al. Tuberculous meningitis: a uniform case definition for use in clinical research. Lancet Infect Dis. 2010;10(11):803-12. Epub 2010/09/09.
8. Sharma P, Garg RK, Verma R, et al. Incidence, predictors and prognostic value of cranial nerve involvement in patients with tuberculous meningitis: a retrospective evaluation. Eur J Intern Med. 2011;22(3):289-95. Epub 2011/05/17.
9. Andronikou S, Smith B, Hatherhill M, et al. Definitive neuroradiological diagnostic features of tuberculous meningitis in children. Pediatr Radiol. 2004;34(11):876-85. Epub 2004/09/21.
10. Andronikou S, Wilmshurst J, Hatherill M, et al. Distribution of brain infarction in children with tuberculous meningitis and correlation with outcome score at 6 months. Pediatr Radiol. 2006;36(12):1289-94. Epub 2006/10/13.
11. Andronikou S, Wieselthaler N, Smith B, Douis H, Fieggen AG, van Toorn R, et al. Value of early follow-up CT in paediatric tuberculous meningitis. Pediatr Radiol. 2005;35(11):1092-9. Epub 2005/08/05.
12. Thwaites GE, Chau TT, Farrar JJ. Improving the bacteriological diagnosis of tuberculous meningitis. J Clin Microbiol. 2004;42(1):378-9. Epub 2004/01/13.
13. Pai M, Flores LL, Pai N, Hubbard A, Riley LW, Colford JM, Jr. Diagnostic accuracy of nucleic acid amplification tests for tuberculous meningitis: a systematic review and meta-analysis. Lancet Infect Dis. 2003;3(10):633-43. Epub 2003/10/03.
14. Patel VB, Theron G, Lenders L, Matinyena B, Connolly C, Singh R, et al. Diagnostic Accuracy of Quantitative PCR (Xpert MTB/RIF) for Tuberculous Meningitis in a High Burden Setting: A Prospective Study. PLoS Med. 2013;10(10):e1001536. Epub 2013/10/30.
15. Solomons RS, van Elsland SL, Visser DH, Hoek KG, Marais BJ, Schoeman JF, et al. Commercial nucleic acid amplification tests in tuberculous meningitis—a meta-analysis. Diagn Microbiol Infect Dis. 2014;78(4):398-403. Epub 2014/02/08.
16. Guidance for national tuberculosis programmes on the management of tuberculosis in children. [Internet] 2014 [updated 15 May 2015]; Second:[Available from: *http://apps.who.int/medicinedocs/documents/s21535en/s21535en.pdf*.
17. Rana SV, Chacko F, Lal V, Arora SK, Parbhakar S, Sharma SK, et al. To compare CSF adenosine deaminase levels and CSF-PCR for tuberculous meningitis. Clin Neurol Neurosurg. 2010;112(5):424-30. Epub 2010/03/30.
18. Prasad K, Singh MB. Corticosteroids for managing tuberculous meningitis. Cochrane Database Syst Rev. 2008(1):CD002244. Epub 2008/02/07.
19. Bruwer GE, Van der Westhuizen S, Lombard CJ, et al. Can CT predict the level of CSF block in tuberculous hydrocephalus? Childs Nerv Syst. 2004;20(3):183-7. Epub 2004/02/18.
20. Tandon V, Mahapatra AK. Management of post-tubercular hydrocephalus. Childs Nerv Syst. 2011;27(10):1699-707. Epub 2011/09/20.
21. Thwaites GE, Tran TH. Tuberculous meningitis: many questions, too few answers. Lancet Neurol. 2005;4(3):160-70. Epub 2005/02/22.
22. Thwaites G, Fisher M, Hemingway C, Scott G, Solomon T, Innes J. British Infection Society guidelines for the diagnosis and treatment of tuberculosis of the central nervous system in adults and children. J Infect. 2009;59(3):167-87. Epub 2009/08/01.
23. World Health Organization. Treatment of tuberculosis: Guidelines. 2010 [updated 15 May 2015]; Available from: *http://www.who.int/tb/publications/2010/9789241547833/en/*.
24. Gupta R, Thakur R, Gupta P, Jalan N, Kushwaha S, Gupta M, et al. Evaluation of Geno Type MTBDRplus Line Probe Assay for Early Detection of Drug Resistance in Tuberculous Meningitis Patients in India. Journal of global infectious diseases. 2015;7(1):5-10. Epub 2015/02/28.

25. Medical Research Council Streptomycin in Tuberculous Trials Committee. STREPTOMYCIN treatment of tuberculous meningitis. Lancet. 1948;1(6503):582-96. Epub 1948/04/17.
26. van Well GT, Paes BF, Terwee CB, Springer P, Roord JJ, Donald PR, et al. Twenty years of pediatric tuberculous meningitis: a retrospective cohort study in the western cape of South Africa. Pediatrics. 2009;123(1):e1-8. Epub 2009/04/16.
27. Karande S, Gupta V, Kulkarni M, et al. Prognostic clinical variables in childhood tuberculous meningitis: an experience from Mumbai, India. Neurol India. 2005;53(2):191-5; discussion 5-6. Epub 2005/07/13.
28. National guidelines on diagnosis and treatment of Pediatric Tuberculosis. [Internet] 2012 [updated 15 May 2015]; Available from: *http://tbcindia.nic.in/Paediatric%20guidelines_New.pdf*.
29. World Health Organisation. Rapid Advice: Treatment of tuberculosis in children [Internet] 2010 [updated 15 May 2015]; Available from: *http://whqlibdoc.who.int/publications/2010/9789241500449_eng.pdf*.
30. Palur R, Rajshekhar V, Chandy MJ, Joseph T, Abraham J. Shunt surgery for hydrocephalous in tubercular meningitis: A long-term follow-up study. 1991;74:64-9.

CHAPTER 12

Cerebrospinal Fluid Examination in Bacterial Meningitis: Common Pitfalls

TM Ananda Kesavan

Acute bacterial meningitis (ABM) is the most common central nervous system (CNS) infection in children. There are certain peculiarities of nervous system, making it more vulnerable to infection **(Table 12.1)**.

Acute bacterial meningitis is often devastating leading to death or serious neurologic sequelae. One of the important factor determining the prognosis is early treatment, so early diagnosis and prompt treatment is crucial.

Even though meningitis is a common infection, under diagnosis of this disease is not uncommon. It may be due to atypical signs in infant (unfortunately in infants, the infection is more common and serious) and altered clinical features due to prior antibiotic use. False negative signs of meningeal irritation also seen in critically ill child, meningitis in a child with severe protein-energy malnutrition (PEM), severe immunodeficiency conditions, such as HIV.

On the other hand, an anxious physician may overdiagnosis ABM in any child with fever, headache and vomiting. It may lead to unwanted and prolonged treatment. Sometimes clinician even more confused with false signs of meningeal irritation **(Table 12.2)**.

In the following section, we will discuss the common dilemmas in the CSF examination in a case of ABM in children.

CEREBROSPINAL FLUID IN BACTERIAL MENINGITIS

Stabilize the patient [care of airway, breathing and circulation (ABC)] before doing lumbar puncture (LP). Contraindication for doing LP is not common in children **(Table 12.3)**. In uncomplicated meningitis where cerebral edema is symmetrical the chance for coning is less (where as in a case

Table 12.1 Factors leading to vulnerability to nervous system infection

- Deficient local host defenses that do not suppress the multiplication of pathogen
- Detrimental effects of cerebral blood flow alterations
- Harmful effects of increased intracranial pressure caused by brain swelling
- Limited repair mechanism of neuronal tissue
- Insufficient lymphatic drainage
- Poor concentration of immunoglobulin, complement, deficient opsonization and macrophages in CSF

Abbreviation: CSF, cerebrospinal fluid

Table 12.2 Causes of false positive neck sign

Intracranial causes	Extracranial causes
• Encephalitis	• Meningism
• Cerebral malaria	• Upper lobe pneumonia
• ICSOL-Post fossa tumors	• Tonsillitis
• Brain abscess	• Retropharyngeal abscess
• Benign intracranial tension	• Cervical vertebral problems
	• Cervical lymphadenitis

Table 12.3 Contraindication to lumbar puncture
• Obvious signs of increased ICP
• Clinically relevant cardiorespiratory compromise
• History or signs of bleeding disorder
• Infection at puncture site

Abbreviations: ICP, intracarnial pressure

Table 12.4 Causes for xanthochromic CSF
• Subarachnoid hemorrhage (after 12 hours)
• Blood in the CSF (traumatic LP with >1 Lakh RBC per cmm)
• Increased protein (>150 mg%)
• Hyperbilirubinemia (>15 mg% in newborn)
• A child taking rifampicin

Abbreviations: CSF, cerebrospinal fluid; LP, lumbar puncture; RBC, red blood cell

Table 12.5 Conditions associated with low CSF sugar
• Mumps
• HSV infection
• Varicella-zoster
• Lymphocytic choriomeningitis
• Fungal meningitis
• Widespread neoplastic involvement of the meninges
• Subarachnoid hemorrhage

of tumor or abscess where the pressure effect is unilateral and not uniform and chance for coning is high). In suspected case of ABM, start empirical antibiotics without waiting for CSF examination. Do not forget to do fundus examination and blood sugar estimation before LP.

Cerebrospinal fluid should be collected in 4 bottles–one each for biochemistry, cell count and Gram stain culture test and for other tests (CRP, CSF Ag detection test, etc.). In a well defined case of ABM, CSF is under high pressure, proteins will be high and sugar will be less than two third of the blood sugar. Gram stain (positive in 60–80% in untreated child) will help to identify the organism and culture will help to select the proper antibiotics. Nowadays, CSF C-reactive protein (CRP), rapid antigen detection tests, etc. are available even in remote areas and many of these tests are useful in children previously treated with antibiotics. Even though all these facilities are available, rarely a practicing pediatrician may find it difficult to interpret a CSF result in his office practice.

DIAGNOSTIC DILEMMAS IN CEREBROSPINAL FLUID EXAMINATION

The CSF appearance may be turbid due to cells, bacteria, or blood. CSF will be turbid, when the white blood cell (WBC) count is more than 200 per cmm or red blood cell (RBC) count of more than 400 per cmm.

Xanthochromic CSF

It will appear as early as 2–4 hours (oxy Hb) or in a child with subarachnoid hemorrhage by 12 hours (bilirubin). Xanthochromic CSF seen due to blood in the CSF, increased protein more than 150 mg%, hyperbilirubinemia of more than 15 mg% (in a newborn). Causes for xanthochromic CSF are given in **Table 12.4**.

CSF Glucose

Normal CSF glucose is 40–80 mg and a ratio less than 0.5 abnormal. In a neonate, CSF glucose 34–112 mg (ratio 0.7 : 0.9) and a ratio less than 0.6 is abnormal. Blood glucose should be estimated ideally 2–4 hours prior to performing LP.

In severe hyperglycemia [if the child had received glucose containing fluids before LP or in diabetic ketoacidosis (DKA)] the ratio is 0.4 and a ratio less than 0.3 abnormal. Very low CSF glucose is associated with high incidence of hearing defect and is a poor prognostic sign in ABM.

Cerebrospinal fluid glucose can be decreased in 3.5% of children with aseptic meningitis. Other conditions where one will get low CSF sugar is given in **Table 12.5**.

CSF Protein

Normally, protein content in the CSF is less than 40 mg% and in neonate it may as high as 150 mg%. A protein level of above 150 mg per dL can cause xanthochromia. "Cob-web" appearance of CSF is due to high level of CSF protein, i.e. 1.5 gm/L. It may be normal in initial stages of ABM and misleading in traumatic tap. Protein may be high in Guillian-Barré syndrome, multiple sclerosis, in spinal block (TBM) and parameningeal infiltrations.

In viral meningitis, CSF protein is less than 100 mg/dL, almost never more than 250 mg%.

CSF Cell Count

In normal child, the CSF cell count is less than 5 cells per cmm with no polymorph. In a newborn the normal cell count may be as high as 30 cells per cmm and up to 60% polymorphs. Presence of plasma cells and eosinophils in the CSF is always abnormal.

Very low count indicates severe meningitis. Cell count tends to fall over time and decreased if measured after 1 hour. So a physician doing a lumbar puncture should examine his patients's CSF without delay.

After a generalized seizure, there is chance for CSF pleocytosis. But the rise in cell count is usually less than 80 cells per cmm. CSF pleocytosis may confuse a treating pediatrician, especially when he does CSF study in a child with fever and seizure. Anyway one has to rule out CNS infection, before attributing CSF pleocytosis due to seizure.

Cerebrospinal fluid lymphocytosis (of more than 50%) can occur in 13–32% of bacterial meningitis. So, if general condition of the patient is not improved in 24–48 hours of antibiotic treatment, repeat LP. If there is polymorph, treat it as pyogenic meningitis. In 1–13% of TBM, a predominant polymorphic picture may be seen.

In viral meningitis, a predominant polymorphonuclear leukocytosis seen in 1/3 of children and usually gets converted to lymphocytosis in 24–48 hours. The CSF cell count in viral meningitis is seldom exceeds 1000 per cmm (except in mumps).

Gram Stain

This is one of the most useful part of CSF examination, but unfortunately not performed routinely. We can identify the organism and can start appropriate antibiotic while awaiting for the culture and sensitivity test. The positivity is 60–80% in untreated bacterial meningitis. Positivity is less in pretreated patients.

CSF Culture

Culture will be positive in CSF is up to 80% in good centers. Send blood also for culture. It will be positive in 60–80% in untreated children. Always send CSF for culture even when the fluid appears to be crystal clear and acellular. Similarly one can do CSF culture and sensitivity test in a case of traumatic LP (one useful test in a case of blood-stained CSF).

Metabolic Changes in CSF in Bacterial Meningitis

Various metabolic changes will occur in CSF in ABM **(Table 12.6)**.

All these tests are not readily available or not reliable, but can be done in specific cases or in research institutions.

Tests to Differentiate Septic from Aseptic Meningitis

Many tests are available, but none of them are uniformly reliable. Bacterial antigen tests are very useful. Latex agglutination test has a sensitivity 81% for detecting Hemophilus influenzae type b (Hib), 50–70% for pneumococcal and 30–70% for *Neisseria meningitis*. The specificity for these 3 antigens are about 90–96%. Antigen tests are useful when the child had received prior antibiotic treatment.

Detection of bacterial deoxyribonucleic acid (DNA) by polymerase chain reaction (PCR) is very sensitive, but is very costly and not freely available. Limulus lysate test (useful in gram-negative infection, with a positive rate: 70–90%)

Table 12.6 Metabolic changes in CSF in ABM

Increased
• CSF lactate
– LDH
– CRP
– CPK
– Aspartate transaminase
– Vasopressin
– Ferritin
Decreased
• CSF pH

Abbreviations: CSF, cerebrospinal fluid; ABM; acute bacterial meningitis; LDH, lactic dehydrogenase; CRP, C-reactive protein; CPK, creatine phosphokinase and CSF lactic acid (more than 35 mg% in bacterial meningitis with a predictive value of less than 30%) are rarely performed.

CSF CRP Level

It is one of the tests commonly performed nowadays. It is nonspecific and is elevated in 95–100% of ABM. It elevated in 60% of nonbacterial meningitis also. CRP also elevated in inflammatory and necrotic conditions. A negative CRP excludes bacterial meningitis, while a positive test need not always indicate a bacterial infection. High CRP value both in blood and CSF has got very high sensitivity and specificity.

Two other situations where CSF may confuse the pediatricians are:
1. CSF changes in partially treated pyogenic meningitis and
2. Problem of traumatic tap in a suspected case of bacterial meningitis.

CSF Changes in Partially Treated Pyogenic Meningitis

The first changes that will happen after antibiotic use in a case of ABM is negative Gram stain and sterile CSF culture. These changes can happen with in 24 hours of antibiotic treatment. CSF glucose reaches normal on the 3rd day in 80% of patients but protein remains elevated even after 10th day, in up to 40% of patients.

Prior antibiotic use does not affect total WBC count, CSF protein and CSF glucose. So, even if the child had received antibiotic, all these investigations should be done. Same is almost true in a case of traumatic CSF. Oral antibiotics with poor blood brain penetration usually does not affect the CSF results.

Prior antibiotic use decrease the percentage of polymorph in CSF. In this situation, bacterial antigen tests have certain advantages–antigen tests do not depend upon viable organism in the CSF. So, they may give positive results even when Gram stain and culture are negative.

CSF may be normal in ABM (up to 6%) and in such cases, CSF becomes abnormal in 24 hours. So, it is important to do repeat LP, if one strongly suspecting ABM clinically.

Problem of Traumatic Tap in a Suspected Case of Bacterial Meningitis

It is a known fact that holding the child in a perfect position is more difficult than inserting the LP needle. Even an experienced person sometimes find it difficult to get CSF sample without trauma. Correction in the form of subtracting 1 WBC for every 700 RBCs and subtracting 1 mg/dL from total protein for every 1000 RBCs are some common methods used. Always remember that CSF glucose, Gram-stain and culture are not altered by traumatic tap, provided contaminant is less than 2 lakhs RBC/cmm. One may get red blood cells in CSF as in case of herpes simplex meningitis even without trauma.

WHEN TO DO REPEAT LUMBAR PUNCTURE?

In uncomplicated case of ABM, there is no indication for repeat LP. The various indications to repeat LP is given in **Table 12.7**.

CSF Findings and Prognosis

Various parameters in CSF will give an idea about the prognosis. It will give a rough idea about the overall outcome to the treating physician. CSF factors associated with poor prognosis is given in **Table 12.8**.

Table 12.7 Indication for repeat LP

- Lack of clinical improvement in 24–48 hours
- Gram-negative meningitis
- Beta lactam resistant organism
- Recurrent meningitis
- Meningitis in a newborn

Table 12.8 CSF findings associated with poor outcome in ABM

- High bacterial count in CSF
- Very low or high CSF leucocyte count
- High CSF protein level
- Very low CSF sugar
- Delay in CSF sterilization

Abbreviations: CSF, cerebrospinal fluid; ABM, acute bacterial meningitis

Complete and careful CSF examination without delay is the rule. Sometimes CSF results may confuse the physician especially in partially treated case of meningitis. A repeat LP is rarely indicated and neuroimaging has limited value in uncomplicated meningitis.

BIBLIOGRAPHY

1. Dougherty JM, Roth RM. Cerebral spinal fluid. Emerg Med Cli North Am. 1986;4:281-97.
2. Feign and Cherry. Textbook of Pediatric Infectious Diseases, 6th Edn. Saunders; 2009. pp. 481-99.
3. Seehusen DA, Reeves MM, Fomin DA. Cerebrospinal fluid analysis. Am Fam Phys. 2003;68:1103-9.

CHAPTER 13

Cerebral Malaria

Ketan H Shah

INTRODUCTION

Malaria is very common disease in tropical country.[1] India has very high incidence of malaria. Peak incidence is seen during monsoon season. WHO recommends 'test, treat and track' to control malaria.

ABOUT PATHOGEN

Malaria is caused by infection of red blood cells with protozoan parasites of genus *Plasmodium*. It is transmitted to human being by female anopheles mosquitoes. The genus *Plasmodium* includes *Plasmodium vivax*, *Plasmodium falciparum*, *Plasmodium malariae* and *Plasmodium ovale*. Out of all *Plasmodium falciparum* is most serious type. More than one species can infect person at a time. *Plasmodium knowlesi* malaria is also reported to be pathological. *Plasmodium falciparum* can cause parasitemia up to 60%, while other malarial parasites have less than 2% of parasitemia. *Plasmodium vivax* malaria causing cerebral malaria is reported occasionally.

Life cycle of malaria parasite is complex.[2] Human host has asexual phase and mosquito has sexual phase. In human, two step process is seen, exoerythrocytic (hepatic) and erythrocytic (red cells) phase. Sporozoites enter in human blood after mosquito bite and then in liver they multiply asexually to form schizont. After rupture of liver cell thousands of merozoites are released. These merozoites enter RBC. Various stages of development occur in RBCs—ring form, trophozoites and then erythrocytic merozoites. Once erythrocyte membrane ruptures, thousands of merozoites are released. During release of merozoites fever appears. These merozoites develop into male and female gametocytes. This is ingested by female anopheles mosquito and in the stomach of mosquito these gametocytes fuse to form zygote. Zygote undergoes series of transformation to form sporozoites. These sporozoites enter into salivary gland and with mosquito bite they enter into human blood stream. This completes the life cycle.

Pathophysiological Sequence of Cerebral Malaria/Complicated Malaria

Heavy parasitemia occurs in *P. falciparum* malaria. It causes many changes in human host.
- There is excessive production of cytokines. Various inflammatory markers are released and they are responsible for many pathological changes.
- Polyclonal activation causes hypergamma-globulinemia and formation of immune complexes.
- There is immunosuppression.
- Cytoadherance of infected RBCs causes blockage, leakage of blood and blood products.

- Tissue anoxia occurs because of cytoadherance and inflammatory changes.
- Hypoglycemia and lactic acidosis are common complications.[2]
- Cumulative effect of all causes multiorgan damage including brain dysfunction.[1]

Clinical Features of Cerebral Malaria

Cerebral malaria may be isolated presentation or may be part of multiorgan involvement. In young child, it may present with fever, poor feeding and lethargy. It starts with fever and in no time leads to convulsion and coma. Convulsion may be generalized or subtle. Nystagmus may be present. Every effort should be taken to rule out other treatable metabolic, nonmetabolic and infectious causes.[3] If not diagnosed in time it may progress very fast to cause lethal malaria. Young children, pregnant lady (as immunity is weaned off), immunocompromised child and child staying in nonendemic zone are at risk of sever malaria. Nonimmune person traveling to endemic area is also at high-risk of sever-malaria.

Other features of severe malaria are:
- *Impaired consciousness*: A Glasgow coma score <11 in adults or a Blantyre coma Score <3 in children.
- *Prostration*: Generalized weakness so that the person is unable to sit, stand or walk without assistance.
- *Multiple convulsions*: More than two episodes within 24 hours.
- *Acidosis*: A base deficit of >8 mEq/L or, if not available, a plasma bicarbonate.
- Level of <15 mmol/L or venous plasma lactate ≥5 mmol/L. Severe acidosis manifests clinically as respiratory distress (rapid, deep, labored breathing).
- *Hypoglycemia*: Blood or plasma glucose < 2.2 mmol/L (< 40 mg/dL).
- *Severe malarial anemia*: Hemoglobin concentration ≤5 g/dL or a hematocrit of ≤15% in children <12 years of age (<7 g/dL and <20%, respectively, in adults) with a parasite count >10 000/μL.
- *Renal impairment*: Plasma or serum creatinine >265 μmol/L (3 mg/dL) or blood urea >20 mmol/L.
- *Jaundice*: Plasma or serum bilirubin >50 μmol/L (3 mg/dL) with a parasite count 100 000/μL.
- *Pulmonary edema*: Radiologically confirmed or oxygen saturation <92% on room air with a respiratory rate >30/minute, often with chest indrawing and crepitations on auscultation.
- *Significant bleeding*: Including recurrent or prolonged bleeding from the nose, gums or venipuncture sites; hematemesis or melena.
- *Shock*: Compensated shock is defined as capillary refill ≥3 seconds or temperature gradient on leg (mid to proximal limb), but no hypotension. Decompensated shock is defined as systolic blood pressure <70 mm Hg in children or < 80 mm Hg in adults, with evidence of impaired perfusion (cool peripheries or prolonged capillary refill).
- *Hyperparasitemia*: *P. falciparum* parasitemia >10%.

Laboratory Tests

Peripheral smear examination and rapid antigen tests are diagnostic. However, in initial stage parasites may not be detected. But low Hb, normal WBC count and low platelet will give us idea of possibility of malaria. Peripheral smear examination can be done in thick and thin smear preparation. Smear preparation can be done at any time of the fever, not necessarily at peak or at rigors. Fingertips and earlobules are highly vascular area. Chances of parasites density are high in these two areas. Microscopy can detect number of parasites, stage and, type of parasite **(Table 13.1)**. This will help in type of drug selection (although in cerebral malaria it is always artemisinin derivatives not chloroquine) and for prognosis purpose also. Heavy parasitemia of more than 5% will have poor prognosis. Quantitative buffy coat (QBC) smear method is another preparation, where in quantitative buffy coat smear is taken (centrifugation of blood and buffy coat is examined). The chances of seeing parasites are high with buffy coat smear. Parasites can be seen in fluorescent microscopy by using flurochromes. Acridine orange is one of them. Parasites will pick up this stain and can be seen in fluorescent microscopy. However, this method needs special instrument and it is costly.

Table 13.1 Advantages and disadvantages of thick and thin smear examination

Thick smear	Thin smear
RBCs are lysed	Single layer of blood film
Many layers of blood film are seen	Fixed RBCs are seen
Large volume of blood smear can be examined	Smaller volume of blood is screened
Good screening test	Good species differentiation
Low density infection can be detected	Low density infection can be missed

Abbreviation: RBC, red blood cell

Ideal thin film
- Surface is even and uniform.
- Margin do not extend to the side of the slide.
- Tail ends near the center of the slide.
- Consist of a single layer of red cells.

Ideal thick film
- Uniform thickness so, newsprint can be read through.
- *In thick film:* Parasite, WBC and platelet are seen.
- *In thin film:* Parasite, WBC, platelet and RBC are seen.
- The advantages and disadvantages of thick and thin smear examinations are shown in **Table 13.1**.

Rapid Diagnostic Test

RDT (rapid diagnostic test of malaria or malaria antigen test) if available, will give us fast result. Selection of RDT and its interpretation is important. It detects various parasites antigens or enzymes that are species or genus specific.

Antigens targeted by RDTs:
- Histidine rich protein II (HRPII)—Produced by trophozoites and young (not mature) gametocyte of *P. falciparum*.
- Parasite lactate dehydrogenase (pLDH).
 This enzyme is produced by asexual and sexual stages (gametocyte) of malaria parasite. Test kits currently detect pLDH from all four *Plasmodium* species:
- Parasite lactate dehydrogenase (pLDH)- *P. falciparum* specific.
- Parasite lactate dehydrogenase (pLDH)- *P. vivax* specific isomer.
- Plasmodium aldolase—all four species.
- Different malarial antigens available in test kit **(Table 13.2)**.
- HRPII: Specific for *P falciparum*.

Table 13.2 Types of antigen and their diagnostic utility

Species	HRP2	LDH	Aldolase
P falciparum	✓	✓	✓
P vivax	✗	✓	✓
Pan (for all four types)	✗	✓	✓

- pLDH for *P. falciparum:* Specific for *P. falciparum*.
- pLDH for *Plasmodium* species (PAN)-specific for *P. falciparum, P. vivax, P. ovale* and *P. malariae*.
- pLDH for *P. vivax*-Specific for *P. vivax*.
- pAldolase: Specific for all four species.

In partially treated case, pf HRP2 (*Plasmodium falciparum* Histidin rich protein 2 antigen tests) will be positive. This test remains positive for long time 2-3 weeks even after treatment. So, in acute setting, this antigen –pf HRP2 is useful. In relapse or recurrence it may not be useful. pLDH is available in species specific and all four type specific enzyme tests also. pAldolase is same way for all four types. In case of negative smear and negative RDT, repeat smear after 6–12 hours is recommended. If smear is negative after 6–12 hours than chances of having malaria are extremely less. PAN aldolase test is more specific and sensitive than HRP test (Histidine-rich protein antigen). (PAN indicates all four types of malarial parasites). Clinician should be aware about the test used for the diagnosis. Associated other system involvement will also give clue to the diagnosis of malaria.

TREATMENT

Objective: "Save the life" is primary objective. Secondary objective may be prevention of disability and prevention of recrudescence.

Clinical Assessment of the Patient

- Airway, breathing and circulation are established.
- Glasgow coma scale/Blantyre coma score is recorded.
- Hematocrit, parasite count, renal function tests, hepatic function, blood glucose, lactate and blood gases analysis are done. Hypoglycemia and severe acidosis needs correction. Hepatic and renal dysfunction need more aggressive management in intensive care unit (ICU) setup.
- Rehydration depending upon degree of dehydration is done. In adult patient over hydration can cause pulmonary edema. Judicious use of IV fluid is recommended.
- Lumbar puncture is done if bacterial meningitis is suspected. Cerebral malaria is not associated with meningeal signs or photophobia. Along with cerebral malaria or severe malaria, bacterial sepsis is known. Blood can be drawn for bacterial culture and if needed antibiotic can be started. Gram negative infection do accompany severe malaria.

Specific Antimalarial Treatment

According to World Health Organization (WHO) and Indian Academy of Pediatrics (IAP) guidelines.[1,3] Artesunate is preferred drug for cerebral malaria and all complicated malaria. Various artemisinin derivatives are available. Various trails have favored use of artesunate as first line of treatment for severe complicated malaria. (AQUAMAT trial).[4] Amongst all derivatives artesunate is superior drug. It is superior to quinine. The incidence of convulsion, coma and hypoglycemia developing after hospitalization are significantly reduced.

Dose: Revised guidelines from WHO states 3 mg/kg/dose for below 20 kg child. Second dose after 12 hours and then once in 24 hours till patient can tolerate oral artemisinin combination therapy (ACT).

Intravenous access, if not available than rectal suppository of artesunate can be tried. There is no sufficient evidence for recommendation of rectal suppository of artesunate above 6 years of age. Below 6 years of age 10 mg/kg dose suppository of artesunate can be kept. If suppository expels out within 30 minutes of insertion, it should be repeated.

Outcome is good with IV artesunate than quinine. There are reports of postartesunate hemolysis and anemia after a week. It is because of killing of ring forms of parasites in RBC by artesunate. These RBC have short life span. They are taken by spleen and resend to circulation. They have shortened life span so destruction of RBC causes anemia.

If artesunate is not available than IM artemether can be used.

Intramuscular artemether is another alternative if IV artesunate cannot be given. It is oil based injection, given on anterolateral side of thigh. 3.2 mg/kg first dose and then 1.6 mg/kg/2nd, 3rd day, till patient can take oral artemisinin combination therapy (ACT). All injectable artemisinin derivatives should be followed by oral ACT as soon as patient starts taking oral drugs. Oral ACT is of various combinations.

- Artesunate + mefloquine should be avoided as mefloquine has neurotoxicity.
- Artemether + lumefantrine combination is better option **(Table 13.3)**.
- Artesunate + amodiaquine (not available in India)
- Dihydroartemisinin + Piperaquine (not available).
- Artesunate + sulfadoxine-pyrimethamine combination has inferior choice than artemether + lumefantrine combination. As in India resistance to sulphadoxine-pyrimethamine is found in *P. falciparum*.

Artemisinin drug clears parasites very fast and partner drug having long duration of action clears remaining parasites. Partner drug prevents development of resistance to artemisinin drug. It gives period of post-treatment prophylaxis for many days.

Single dose of Primaquine 0.25 mg/kg is recommended to reduce transmissibility.

Table 13.3 Dosage guidelines for artemether+lumefantrine combination[1]

Body weight	Dose (artemether+lumefantrine)
5 to < 15	20+120
15 to <25	40+240
25 to <35	60+360
>35	80+480

Quinine

If artemisinin derivatives are not available then quinine can be used. However, quinine is inferior option. It is available in various salt formulations. Dihydrochloride is standard salt use for IV preparation. It is always given in diluted form with 5% dextrose and slow infusion over 3-4 hours. Loading dose of 20 mg/kg is recommended. Followed by 10 mg/kg/dose eight hourly. IM quinine dihydrochloride salt is painful. It can be given in diluted form of 60-100 mg/mL (available preparation has 300 mg/mL). 10 mg/kg dose in each thigh is given. Gluconate salt is less painful. Quinine causes serious hypotension. It is always given as slow IV infusion and never as bolus. Quinine can be combined with clindamycin or doxy/tetracycline.

Incorrect Approach to Treatment[1]

- Artesunate and quinine both together is not recommended. Artesunate + doxycycline (3.5 mg/kg once a day) or artesunate + clindamycin (10 mg/kg/dose twice a day) are reserved in rare occasions of artemisinin-based combination therapy (ACT) treatment failure. Doxycycline not recommended in child below 8 years.
- Artemisinin should not be used as alone drug it should be always followed by ACT combination.
- In undiagnosed case if parasites are not found and treatment is started it should be completed and never left in between.
- Heparin, prostacyclin, deferoxamine, pentoxifylline, low molecular weight dextran, urea, high dose corticosteroids, acetylsalicylic acid, deferoxamine, antitumor necrosis factor antibody, cyclosporine, dichloroacetate, adrenaline, and hyperimmune serum are not recommended.

Management of Other Complications Related to Malaria

Hypoglycemia, convulsions and fluid management are important adjuvant treatment. Anemia can be managed with blood transfusion. Acidosis, renal failure needs correction. Bleeding diathesis needs Vitamin K supplements and if needed transfusion. Antipyretic, antiemetic are needed as adjuvant treatment. Exchange transfusion is not an established therapy. Anticonvulsant drugs are used as per need. Prophylactic use of anticonvulsant is not recommended. Bacterial infection does coexist. Judicious decision of using broad spectrum antibiotic is recommended.

REFERENCES

1. World Health Organization. Treatment of severe malaria in guidelines for the treatment of malaria, 3rd edn. Geneva. WHO: 2015. Accessed on 8th July 2015.
2. Uttam KG. Protozoal, parasitic and fungal infections. Text book of pediatric infectious diseases. Volume 2 .pp.346-50.
3. Sukumaran TU. IAP guidelines/Protocols. In: Text book of pediatric infectious diseases. Volume 2.pp.404-10.
4. Artesunate vs. quinine in the treatment of severe Falciparum malaria in African children (AQUAMAT). Lancet. 2010;376(9753):1647-57.

CHAPTER 14

Neurocysticercosis

Anoop Verma

INTRODUCTION

Cysticercosis, the most common cause of adult onset epilepsy in the third world,[1,2] is due to infection with the cystic larval form of the tapeworm, *Taenia solium*. The intestinal dwelling tapeworm stage develops following the ingestion of raw or poorly cooked pork containing cystic larvae. The tapeworm releases infectious ova into the feces and when ingested by free roaming pigs, hatch, migrate and develop into cystic larvae in the muscles, brain and other tissues of the pig. Like the pig, humans also develop larval cysts in their tissue after accidental ingestion of ova. Most of the symptoms and disease in humans results from infection of the central nervous system by larval cysts. Presenting symptoms and signs can be particularly varied due to differences in location, number of cysts and associated inflammation.[1,3]

Neurocysticercosis is central nervous system (CNS) infection with *T. solium*. It is perhaps the most common parasitic infestation of the CNS and has received attention in the last two decades because of the availability of MRI and CT scanning in the countries where cysticercosis is endemic.

THE INDIAN FACTS

- In Indian subcontinent, Pork eaters contribute to less than 1–2% of neurocysticercosis (NCC), and vegetarian contribute to more than 95% of NCC.[4]
- In Indian subcontinent, single cyst infection contributes to 47.7–53.4% of NCC.[5,6]
- Prevalence of taeniasis was 18.6% in Mohanlalganj block of Lucknow district and active epilepsy was confirmed in 5.8% of the population and 48.3% of people with epilepsy fulfilled either definitive or probable criteria for NCC.[7]
- Prevalence of taeniasis ranged from 0.5% in hospitalized in northern India to 12–15% in labor colonies where pigs are raised.[8]
- *Vellore*: Prevalence of NCC causing active epilepsy was 1.3 per 1000 population.[9]
- *Puducherry*: Cysticercosis seroprevalence among the healthy blood donors was 6.5% using both antigen and antibody detection methods.[10]
- *Bengaluru*: NCC is seen in 2% of unselected patient of epilepsy.[11]
- *New Delhi*: NCC accounts for 2.5% of all intra-cranial lesion.[12]
- Solitary cystic granuloma (SCG) contributes to two-third of all patients with NCC.[13] SCG contributed 26–50% patients with partial seizures.
- *Patiala*: Solitary lesion contributes 88% in a pathologically proven cases of cysticercosis.[14]
- *Chandigarh*: In a seroprevalence study, anti-cysticercus antibody was found in 17.3% with high prevalence 24% reported from slums, however 8% of seropositives had previous history of seizures.

Table 14.1 Anatomical classification of neurocysticercosis

Anatomical classification
- Parenchymal
- Extraparenchymal
  - Ventricular
  - Subarachnoid
- Mixed

Table 14.2 Classification of neurocysticercosis into active and inactive forms

Active forms of NCC
- Arachnoiditis
  - Hydrocephalus secondary to meningeal inflammation
  - Parenchymal cysts
  - Brain infarct secondary to vasculitis
  - Mass effect due to large cyst or the cyst lumps
- Intraventricular cyst
  - Spinal cyst

Inactive forms of NCC
- Parenchymal calcifications
- Hydrocephalus secondary to meningeal fibrosis

Source: Adapted from Arch Intern Med. 1985;145: 442-5.

- *Ludhiana*: Around 27 of 106 cases were EITB assay positive in patients with active epilepsy in a community based survey in slums of Ludhiana.[15]

CLASSIFICATION OF NCC (TABLES 14.1 AND 14.2)

Anatomical classification is important for clinician, radiologist and pathologist, but it does not take into consideration to the evolutionary stages, which has influence on presentation of disease.

Seizure Genesis

The risk of seizures is greatest in disease associated with viable or degenerating cysts but continues to occur to a lesser extent in chronic calcific cysticercosis. Little is known about why and how seizures and epilepsy develops in this infection. *The probable mechanism to explain are:*
- The seizure activity is localized to inflamed and degenerating cysts. The disruption of blood brain barrier with leakage of serum component to the brain is sufficient to cause seizure.[16]
- Antihelmintic treatment initiates a host inflammatory response around cysts that mimics histological and radiological findings typical of naturally degenerating cysts and also associated along with an increased risk of seizures.
- In a small animal model, seizures were induced by the host response rather than the parasite itself.[17] The rational for using corticosteroids during treatment is an attempt to control the inflammation and accompanying seizures.

CLINICAL FEATURES

The clinical feature depends on number and the site of neurocysticercus cysts in the brain.

SOLITARY CEREBRAL CYSTIC GRANULOMA

Etiology

The etiology of solitary cerebral cystic gramuloma (SCCG) as neurocysticercosis was detected in biopsy taken from the excised lesion at vellore.[18]

Seizures

The presence of seizure is the most important presentation of NCC. This can be either acute symptomatic or they may be remote symptomatic. Partial seizures, with or without secondary generalization, or generalized seizures are more common than complex partial seizures. NCC is the cause of status epilepticus seen in less than 1% cases is single lesion cases.

The natural history of neurocysticercosis is either they resolve completely or it leaves a punctate calcification. The chances of seizure recurrence are there till the lesion is enhancing on CT. Majority of granuloma disappears by one year.

Meningeal Cysticercosis

The entrapment of granuloma between two convolutions of cerebral hemisphere is called "cysticercus cellulosae", and the cyst lying in the basal cistern is called as "cysticercus recemosus". There can be visual field defect, decreased visual activity and third nerve entrapment presenting as diplopia. These features explains the brain stem nerve entrapment due to arachnoiditis.

Table 14.3 Clinical and radiological features consisting with a diagnosis of solitary cystic granuloma (SCG)[19]

- *Clinical features that are supportive of a diagnosis of SCG*
  - Focal seizures with or without secondary generalization
    Note: Seizures may be new-onset or longer duration; may be generalized at onset; may occur in cluster (2 or more seizures over 2–3 days); may be followed by unilateral or diffuse headaches lasting for a few hours to days; or may be followed by transient and mild postictal neurologic deficits.
- *Clinical features that make a diagnosis of SCG unlikely*
  - Persistent and severe neurologic deficit
  - Clinical evidence of intracranial hypertension
  - Evidence of neurologic deficit, other systemic disease (e.g. systemic infection such as AIDS) that account for imaging finding
  - Age 2 years and 60 years
- *CT features compatible with a diagnosis of SCG*
  - Single, small (20 mm), well defined
  - Contrast-enhancing (closed ring, disc, nodular type)
  - With or without surrounding lesion
  - Associated with minimal mass effect and no midline shift
- *MRI features compatible with a diagnosis of SCG*
  - Single, small (20 mm) lesion with fluid contents
  - *T1 sequence:* Intensity slightly greater than or isointense to CSF
  - *T2 sequence:* Hyperintense or isohypointense with central hyperintensity
  - Ring or nodular type enhancement after contrast
  - Scolex may or may not be visible as an eccentric nodule within the fluid cyst contents
  - T1 isointense and T2 iso/hypointense
  - Mild-to-moderate surrounding edema bit no midline shift

Source: Singh GD. Neurocysticercosis Indian scenario. Medicine update. 2012;22

Disseminated Disease

The syndrome is characterized by pseudo muscular hypertrophy, palpable subcutaneous nodules, seizures and abnormal mentation. There is diffuse symmetrical painful or painless enlargement of all groups of muscles associated with weakness and easy fatigability.

Intraventricular Cyst

The sign and symptom of ventricular involvements are hydrocephalus and raise intracranial pressure and ventriculitis.

DIAGNOSIS

The diagnosis of cysticercosis is objective evaluation of clinical, radiological, immunological and epidemiological parameters. The revised criteria for Indian patient are as given in **Table 14.3**.

Serological Diagnosis

The complement fixation test, indirect hemagglutination tests and enzyme-linked immunosorbent assay (ELISA) are tried for the diagnosis of NCC. The gold standard in the diagnosis of NCC is EITB. This has specificity to 100% and sensitivity of 94–98% for patient with two or more cystic enhancing lesion.[20] Western blot positivity depends on number of cysticerci.

Neuroimaging Diagnosis

The stages and neuroimaging correlates are given in **Table 14.4**.
- MRI is considered the best neuroimaging tool for the diagnosis of degenerating cyst and viable cyst, CT is best for calcified lesion.
- MRI can detect the various stages of cyst whereas CT fails to do so.

Table 14.4 Stages and imaging correlates

Oncosphere		Parenchyma	Various stage
Vesicular phase Viable cysticerci NCCT	↑ Transitional phase ↓	Circumscribed, rounded hypodense are—10 mm (4–20 mm) No perifocal edema	
Colloidal phase Nonviable cysticerci (CECT)		Annular enhancement surrounded by irregular perilesional edema	
Nodular-granular phase Nonviable cysticerci		Hypodense area with (NCC) hyperdense rounded nodular image with edema (CECT)	
Calcification Dead (sequelae)		Rounded homogenous hyperdense area, no enhancement of contrast (NCCT)	

- Magnetic resonance spectroscopy can be performed in MRI to pick up various metabolite from the lesion and possible to differentiate tuberculoma with NCC.
- Repeat contrast CT or MRI after six month should be done all individuals with solitary cystic granuloma.
- Repeat CT at 3 month can be considered in situation where alternate etiologies are considered like neoplasm, tuberculoma, fungal granuloma, to see enlarging lesion or change in morphology of the lesion.

CONCEPTS OF TREATMENT

- Guidelines for treatment of neurocysticercosis must be individualized in terms of number and location of lesions, as well as based on the viability of the parasites within the nervous system
- Growth of a parenchymal cysticercus is not a common event and may be life-threatening. A growing parasite deserves active management, either with antiparasitic drugs or by surgical excision.
- In patients with intracranial hypertension secondary to neurocysticercosis, the priority is to manage the hypertension problem before considering any other form of therapy. Antiparasitic drug treatment is never the main priority in the setting of elevated intracranial pressure.
- Antiepileptic drugs are the principal therapy for seizures in neurocysticercosis. In general, seizures should be managed in a similar manner to other causes of secondary seizures (remote symptomatic seizures), since they are due to an organic focus that has been present for a long time. However, after resolution of the parasitic infection with normalization of imaging studies, most patients who are seizure-free can eventually discontinue antiepileptic drugs. Antiparasitic drugs should not be regarded as an alternative for antiepileptic drug therapy.

Treatment Guidelines

- Guidelines for treatment of neurocysticercosis must be individualized in terms of number and location of lesions, as well as based on the stage of the parasites within the brain.
- A growing parasite deserves active management, either with antiparasitic drugs or by surgical excision. Current consensus suggests that albendazole and praziquentel both are effective reducing the cyst load. The presence of type, location, number of cyst will decide the need for cysticidal drugs. Before starting these drugs ensure that intracranial hypertension and cerebral edema is not present.
    - Albendazole is better tolerated with fewer side effect, has increased bioavailability with concomitant steroid administration, the serum level is not affected with antiepileptic drugs along, as against use of praziquentel where the drug level is affected with steroid and antiepileptic drugs. Albendazole is used in the dose of 15 mg/kg divided in two doses for either 7 days or 28 days, both schedule appears equally effective for parenchymal NCC. Fundus examination is done to rule out choroidal cysticercus before starting the cysticidal drugs.
    - Steroids are used on short-term basis along with cysticidal drugs, two days before the cysticidal drugs, to reduce the host inflammatory response. Dexamethazone can be started in acute stage and can be shifted to prednosolone 1-2 mg/kg/day.
    - Hector Garcia and colleagues, in a double-blind, randomized, controlled trial, reported that combined treatment with albendazole and praziquantel resulted in an increased antiparasitic efficacy in patients with multiple brain cysticercosis cysts without increased side-effects.[21]
- In patients with intracranial hypertension secondary to neurocysticercosis, the priority is to manage the hypertension problem before considering any other form of therapy.
- Antiepileptic drugs are the principal therapy for seizures in neurocysticercosis, as they are due to an organic focus that has been present for a long time. As soon as lesion disappears on CT, the antiepileptic drugs can be tapered off. Antiparasitic drugs should not be regarded as an alternative for antiepileptic drug therapy.
- Surgery is indicated especially endoscopic removal of the cyst of ventricular cyst. Post obstructive hydrocephalus has to be dealt surgically.

REFERENCES

1. Garcia HH, Del Brutto OH. Neurocysticercosis: updated concepts about an old disease. Lancet Neurol. 2005;4(10):653-61.
2. Relationship between epilepsy and tropical diseases. Commission on Tropical Diseases of the International League Against Epilepsy. Epilepsia. 1994;35(1):89-93.
3. White AC, Jr. Neurocysticercosis: a major cause of neurological disease worldwide. Clin Infect Dis. 1997;24(2):101-13; quiz 114-105.
4. Nash TE. Human case management and treatment of cysticercosis. Acta Trop. 2003;87(1):61-9.
5. Prasad A, Gupta RK, Nath K, Pradhan S, Tripathi M, Pandey CM, et al. What triggers seizures in neurocysticercosis?—A MRI based study in pig farming community from a district of North India. Parasitol Int. 2008;55:166-71.
6. Tsang VCW, Garcia HH. Immunoblot diagnostic test (EITB) for *Taenia solium* cysticercosis and its contribution to the definition of this under-recognized but serious public health problem. In: Garcia HH, Martinez SMM (Eds), *Taenia solium* Taeniasis/Cysticercosis. Editorial Universo, Lima, Peru 1999;245_/254.35.
7. Prasad KN, Prasad A, Gupta RK, et al. Prevalence and associated risk factors of *T. solium* taeniasis in a rural pig farming community of north India. Trans R Soc Trop Med Hyg. 2007;101:1241-7.
8. Khurana S, Aggarwal A, Malla N. Prevalence of anticysticercus antibodies in slum, rural and urban populations in and around Union territory, Chandigarh. Indian J Pathol Microbiol. 2006;49:51-3.
9. Jayaraman T, Prabhakaran V, Babu P, Raghava MV, Rajshekhar V, Dorny P, et al. Relative seroprevalence of cysticercus antigens and antibodies to Taenia ova in a population sample in south India suggests immunity against neurocysticercosis. Trans R Soc Trop Med Hyg. 2011;105:153-9.

10. Parija SC, Balamurungan N, Sahu PS, et al. Cysticercus antibodies and antigens in serum from blood donors from Pondicherry, India. Rev Inst Med Trop Sao Paulo. 2005;47:227-30.
11. Wadia RS, Makhale CN, Kelkar AV, Grant KB. Focal epilepsy in India with special reference to lesions showing ring or disc-like enhancement on contrast computed tomography. J Neurol-Neurosurg Psychiatry. 1987;50:1298-301.
12. Mani A, Ramesh CK, Ahuja GK. Cysticercosis presenting as epilepsy. Neurol. 1974;22:30.
13. Wani MA, Banerjee AK, Tandon PN. Neurocysticercosis some uncommon presentations. Neurol. 1981;29:58-63.
14. Saigal RK, Sandhu SK, Sidhu PK, et al. Cysticercosis in Patiala (Punjab). J Postgrad Med. 1984;30:46-8.
15. Singh G. Association between Toxocara canis and epilepsy, collaborative, community prevalence and hospital-based incidence case - control study.
16. Seiffert E, Dreier JP, Ivens S, Bechmann I, Tomkins O, Heinemann U, et al. Lasting blood-brain barrier disruption induces epileptic focus in the rat somatosensory cortex. J Neurosci. 2004;24(36):7829-36.
17. Stringer JL, Marks LM, White AC Jr., et al. Epileptogenic activity of granulomas associated with murine cysticercosis. Exp Neurol. 2003;183(2):532-6.
18. Chandy MJ, Rajshekhar V, Prakash S, Ghosh S, Joseph T, Abraham J, et al. Cysticercosis causing single, small CT lesions in Indian patients with seizures. Lancet. 1989;1:390-1.
19. Singh GD. Neurocysticercosis Indian scenario. Medicine update. 2012;22.
20. Richards F Jr, Schantz PM. Review laboratory diagnosis of cysticercosis. Clin Lab Med. 1991;11(4):1011-28.
21. Garcia HH, Gonzales I, Lescano AG, et al. for the cysticercosis working group in Peru. Efficacy of combined antiparasitic therapy with praziquantel and albendazole for neurocysticercosis: a double-blind, randomized controlled trial. Lancet Infect Dis. 2014.

CHAPTER 15

Neurological Manifestations in Human Immunodeficiency Virus Infection

Latika Nayar

INTRODUCTION

Nervous system is a major target for human immunodeficiency virus (HIV) affecting both central nervous system and peripheral nervous system. Neurological disease is the first manifestation of HIV infection in as many as 10–20% and 60% have neurological dysfunction sometime in the course of illness. Autopsies done in HIV positive patients reveal pathological abnormalities in 75–90%. *HIV infection affects nervous system in the following ways*:[1]
- Direct effects of the virus often seen as HIV encephalopathy
- Opportunistic infections
- Adverse effects of antiretroviral (ARV) drugs.

PATHOGENESIS

The HIV virus crosses blood brain barrier and enters nervous system probably during the initial systemic infection itself. Three pathways have been described for viral entry into the brain.[2]
1. Virus may be carried by the infected macrophages and monocytes (Trojan Horse Effect)
2. Cell free virus may pass from the vascular compartment to brain tissue
3. Direct HIV infection of specialized endothelial cells of blood-brain barrier (BBB).

Once the virus enters the central nervous system (CNS) compartment, virus primarily infects perivascular macrophages and microglia, and activate several cell types like the macrophages, microglia oligodendroglia and astrocytes resulting in inflammatory response and release of TNFα, nitric oxide, etc. and several cytokines which impair the neuronal function. Neurons are not directly infected by the HIV virus at any stage of the infection. HIV can also cause increased permeability of BBB to other substances.[3]

Development of neuroAIDS depends on:
- Degree of immunosuppression
- Neurovirulence of the viral strain
- Genetic makeup of the host
- ARV drug intake.

Neurological disorders in HIV-infected persons include encephalopathy, seizures, vascular abnormalities, opportunistic infections of CNS, focal mass lesions, myelopathy, myopathy and peripheral neuropathy. Though children and adults have similar manifestations, because of the effect of infection on the growing brain, neurodevelopmental problems are more common in children who acquire infection in the perinatal period. As these children become more immunosuppressed later in life. They also develop opportunistic infections and CNS neoplasms. Early detection and initiation of treatment often lead to favorable outcomes.

HIV ENCEPHALOPATHY

The HIV encephalopathy is defined by CDC as characterized by the following features.[4,5]
- Microcephaly
- Failure to attain/loss of neurodevelopmental milestones or loss of intellectual abnormalities
- Acquired symmetrical motor deficits.

Prior to the introduction of highly active antiretroviral therapy (HAART), 30–50% of symptomatic children developed progressive encephalopathy and the incidence has decreased to 5–10% with early initiation of HAART.[4,6]

In children with perinatal infection, clinical features of neurological dysfunction is seen as early as 2 months or as late as 5 years. Manifestations may be quite apparent when they present with developmental delays or regression, spasticity, hyperreflexia, etc. or may be very subtle when they present with subtle cognitive problems like mild attention deficits, poor handwriting, difficulty in problem solving, mathematics, etc. Language delay (receptive and expressive) is found to be very frequently associated with early HIV infection **Table 15.1**.

Health care provider should be vigilant about the appearance of the following abnormalities:
- Microcephaly/deceleration in head growth
- Abnormal tone and reflexes
- Focal signs
- Speech and language delay.

Investigations

The CSF study may be done in the rapidly progressive type to rule out CNS infections. HIV infection itself causes lymphocytic pleocytosis and increase in protein up to 100 mg/dL. Changes in neuroimaging may precede or follow clinical manifestations. Diffuse cerebral atrophy, white matter hyperintensities in parietooccipital and frontal lobes, basal ganglia calcifications are the common findings **(Fig. 15.1)**.

Early initiation of HAART and other developmental interventions help to arrest the progress of HIV encephalopathy.[6]

OPPORTUNISTIC INFECTIONS OF NERVOUS SYSTEM

Frequency of opportunistic infections in children is significantly less when compared to adults.[7] These infections are seen in advanced HIV infection and may not be easily recognizable due to lack of inflammatory response in the severely immunosuppressed children. Hence, opportunistic infections should be ruled out when an HIV-infected persons develop any change in mental status or behavior or seizures or persistent headache or fever or malaise. Common opportunistic infections of CNS are given in **Table 15.2**.

Neurosyphilis is another CNS infection common in adults with early presentation as meningovascular syphilis or late presentation as Tabes Dorsalis or general paresis or optic atrophy.

Table 15.1 Three distinct courses are identified in human immunodeficiency virus encephalopathy

Type	Course
Static	Developmental arrest/delay (presents as cerebral palsy)
Progressive	Acute—Rapidly progressive course with loss of acquired milestones (resembles white matter degenerative disorder) **(Fig. 15.1)** Subacute—Slowly progressive (resembles neurodegenerative disorder)

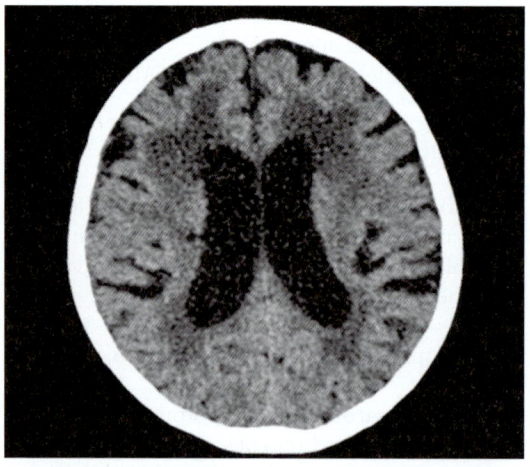

Figure 15.1 CT brain in HIV encephalopathy showing generalized brain atrophy
Courtesy: Dr Ajith MS

Table 15.2 Common opportunistic infections of central nervous system in human immunodeficiency virus infection[1]

Disorder	Common clinical findings	Diagnosis
Bacterial meningitis	• Fever • Nuchal rigidity • Nausea, vomiting • Irritability • Poor feeding • Headache/Bulging fontanelle • Confusion or change in behavior • Photophobia	*CSF:* Usually elevated opening pressure, leukocytosis with neutrophil predominance, elevated protein, low glucose, organisms on Gram stain and culture
Mycobacterium tuberculosis	Meningitis with subacute onset, not responding to standard antibiotics; Focal findings due to CNS tuberculoma Other signs suggestive of TB: • Persistent and unremitting cough • Failure to gain weight or weight loss • Fever	CSF usually elevated opening pressure with lymphocytosis, elevated protein, low glucose AFB/TB culture insensitive Evidence of TB elsewhere (by CXR, sputum/gastric aspirate, etc.) *CT:* Obstructive hydrocephalus, basilar meningeal enhancement **(Fig. 15.2)** TB skin test and history of TB contact can be helpful
Cryptococcal meningitis	• Subacute onset • Fever • *Headache:* Often intense and persistent May also have: • Nuchal rigidity and Kernig's sign often absent • Nausea and vomiting mass lesions • Altered level of consciousness • Impaired mental function • Cranial nerve lesions • Visual deficits • Extraneural lesions in skin (molluscum like lesions), lungs, etc. • Occurs in patients with CD4 <100 cells/mL	*CSF:* Elevated opening pressure, predominant mononuclear cell elevated protein, low glucose Positive India ink staining and CSF cryptococcal antigen for rapid diagnosis. Confirmed by CSF fungal culture CSF may appear normal in >50% of cases *CT:* Communicating hydrocephalus, pseudocysts
Toxoplasma encephalitis	Focal neurologic signs (hemiparesis, cranial nerve palsies, ataxia, sensory deficits) are the presenting symptoms accompanied by • Headache • Confusion • Fever • Lethargy May have seizures, associated hepatic involvement, pneumonitis, myocarditis Intracranial mass lesions Ocular: Marked loss of central vision Hazy vision "Floaters" CD4 <100 cells/mL or equivalent percentage for age	Diagnosis is by– • Positive IgG toxoplasma antibody • CT/MRI shows multiple ring enhancing lesions in the basal ganglia and hemispheric corticomedullary junction **(Fig. 15.3)** Differential diagnosis of ring enhancing lesions: • CNS lymphoma • Tuberculoma • Cryptococcoma, neurocysticercosis • Brain abscess In patients with HIV infection, TE is the most common cause for ring enhancing lesion • Response to treatment *Ophthalmologic exam:* White or yellowish foci with elevated, edematous margins, surrounded by a zone of hyperemia (active lesion)

Contd...

Contd...

HSV encephalitis	Acute or subacute encephalitis • Fever • Altered level of consciousness • Headache • Seizures • Behavior changes • Associated vesicles or ulcers • Keratitis, retinitis, conjunctivitis	*CSF:* Elevated WBC, RBC present, elevated protein, normal glucose, HSV DNA PCR *EEG:* PLED *CT/MRI:* Temporal lesions, mass effect, hemorrhage
CMV	Retinitis: • Changes in visual acuity areas • Sees "floaters" • Acquired inability to fix and follow (small infants) • Abnormal light reflexes (small infants) Subacute or chronic encephalitis/ventriculitis: • Weakness • Confusion • Loss of developmental milestones Axonal polyradiculopathy • Painful, ascending weakness • Loss of deep tendon reflexes • Loss of bladder/bowel control CD4 <50 cells/mL or equivalent percentage for age	*Ophthalmologic exam:* Yellowish–white granular with perivascular exudates and hemorrhage *Histology:* Coagulation necrosis, microvascular abnormalities Confirms infection but not disease: Anti-CMV antibodies if >12 months CSF pleocytosis in 50%, frequently PMN predominance, elevated protein, occasionally with low glucose, CMV DNA by PCR
Progressive multifocal leukoencephalopathy	Subacute onset leukoencephalopathy • Weakness, hemiparesis • Cognitive impairment enhancement • Speech impairment • Vision impairment • Ataxia • Sensory abnormalities	*CT:* Multiple radiolucent areas in white matter without edema **(Fig. 15.4)**, mass effect CSF PCR for JC virus

Treatment and prophylaxis of opportunistic infections should be based on standard guidelines.

CNS Neoplasms

Primary CNS lymphoma, though rare in children, is the most common CNS neoplasm associated with HIV infection. It is a high grade B cell lymphoma attributed to Ebstein Barr virus infection. Child presents with altered mental status, confusion, memory loss and seizures.[1,6] CT shows isodense or hypodense lesion with ill defined borders with contrast enhancement. HAART and antineoplastic chemotherapy are helpful.

Leiomyosarcoma is a rare CNS neoplasm associated with HIV infection, often seen along with lesions in other sites like lung, spleen, GIT, etc.

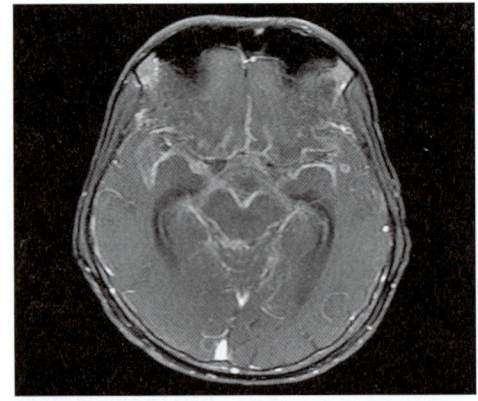

Figure 15.2 MRI showing basal exudates and ring-enhancing lesions in tuberculosis
Courtesy: Dr Ajith MS

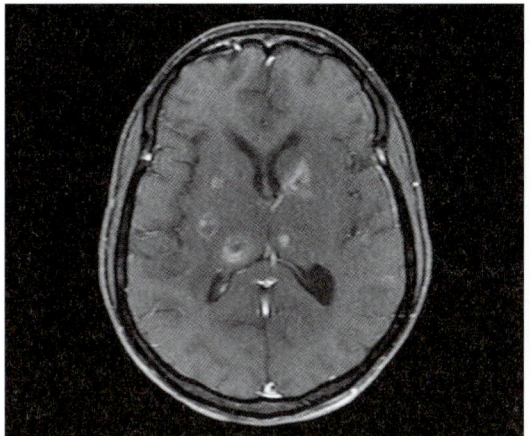

Figure 15.3 Ring enhancing lesions in gray–white junction and showing basal ganglia with eccentric nodules
Courtesy: Dr Ajith MS

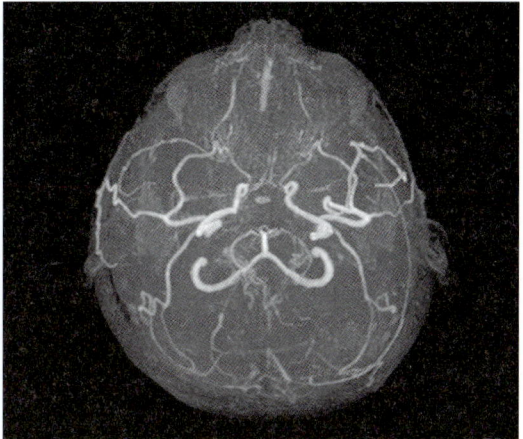

Figure 15.5 MR angiogram showing bilateral MCA and ACA narrowing with multiple collaterals in moyamoya disease in an HIV-infected child who presented with stroke
Courtesy: Dr Ajith MS

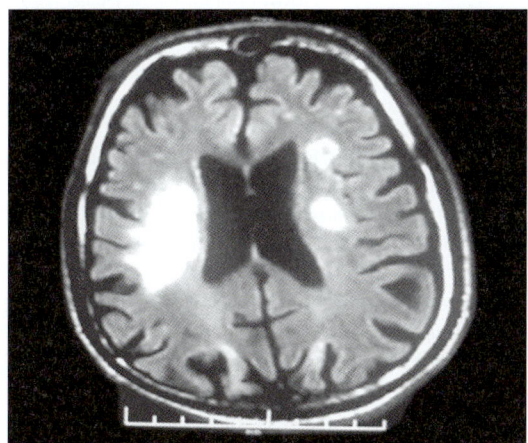

Figure 15.4 MRI of progressive multifocal leukoencephalopathy showing periventricular asymmetric hyperintensities in T2
Courtesy: Dr Rakesh TP

- Hypercoagulable state due to antiphospholipid antibody, decrease in protein S, dyslipidemia due to drugs (protease inhibitors, stavudine, etc.)
- Rarely moyamoya disease **(Fig. 15.5)**.

HIV Myelopathy

Rarely seen in children. HIV virus causes demyelination and vacuolar changes in the cord resulting in weakness without cognitive impairment or seizures.[1,6,7]

Peripheral Neuropathy

Peripheral neuropathy is very common in HIV-infected persons, most often due to the mitochondrial toxicity of NRTIs, presenting as polyneuropathy with burning sensation of soles, areflexia, etc. which responds to substitution of the offending drug. *HIV virus also can affect peripheral nerves presenting as either:*
- Distal sensory neuropathy which responds to HAART
- Acute inflammatory demyelinating polyneuropathy presenting as Guillain Barre syndrome for which IVIg or plasmapheresis are also needed.

Stroke

This is more often seen in advanced HIV infection. Different causes for stroke are the following:[1,4,6]
- HIV-associated vasculitis
- Thrombocytopenia

Table 15.3 Syndromic approach to neurological symptoms in human immunodeficiency virus infection

Syndrome	Clinical features	Etiology
Global cerebral syndrome (meningitis/meningoencephalitis)	• Headache • Fever • Nausea, vomiting • Cognitive impairment • Altered consciousness • Neck stiffness	• Cryptococcosis • Tuberculosis • CMV • Bacterial meningitis • HSV encephalitis • Neurosyphilis
Focal cerebral lesions	• Headache • Focal neurological deficits (hemiplegia, hemianopia, focal seizures)	• Toxoplasma encephalitis • Tuberculoma • Neurocysticercosis • PML • Primary CNS lymphoma
Dementia	• Cognitive impairment • Psychomotor slowing • Behavioral disturbances	HIV
Myelopathy	• Paraparesis • Sensory changes • Sphincter problems	• CMV • HIV
Peripheral neuropathy	• Burning pain • Tingling • Numbness • Hyporeflexia	• Drugs-NRTI • Nutritional deficiency-B12 • HIV • Alcohol in adolescents

Diagnosis is by nerve conduction studies, lumbar puncture, EMG, nerve biopsy, etc.

Myopathy

The HIV-associated myopathy is characterized by muscle pain and proximal weakness. It can be due to the direct effect of HIV virus or opportunistic infections (e.g. CMV), but more commonly due to ARV drugs like zidovudine.

A syndromic approach is very useful in the diagnosis of HIV-related CNS symptoms **(Table 15.3)**.

Psychiatric Manifestations of HIV Infection

Human immunodeficiency virus and psychiatric disorders have complex relation and recognition of psychiatric diseases in HIV positive persons is more difficult in the presence of neurological dysfunction. Psychiatric disorders can be due to the psychological consequence of the infection or due to the direct effect of HIV virus on the brain.[5,9]

Depression has been identified to be the most common psychiatric disorder associated with HIV infection in many studies. Attention deficit hyperactivity disorder, oppositional defiant disorder, conduct disorder, anxiety disorders, etc. are also more common in these children, the exact reason for which is not known. Opportunistic infections and CNS neoplasms also can have psychiatric symptoms.[10] Moreover, disclosure of the disease state, orphan status, and fear about stigma, future life options all negatively affect the psyche of the HIV-infected child. Drugs also can produce psychiatric manifestations especially efavirenz which can cause sleep disturbances, hallucinations, vivid dreams, etc.

SUMMARY

The HIV-related neurological abnormalities, though less in children, are varying and may be the initial presentation of HIV infection itself. HIV-affected children have significant developmental delays and hence healthcare workers should assess these children at frequent intervals for early recognition and intervention. Early initiation of HAART has gone a long way in reducing the frequency and severity of neurological problems.

REFERENCES

1. Elizabeth LD, Cruz N, Yin D. Neurological and Psychiatric Manifestations of Pediatric HIV infection. HIV curriculum for the health professional. *http://www. bipai. org/ curriculum/HIV curriculum.*
2. Resnick L, Berger JR, Shapshak P, et al. Early penetration of blood brain barrier in HIV. Neurology. 1988;38(1):9-14.
3. Neurological complications in HIV infected children and adolescents. HIV clinical resource. Office of the Medical Director, New York State, Department of Health AIDS Institute, 2003.
4. Tardieu M, Le Chenedac J, Persoz A, et al. HIV-1 related encephalopathy in infants compared with children and adults. French Pediatric HIV infection Study and the SEROCO group. Neurology. 2000;54:1089-95.
5. Nozyce M, Hittelman J, Muenz L, et al. Effect of perinatally acquired human immunodeficiency virus infection on neurodevelopment in children during the first two years of life. Pediatrics. 1994;94:883-91.
6. van Arnhem LA, Bunders MJ, Henriette JS, Charles BLM Majoie. Neurological abnormalities in HIV-1 infected children in the era of combination ARV therapy. Journal. 2010.
7. Bossi G, Maccabruni A, Caselli D, et al. Neurological manifestations in HIV-infected child. Minerva Pediatrics. 1995;47(7-8): 285-95.
8. Vardhman S, Udgirhar, Milind S, Tullu, Sandeep B, Bavdekar, Vijayaylaxmi B, Shahrao, Kamat JR, Priya R. Neurological manifestations in HIV infection. Indian Pediatrics. 2003;40:230-4.
9. Dube B, Benton T, Cruess DG, et al. Neuro-psychiatric manifestations of HIV Infection and AIDS. J Psych Neurosci. 2005; 30(4):237-46.
10. Chandra PS, Desai G, Ranjan S. HIV and psychiatric disorders. Indian J Med Res. 2005;121.p.445-67.

CHAPTER 16

Febrile Seizures

KP Sarabhai

Febrile convulsions have long been recognized, but only in recent years more fully understood. Hippocrates, writing in the 4th century BC, described such a convulsion, clearly differentiating it from rigors and breath holding attacks. Hippocrates noted that both generalized and partial seizures can occur, and realized that there was a strong association with age, high fever and a precipitating infection.

DEFINITION

"An event in infancy or childhood, usually occurring between 3 months and 5 years, associated with fever, but without evidence of intracranial infection or defined cause." This definition was given by National Institutes of Health (NIH) consensus conference 1980.

Definition by International League Against Epilepsy (ILAE): "A seizure occurring in child after 1 month of age, associated with febrile illness not caused by an infection of central nervous system (CNS) without previous neonatal seizures or a previous unprovoked seizures, and not meeting criteria for other acute symptomatic seizures".

Fallacies: Both definitions do not exclude children with prior neurological impairment. Do not provide specific temperature criteria. Do not define a "seizure" as well.

In both the definitions, three components—age, fever and seizure are critical elements.

Incidence:
- 2–5% in Western countries
- 7% in Japan
- 8–10% in our country.

Race: Febrile seizure (FS) occurs in all races with no discrimination.

Sex: Some studies demonstrate slight male predominance.

HOW COMMON ARE FEBRILE SEIZURES?

Approximately one in every 25 children will have at least one febrile seizure, and more than one-third of these children will have additional febrile seizures before they outgrow the tendency to have them.

PATHOPHYSIOLOGY

In young children, seizure threshold is low. Further infants and children are susceptible to frequent childhood infections like upper respiratory infection (URI), otitis media, viral syndromes, and they respond to these infections with higher body temperatures. This leads to precipitation of febrile seizures. It is possible that endogenous pyrogens such as interleukin 1 plays a role by increasing neuronal excitability. There is a hypothesis that activated cytokine network may have a role in the pathogenesis of febrile seizures.

In one study, average zinc level was found significantly lower in children with febrile seizures as compared to controls.[1] It helps in synthesis of gamma-amino butyric acid (GABA) which is an inhibitory neurotransmitter. It has inhibitory effect on excitatory N-methyl-D-aspartate receptors. When a patient develops low levels of zinc, N-methyl-D-aspartate receptors become activated and induce an epileptic discharge in children with high fever. Role of zinc in reducing the incidence and severity of febrile seizures needs further investigations.

Iron status is considered a possible risk factor for first febrile seizure (FFS). Children with FFS have a significantly low level of plasma ferritin. Exact explanation however remains speculative.[1]

A number of studies show that iron deficiency affects virtually every organ system including CNS. Iron deficiency leads to developmental abnormalities, ischemic strokes, venous thrombosis, breath holding spells and other neurologic problems including FFS.[2]

It is obvious now that deficiency of iron during gestation and lactation results in abnormality of brain development which is often irreversible. It is therefore imperative to prevent Fe deficiency in women of child bearing age, during gestation, throughout infancy and childhood. First febrile seizure and breath holding spells are important consequences of iron deficiency.

Human herpes simplex virus 6 and 7 have been found in 20% children presenting with their first febrile seizure. Shigella gastroenteritis also has been associated with febrile seizures.

A relationship between recurrent febrile seizure and influenza A and B has also been suggested in one study.

GENETICS

Febrile seizure is an extremely heterogenous condition with a complicated and as yet, unclear genetic basis. A positive family history is elicited in 25–40% of patients.

In a child with FS, risk is 10% for the other sibling and risk is almost 50% for the sibling if a parent had FS as well. Although clear evidence exists for a genetic basis of febrile seizures, the mode of inheritance is still not very clear.

Recently a locus has been linked to FS. Linkage studies have reported linkages on numerous chromosomes (2q,5q,8q,19p,and 19q). Strongest linkage being on 2q and specifically linkage to the gene responsible for Na channel receptors. A locus for simple pure febrile seizures maps to chromosome 6q22–q24.[3]

The linkage on chromosome 2q and 19q is associated with phenotype of FS, generalized epilepsy (tonic, clonic, absences, and myoclonus), and a continuation of FS beyond 5 years of age (GEFS+) shows evidence of Na channel involvement.

Data indicate an association with the 3/4 genotype of the apolipoprotein E gene with a milder phenotype. Apolipoprotein E is effective in regard to prognosis.

Recently, mutations in GABA receptor and sodium channel genes have been identified that are associated with febrile seizures and generalized seizures.

In GABA receptors, the 2 subunit is critical for receptor trafficking, clustering, and synaptic maintenance, and mutations in the 2 subunit have been monogenically associated with autosomal dominant transmission of febrile seizures. Autosomal dominant pattern of inheritance has been demonstrated in quite a few families.[3]

TYPES OF FEBRILE SEIZURES

- Simple febrile seizures (typical)
- Complex febrile seizures (atypical).

Simple Febrile Seizures

- Seizures are generalized.
- Duration of seizure is <15 minutes.
- Do not recur within 24 hours.

Complex Febrile Seizures

- Seizures are usually focal.
- Duration of seizure is prolonged beyond 15 minutes.
- Recur more than once within 24 hours.

Symptomatic Febrile Seizure

When the child has a preexisting neurological abnormality or acute illness and suffers febrile seizure, it is labeled as symptomatic febrile seizure. Age and fever are the same as for simple febrile seizure.

Clinical Evaluation

- Look for the type of seizures whether generalized/focal.
- Duration of seizure.
- History of fever, duration of fever, potential exposure to illness.
- History of the cause of fever (e.g. viral illnesses, gastroenteritis, etc.).
- Recent use of antibiotic.
- Past history of seizures.
- Any neurological problems.
- Developmental delay.
- History of trauma.
- History of toxic ingestion.
- Fits occurring more than 12 hours after the onset of an illness are almost certainly not febrile convulsions, unless there is a complication such as otitis media developing after a sore throat, and causing a new rise in temperature. FS only occur with a rapid rise of temperature, and there must be a history of the child having been off color and probably off his food for a few hours before the fit occurred.
- Underlying cause for fever should be sought.
- Physical examination often reveals otitis media, pharyngitis, or a viral exanthem.
- Serial evaluation of neurological status of patient is essential.
- Check for meningeal signs/signs of trauma/or toxic ingestion.
- Take a history of vaccination. One in a thousand children may suffer a FS after receiving the measles, mumps, and rubella (MMR) vaccine. It occurs 8-10 days after the vaccination and is caused by the measles component of the vaccine. Fever following diptheria, tetanus toxoids and pertussis (DPT) vaccination may also lead to FS.
- Children who are prone to FS should follow the same program of vaccination as implied for all other children.

RISK FACTORS

The children who have following risk factors have a greater possibility of getting FS:
- Family history of febrile seizures.
- High temperature.
- Parental report of developmental delay.
- Rapid rise in temperature is a cause of febrile seizure.

Some studies suggest that women who smoke or drink alcohol during their pregnancies are more likely to have children with febrile seizures, but more research needs to be done before this link can be clearly established.

Iron status is considered a possible risk factor for FFS.

Zinc deficiency is also a risk factor for FS.

LAB STUDIES

Not recommended unless they are performed as a part of the search for the cause of the fever. Electrolyte assessment are rarely helpful in evaluation of febrile seizure. Patients who have fever alone or fever with seizure have similar incidence of bacteremia. During evaluation the most important responsibility of physician is to rule out possibility of meningitis or encephalitis.

IMAGING STUDIES

Computed tomography (CT) scan is not necessary in evaluation of a child with simple febrile seizure but may be considered for children with atypical features including focal neurologic signs or preexisting neurologic deficits.[4]

ELECTROENCEPHALOGRAM

Not necessary in routine evaluation of a child with a first simple febrile seizure.

The electroencephalogram (EEG) between fits is normal. It may however be useful in evaluation of patient with complex FS, febrile seizure with atypical features or febrile seizure with other risk factors for later epilepsy.

LUMBAR PUNCTURE

Controversy exists regarding need for lumbar puncture (LP) in child with a simple FS.

Patients who have a first time febrile seizure and do not show a rapidly improving mental status (short postictal period) should be evaluated for meningitis and LP is done. American Academy of Pediatrics (AAP) strongly recommends (1996) LP in patients younger than 12 months presenting with FS because signs and symptoms of meningitis may be minimal or absent in this group. LP is considered in patients aged 12–18 months because signs and symptoms of meningitis may be subtle in this group. The LP is not routinely necessary in patients >18 months. Decision rests on clinical suspicion of meningitis.

TREATMENT

Febrile status epilepticus should be treated with airway management, anticonvulsants and supportive care. In postictal period appropriate antipyretic and supportive care should be given.[4]

Simple febrile seizure should have frequent neurologic examination to monitor mental status.

Other causes of seizure should be ruled out. Cause of febrile illness to be treated. Antipyretics to be considered.

Parental anxiety needs to be addressed.

PROPHYLAXIS

Prophylaxis to avoid recurrent FS is controversial.

Opinion against pharmacological prophylaxis has become stronger in last few years.

Indications for prophylaxis are to prevent FS and to allay family anxiety.

We have two options for FS prophylaxis:
1. Intermittent prophylaxis
2. Continuous prophylaxis

Intermittent Prophylaxis

Rectal or oral diazepam 0.3–0.5 mg/kg (max. 10 mg) 8 hourly for the duration of febrile illness, usually 2–3 days. Side effects are minimal except lethargy, ataxia, and irritability. These can be reduced by adjusting the doses. In patients with recurrent complex febrile seizure diazepam gel can be given rectally at the time of seizure approximately 0.5 mg/kg for children aged 2–5 years. This will usually terminate the seizure and prevent recurrence over 12 hours. This, however, does not reduce the risk of later epilepsy in high-risk patients.[5]

Intermittent clobazam 1 mg/kg/day is an effective alternative with minimal side effects which is in the form of ataxia seen in little over 8% cases.

Lorazepam and clonazepam may also be used.

Duration—to be continued till 5 years of age whenever child gets febrile illness.

Continuous Prophylaxis

To be avoided as far as possible but can be instituted if child has recurrent complex FS, has symptomatic FS, or status.

Sodium valproate 20–30 mg/kg/day is preferred choice. Hepatotoxicity may be seen.

Phenobarbitone: Age 2–24 months—5–8 mg/kg/day; Age >2 years—3–5 mg/kg/day. Behavior disorders and cognitive dysfunction may develop.

Hepatotoxicity of sodium valproate is more common in infants so phenobarbitone is the preferred choice.

Carbamazepine and phenytoin are not effective in preventing FS.

Duration of continuous prophylaxis:

If employed it should be used for the shortest period. It is 2 years time without convulsion.

Drug should be withdrawn gradually.

No evidence indicates that antipyretics prevent recurrence of FS.

Indications for Continuous Prophylaxis

Current consensus proposes that patients who have one or more risk factors be considered for continuous prophylaxis.[6]

Risk factors indicating continuous prophylaxis:
- Neurodevelopmental abnormality.
- Complex and atypical seizures.
- Positive family history of epilepsy.
- Multiple febrile seizures.
- Age of onset below 1 year.
- Not responding to intermittent prophylaxis.

RISK FACTORS FOR RECURRENT FEBRILE SEIZURE

- Young age at the time of onset of FFS.
- Relatively low fever at the time of FFS.
- Family history (F/H) of FS in a first degree relative.
- Brief duration between fever onset and FFS.

Patients with all four risk factors have >70% chance of recurrence. With no risk factor chance of recurrence is <20%.

The chance of having another febrile, convulsion in the following year is 30%.

The risk of a second fit reduces every year and it becomes extremely rare after the child turns 6 years old.

It is rare for any child to suffer recurrent febrile convulsions after the age of 4 years.

PROGNOSIS

Febrile seizures are benign events although it is frightening to the parents. Recurrent febrile seizures occur in about 1/3 of children having a first febrile seizure.

Despite the general acceptance that children with febrile seizures have a good prognosis, "the hypothesis persists that febrile seizures are linked etiologically to sudden death in infants and children through a common infectious or environmental agent, anatomical abnormality or genetic susceptibility to fever".

Febrile seizures occurring at temperatures of less than 39°C, or at younger than 1 year of age are particularly associated with mortality.

Mortality rates are similar in children of the febrile seizure group and children in the control group beyond 2 years of age.

In the current study by Vestergaard and colleagues, complex febrile seizures in children were associated with a higher risk for mortality for 2 years but not in the long-term. Simple febrile seizures did not increase the risk for death.

RISK FACTORS FOR EPILEPSY

- Complex febrile seizure.
- Family history of epilepsy.
- Family history of neurologic abnormality.
- Family history of developmental delay.

Patient with two risk factors have up to 10% chance of developing afebrile seizure.[7]

Parent Education

Parents should be taught what to do if their child has another seizure.

Parents are taught to call for assistance if seizure lasts for >10 minutes or if the postictal period lasts >30 minutes.

Parents are counseled for the benign nature of illness.

Simple FS do not lead to neurologic problems.

PARENTAL ANXIETY

If there is a family history of FS and parents are familiar with this history, they tend to be more comfortable with the occurrence of the problem in their own child and there is less over utilization of medical services.

If there is a family history of febrile seizures and a child has FS, parents have a far greater concern about their child medication wise.

One of the key aspects of managing FS is dealing with the anxiety of the family. Parents should be educated and reassured because children with FS do not differ from other children in their intellectual and behavioral outcome even if they have recurrent episodes.

ANALYSIS OF INTELLECTUAL ABILITY OF CHILDREN WITH FEBRILE SEIZURE

It remains same irrespective of age of FFS.

It remains same in children who had one FS as compared to those who had multiple FS.

Proportion of children who need special education remains same in FS group as compared to control group.

Children with simple FS and complex FS do not differ from control group in terms of their academic progress of intellectual abilities.

Antisocial behavior, hyperactivity, in attentiveness and attention deficit have shown same prevalence as in control group.

WHAT RESEARCH IS BEING DONE ON FEBRILE SEIZURES?

The National Institute of Neurological Disorders and Stroke (NINDS), a part of the National Institutes of Health (NIH), sponsors research on all forms of febrile seizures in medical centers throughout the country.

The NINDS-supported scientists are exploring what environmental and genetic risk factors make children susceptible to febrile seizures.

Retrospective studies of patients undergoing surgical evaluation for medically refractory epilepsy have consistently found that approximately 30–40% report prior febrile seizures in childhood. Herpesvirus 6B—has been reported as present in temporal lobe tissue but not in extratemporal tissue from patients undergoing resections for intractable partial epilepsy.

Are these children who have FS precipitated by herpes simplex virus (HSV) infection at higher risk for subsequent mesial temporal sclerosis (MTS) and temporal lobe epilepsy (TLE)?

REFERENCES

1. Rabbani MW, Ali I Hafiz, Latif HZ, Basit A. Serum zinc level in children presenting with febrile seizures. Pak J Med Sci. 2013;29(4).
2. Daoud A, Batieha A, Ekteish FA, Hijazi A. Iron status: a possible risk factor for the first febrile seizure. Epilepsia. 2002;43(7).740-3.
3. Winawer M, Hesdorffer D. Turning on the heat: The search for febrile seizure genes. Neurology. 2004;63(10):1770-1.
4. Riemenschneider TA, Baumann RJ, Duffner PK, et al. Practice parameter: the neurodiagnostic evaluation of the child with a first simple febrile seizure. American Academy of Pediatrics. Provisional Committee on Quality Improvement, Subcommittee on Febrile Seizures. Pediatrics. 1996;97(5):769-72.
5. Rosman NP, Colton T, Labazzo J, et al. A controlled trial of diazepam administered during febrile illnesses to prevent recurrence of febrile seizures. N Engl J Med. 1993;329(2): 79-84.
6. Baumann RJ, Duffner PK, Schneider S. Practice parameter: long-term treatment of the child with simple febrile seizures. American Academy of Pediatrics. Committee on Quality Improvement, Subcommittee on Febrile Seizures. Pediatrics. Jun 1999;103(6 Pt 1):1307-9.
7. Verity CM, Golding J. Risk of epilepsy after febrile convulsions: a national cohort study. BMJ. 1991;303(6814):1373-6.

CHAPTER **17**

Epileptic Syndromes

Mary Iype

INTRODUCTION

It is long recognized that the approach to epilepsy as focal versus generalized is insufficient for better treatment and prognostication. The epileptic syndrome concept is based on the age at onset, the semiology of the seizures, the electroencephalogram (EEG) pattern, mode of inheritance, chronology of the events, factors activating the seizures, the relation of the seizures to the sleep-wake state, pharmacoresistance, the neurological deficits and co-morbidities, the developmental trajectory of the child and the evolution of the seizures in that child.[1-3] The diagnosis of an epileptic syndrome dictates the management and prognosis. Electroclinical syndromes may be associated with varying etiologies. West syndrome for instance may occur in children with hypoxic-ischemic encephalopathy, intrauterine infection, cortical maldevelopment, tuberous sclerosis complex or a genetic mutation in genes like *ARX* or *STXBP1*.[4] In some cases the etiology may be unknown. Many of these recognized syndromes are self-limiting like the benign familial neonatal convulsions, the benign neonatal convulsions and the benign rolandic epilepsy of childhood; some are pharmaco responsive like childhood absence epilepsy; some are pharmaco resistant like Lennox-Gastaut syndrome and some of these pharmaco resistant syndromes are epileptic encephalopathies where the seizures result in cognitive decline in the patient.[5]

The most salient feature of these syndromes is the age of onset. **Table 17.1** lists the electroclinical syndromes by the age of onset. **Table 17.2** shows the signatory EEG changes in some of these syndromes. **Table 17.3** shows the treatment options available for the epileptic syndromes. Among these epileptic syndromes, the recognized epileptic encephalopathies include Ohtahara syndrome (Early infantile epileptic encephalopathy), Early myoclonic encephalopathy, West syndrome, Dravet syndrome, Lennox-Gastaut syndrome, Epileptic encephalopathy with continuous spike and wave during slow wave sleep (CSWS), Landau-Kleffner syndrome (LKS) and Epileptic encephalopathy (not otherwise specified).

NEONATAL EPILEPTIC SYNDROMES

Benign familial neonatal convulsions (BFNC) typically presents during the first few weeks of life and are characterized by focal, multifocal, or generalized seizures that are brief and occur 20–30 times per day. The seizures may be difficult to control, the EEG may be normal or show the characteristic "theta pointu alternant" pattern (in 50%). A theta pointu alternant pattern consists of runs of theta activity intermixed with sharp waves, seen in awake and asleep states, that often alternates sides and does not change in response to

Epileptic Syndromes

Table 17.1 Types of epileptic syndromes

Idiopathic	Symptomatic
• Generalized	*Infancy* • Early myoclonic encephalopathy (EME) • Early infantile epileptic encephalopathy (EIEE) • Infantile spasms • Dravet syndrome • Malignant migratory partial epilepsy
Infancy • Benign neonatal convulsions (BNC) • Benign neonatal familial convulsions (BNFC)	
Childhood • Childhood absence epilepsy (CAE) • Myoclonic astatic epilepsy (MAE) • Epilepsy with myoclonic absences • Generalized epilepsy with febrile seizure plus (GEFS)	*Childhood onset** Lennox-Gastaut syndrome (LGS) Landau-Kleffner syndrome (LKS) Epileptic encephalopathy with continuous spike and wave in slow wave sleep (CSWS) Devastating encephalopathy in school age children Rasmussen encephalitis Autosomal dominant epilepsy with auditory features (ADEAF)
Adolescent onset • Juvenile absence epilepsy (JAE) • Juvenile myoclonic epilepsy (JME) • GTCS on awakening	
Focal • Benign partial epilepsy of infancy • Benign infantile familial convulsions	*Varying ages* Progressive myoclonic epilepsy (PME)
Childhood onset* • Benign epilepsy with centro temporal spikes (BECTS) • Benign occipital epilepsy (BOE)—early onset • Benign occipital epilepsy (BOE)—late onset • Autosomal dominant frontal lobe epilepsy (ADFLE) • Familial temporal lobe epilepsy	

*Here childhood onset includes adolescent onset also.

various stimuli. The neonate will be neurologically normal. Family history of similar neonatal seizures is important for diagnosis (Autosomal dominant with 85% penetrance). BFNC is linked to voltage gated potassium channels KCNQ2 and KCNQ3 on chromosomes 20q and 8q. The outcome is generally favorable. Resolution of seizures occurs typically in early to mid infancy. Eight to sixteen percent of patients will later develop epilepsy as adults.

Benign idiopathic neonatal convulsions (BINC) is seen in healthy, neurologically normal term neonates. Seizures typically begin on the fifth day of life (fifth day fits). Partial clonic seizures that migrate, increase in frequency and culminate in status epilepticus are common. There is no specific EEG feature. There will be no family history of seizures and seizures typically resolve after 24 hours.

Early infantile epileptic encephalopathy with burst-suppression (EIEE), is a neonatal progressive epileptic encephalopathy. These children have tonic spasms and partial seizures. The seizures are intractable and these children often have an associated cerebral malformation and severe mental retardation. No single cause has been however identified.

Early myoclonic encephalopathy almost always starts in the newborn period. Usually there is an underlying metabolic cause and the major seizure type is the myoclonus which may be multifocal or massive. The seizures are pharmacoresistant and prognosis for survival and psychomotor outcome is bleak.

EPILEPTIC SYNDROMES SEEN AFTER THE NEONATAL PERIOD

Infantile spasms was first described by WJ West in 1841 and is characterized by epileptic spasms or salaam attacks, hypsarrhythmia/variants on EEG and developmental arrest or regression.

Table 17.2 EEG in the different epileptic syndromes

Benign neonatal familial convulsions (BNFC)	Theta pointu alternant
Early myoclonic encephalopathy	Burst suppression pattern
Myoclonic epilepsy in infancy	Nonspecific
Infantile spasms	Hypsarrhythmia
Epilepsy with myoclonic atonic seizures	>3 Hz spikes
CAE	3 Hz spikes
Dravet	4–5 Hz rhythmic theta activity can be noticed over the rolandic areas and the vertex, diffuse spike-waves, generalized spike-waves elicited by intermittent photic stimulation
Epilepsy with myoclonic absence	3 Hz spikes
JAE	>3 Hz spikes
Progressive myoclonus epilepsies	Irregular spikes
Epilepsy with GTC only	>3 Hz spikes
Lennox-Gastaut	<2.5 Hz spikes
JME	>3 Hz spikes
Benign epilepsy with centro temporal spikes (BECTS)	Centrotemporal spikes
Benign occipital epilepsy	Occipital spikes
Epileptic encephalopathy with continuous spike and wave in slow wave sleep (CSWS)	Continuous spike and wave in slow wave sleep

Abbreviations: CAE, childhood absence epilepsy; JAE, Juvenile absence epilepsy; JME, Juvenile myoclonic epilepsy

West syndrome is one of the age-related epileptic encephalopathies with a typical onset is between 3 months and 12 months of age. The epileptic spasms are clusters of sudden, brief, diffuse or fragmented, tonic contractions of axial and limb muscles. Spasms are longer than myoclonic jerks and shorter then tonic seizures in duration. Spasms are usually seen in clusters and may be accompanied by a cry, laughter or autonomic changes. It may be flexor (most common), extensor, mixed or subtle. They usually occur on arousal and in alert states. The etiology is diverse. Hormonal therapy, adrenocorticotrophic hormone (ACTH) or oral prednisolone is the treatment of choice for short-term treatment of epileptic spasms. Vigabatrin an alternative drug preferred in infantile spasms, is the drug of choice when the child has tuberous sclerosis. The ketogenic diet has also been shown to be beneficial. The prognosis is guarded and is governed by the underlying etiology and the treatment. A common mistake that delays initiation of specific therapy is to treat epileptic spasms with phenobarbitone, sodium valproate and other anti-epileptic drugs (AEDs) that are not effective in this context.

Lennox-Gastaut syndrome is characterized by a triad of tonic, atonic, and atypical absence seizures. The EEG pattern of slow spike and wave discharges (1.5–2.5 Hz) on a slow background is classically seen; with paroxysmal fast activity and multifocal spikes in some cases. Cognitive impairment is the rule. The onset is usually between 1 year and 8 years; most cases between 2 years and 5 years. Onset after 10 years is rare. There is a male preponderance.

The tonic seizure is the most characteristic prerequisite, and could be of three types including flexor movement of the head and trunk with apnea preceded by a brief cry (axial), abduction, elevation of limbs, usually arms with clenching of

Table 17.3 Treatment of the recognized epileptic syndromes

Epileptic syndrome	Drugs
Benign neonatal seizures	Not always necessary Phenobarbitone for acute control—self-limiting
Benign neonatal familial seizures	Recurs after neonatal period in less than 15% Taper anticonvulsants after 2 weeks—Retigabine promising
Early myoclonic encephalopathy	There is no effective treatment Identify and treat underlying metabolic problem
Early infantile epileptic encephalopathy	There is no effective treatment surgery for cortical dysplasia
Febrile seizures	AAP- No treatment—reassurance Intermittent oral diazepam if parents are anxious
Migrating partial seizures of infancy	Resistant to treatment Isolated reports—rufinamide, quinidine, potassium bromide
Infantile spasms	FDA recommendation for vigabatrin and ACTH Efforts on to recommend oral steroids
Benign familial infantile seizures	Treatment is not necessary
Benign myoclonic epilepsy in infancy	Excellent response to valproate, which should be withdrawn 3–5 years from onset of treatment
Benign infantile seizures (nonfamilial)	No treatment needed
Benign infantile seizures with mild gastroenteritis	No treatment needed
Dravet's syndrome [severe myoclonic epilepsy of infancy (SMEI)]	It is currently recommended to start Stiripentol as soon as the diagnosis of Dravet syndrome is secure. Topiramate, levetiracetam may be efficient as adjunctive therapies Avoid sodium channel blockers
Benign childhood epilepsy with centrotemporal spikes	Carbamazepine or sodium valproate
Lennox-Gastaut syndrome (LGS)	Pharmacoresistant seizures
Generalized epilepsy with febrile seizure plus (GEFS +)	Usually self-limiting no recommendation
Myoclonic astatic epilepsy of Doose	Only partial response to drugs
Childhood absence epilepsy	Ethosuximide/valproate
Juvenile absence epilepsy	Valproate/lamotrigine
Juvenile myoclonic epilepsy	Levetiracetam/low dose valproate
Early onset benign occipital seizures	Many a time treatment not needed Valproate/carbamazepine
Late onset benign occipital seizures	They usually respond well to carbamazepine which may be needed for two to four years

Abbreviations: AAP, American Academy of Pediatrics; FDA, Food and Drug Administration; ACTH, adrenocorticotropic hormone

the fists (axorhizomelic) and sustained contraction involving most muscles, including distal (global). Atypical absences are the second type of seizure seen as a brief lapse of consciousness. Atonic seizures ("Drop attacks") are particularly hazardous and seen in 56% of patients. Other seizure types that may be seen are generalized, focal and multifocal clonic.

Seizures are resistant to therapy. Drugs are used in combination, mostly guided by anecdotal evidence or personal experience. AEDs may help control one seizure type while worsening another. First line AEDs includes valproic acid and benzodiazepines. The prognosis is unfavorable.

Myoclonic astatic epilepsy of doose is rare and affects 1:10,000. It presents in previously neurologically healthy preschool-aged children. Multiple seizure types are seen including generalized tonic clonic, myoclonic, absence, atonic and myoclonic atonic seizures. Myoclonic atonic seizures are more prominent. The outcome and course are variable with complete remission to intractable epilepsy with poor cognitive outcome. EEG demonstrates 2-3 Hz spike and wave discharges. Up to 32% of children have a family history of epilepsy. The inheritance pattern is unknown.

Dravet syndrome is seen in 1 in 20,000 to 40,000. Approximately 80% of cases have mutation in *SCN1A* (sodium channel) which is usually sporadic. There is often a strong family history of epilepsy. The onset is in the first year of life in a previously well infant. Often prolonged generalized or focal clonic seizures are seen. The seizure is frequently triggered by fever, infection, vaccination or a warm bath. Atypical absence and complex partial seizures with autonomic symptoms occur in 50% in the preschool years. The initial EEG is typically normal. Later there will be slowing that gives way to multifocal and generalized polyspike and wave discharges activated by drowsiness and photic stimulation. Most show photosensitivity with or without associated clinical events (eyelid myoclonia, generalized myoclonic jerks).[6] The MRI may show brain atrophy later in the course of the disease. These children tend to do poorly in visuomotor skill assessment than in tests of language skills. Seizures tend to be pharmacoresistant. The drugs of choice are valproic acid and clobazam. Second line AEDs include Topiramate, Levetiracetam and Zonisamide. Lamotrigine and carbamazepine should be avoided as they can aggravate seizures. Mortality rate is 16-18% (status, sudden unexpected death in epilepsy (SUDEP), drowning).

Generalized (Genetic) epilepsy with febrile seizures plus is characterized by febrile and afebrile seizures. Febrile seizures continue beyond the typical age of remittance (6 years). Afebrile seizures are infrequent, brief, and include generalized tonic-clonic, myoclonic, complex partial and atonic seizures. Seizures start between 4 months and 10 years, with mean onset of 2 years. Prior to the onset of afebrile seizures, GEFS+ can be difficult to distinguish from febrile seizures. Interictal EEG may be normal or may show generalized epileptiform discharges. The inheritance is autosomal dominant. Multiple gene mutations are linked to GEFS+ including 19q13.1 (SCN1B gene), 2q23-24.2 (SCN1A gene) and 5q31.1-33.1. There is excellent prognosis in the majority. Seizures spontaneously remit by age 11 years. Thirty percent continue to have epilepsy.

Childhood absence epilepsy (CAE) comprises 2-15% of childhood epilepsy. Onset is usually between 4 years and 10 years of age as episodic blank stares occurring hundreds of times a day. Girls are 2-5 times more likely to have absences. Most patients with childhood absence have normal neurological examinations and normal intelligence scores. Abnormalities in the T-type calcium channels responsible for rhythmic depolarizing activity in the thalamic neurons is the underlying cause. The seizure usually lasts 5 to 10 seconds. Seizures can be provoked by hyperventilation in approximately 90% of children. The classic EEG finding in typical absence seizures is the sudden onset of 3-Hz generalized symmetrical spike and wave complexes with an abrupt offset. Ethosuximide is the drug of choice. However, sodium valproate should be added in children with associated generalized tonic clonic seizures. Duration of therapy is variable, although the general rule is to taper off therapy after 2 seizure free years.

Juvenile absence epilepsy has an onset typically between ages 9 and 12. The clinical seizures are similar to CAE. Seizures occur less frequently and may be of longer duration. The child is more likely to experience generalized tonic clonic seizures. The interictal EEG shows 3.5-4 Hz spike and polyspike and wave. Response to treatment is good, but may be lifelong.

Juvenile myoclonic epilepsy affects 4 to 10% of all patients with epilepsy. Seizures typically present between 12 years and 18 years. The inheritance is complex. The classic form is likely autosomal dominant and inherited and linked to 6p12-11. Usually the first seizure noted is generalized in the setting of sleep deprivation. A history of myoclonic seizures and possible absence seizures in the preceding months is the usual rule. Seizure types include generalized tonic-clonic, myoclonic, and absence seizures. All have myoclonic seizures, 96% have generalized seizures, and only 20% have absences. Generalized tonic-clonic and myoclonic seizures tend to occur in the morning upon awakening. Seizures are precipitated by sleep deprivation, alcohol ingestion and in women, menstruation.

The interictal EEG in JME consists of generalized spike and polyspike-and-wave discharges of 4 to 6 Hz, usually maximal in the frontocentral regions. Photic stimulation often provokes a discharge (30 to 90%) Traditional treatment was valproic acid with 85-90% response. Newer effective drugs include levetiracetam, lamotrigine, topiramate and zonisamide. Carbamazepine, phenytoin and gabapentin may exacerbate seizures. Response to treatment is excellent but treatment is lifelong.

Benign childhood epilepsy with centrotemporal spikes (BCECTS) is the most common form of idiopathic partial epilepsy and accounts for 13-23% of all childhood epilepsies. Although it is clearly familial, its mode of inheritance is unclear. Onset is between 4 years and 10 years. The peak age of onset is 7-8 years. Children are neurologically and cognitively normal. Nocturnal seizure, usually occurring after falling asleep or before awakening is typical. Seizures are described as unilateral paresthesias of the face, unilateral clonic or tonic activity involving the face, speech arrest and drooling with preserved consciousness. They can have secondarily generalized tonic-clonic seizures. The EEG shows spikes in the midtemporal and central (centrotemporal) head region. Marked activation of spikes in drowsiness and sleep is characteristic, and 30% of cases show spikes only during sleep. If typical history can be elicited, the neurological examination is normal and the EEG findings characteristic, an MRI is not necessary. No treatment is necessary in patients with infrequent, nocturnal, partial seizures. If seizures are frequent (20%) and disturbing to the patient and family, treatment with Sodium valproate or oxcarbazepine is recommended. The prognosis is excellent. Spontaneous remission occurs by age 15 to 17, often much earlier. Some children may develop language, cognitive or behavioral deficits which improve after remission.

Early-onset Benign Childhood Epilepsy with Occipital Paroxysms-Panayiotopoulos Syndrome

The average age of onset is 3-6 years. The child has a normal development. Nocturnal seizures occur in two-thirds, with tonic eye deviation, vomiting (autonomic) and impaired consciousness. Hemiconvulsions are common. Interictal EEG shows normal background with high-amplitude stereotypic occipital spike-wave complexes on eye closure. Seizures are infrequent and one third of patients will only have a single seizure. Paradoxically, seizures are frequently prolonged. The prognosis is excellent. Treatment is not necessary. Rarely, aggravation is known to occur with carbamazepine.

Late-onset Childhood Epilepsy with Occipital Paroxysms-Gastaut Syndrome

This is a rare condition with onset between 6 and 12 years. Family history of epilepsy is seen in 21-37% of cases. Seizures are characterized by visual hallucinations or ictal blindness often with gaze deviation or eyelid fluttering often followed by postictal headache. Focal seizures often evolve into hemiconvulsions or generalized seizures. The EEG shows a normal background, with interictal occipital high amplitude spikes with attenuation on eye opening. Ictal recordings show fast occipital spikes. Seizures respond well to carbamazepine. 50-60% have seizure remission within 2-4 years.

SUMMARY AND CONCLUSION

Knowing a given patient's syndromic diagnosis, helps us to know more about his epilepsy, for example, likely age at onset, EEG patterns, likely responses to medications, and cognitive and developmental status. This information can then be used as the basis to identify potential new "syndromes". We should strive to recognize many more factors to help classify epilepsies into syndromes that better guide treatment.

The concept of epileptic encephalopathy leads to the idea that suppression of epileptic activity may improve cognition and behavior. Early effective intervention may in fact improve seizure control and developmental outcome in some cases.[7,8]

REFERENCES

1. Commission on Classification and Terminology of the International League against Epilepsy. Proposal for classification of epilepsies and epileptic syndromes. Epilepsia. 1985;26:268-78.
2. Commission on Classification and Terminology of the International League against Epilepsy. Proposal for revised classification of epilepsies and epileptic syndromes. Epilepsia. 1989;30:389-99.
3. Berg AT, Berkovic SF, Brodie MJ, Buchhalter J, Cross JH, van Emde Boas W, Engel J, et al. Revised terminology and concepts for organization of seizures and epilepsies: report of the ILAE Commission on Classification and Terminology, 2005-2009. Epilepsia. 2010;51(4): 676-85.
4. Mastrangelo M, Leuzzi V. Genes of early-onset epileptic encephalopathies: From genotype to phenotype. Pediatric Neurology. 2012;46:24-31.
5. Blume WT. Lennox-Gastaut syndrome: potential mechanisms of cognitive regression. Ment Retard Dev Disabil Res Rev. 2004;10:150-3.
6. Bureau M, Bernardina BD. Electroencephalographic characteristics of Dravet syndrome. Epilepsia. 2011;52:13-23.
7. Jonas R, Nguyen S, Hu B, Asarnow RF, LoPresti C, Curtiss S, et al. Cerebral hemispherectomy: hospital course, seizure, developmental, language, and motor outcomes. Neurology. 2004;62:1712-21.
8. Jonas R, Asarnow RF, LoPresti C, Yudovin S, Koh S, Wu JY, et al. Surgery for symptomatic infant-onset epileptic encephalopathy with and without infantile spasms. Neurology. 2005;64: 746-50.

CHAPTER 18

Treatment of Childhood Epilepsy

M Madhusudanan

INTRODUCTION

Epilepsy is a relatively common neurologic disorder in children that has important implications for development, parents, and society. This chapter deals with common dilemmas in the management of epilepsy, i.e. when to start the treatment, which drug to use, and when to stop the medications?

WHEN TO START TREATMENT?

Once the diagnosis of epilepsy has been established clinically, it is important to classify the epilepsy into either a specific syndrome or, when this is not possible, into the type of epilepsy, i.e. partial or generalized and, the latter in to tonic-clonic, absence, myoclonic, atonic, tonic, or clonic. Most epilepsy syndromes are age-related and occur in childhood. In practice, only 45–50% of children will be found to have an identified syndrome.

When a child first presents with a seizure disorder, we have to take into consideration many factors which influence the outcome and thereby decide on starting the anticonvulsant, since antiepileptic drug (AED) once started, should be continued for a prolonged period of time.

The first factor to be decided is whether seizure in question is provoked or not, i.e. induced by an acute insult to the brain (acute symptomatic seizure).

Treatment of Provoked Seizure (Acute Symptomatic Seizures)

It is obvious that one should treat the seizure in the acute phase of the illness. Whether such a patient will require long-term treatment or not is dependent upon the likelihood of recurrence of inducing factors. If the provoking factor or inducing factor does not recur, the risk of subsequent seizures is very low and long-term therapy with AED is unwarranted.

In the majority of patients with first acute symptomatic seizure, the associated illness responsible for the seizure is usually apparent. Thus, patients with hypoglycemia, head injury, encephalitis, cerebrovascular disease, etc. can all present with seizure. Such patient with provoked seizures needs treatment with anticonvulsant only for the duration of illness.

Management of First Unprovoked Seizure

If the child presents with first unprovoked seizure and the clinical finding and if necessary, investigations do not suggest any underlying structural lesion, what is his chance of having another seizure? Finding the chance of recurrence is important since once AEDs are instituted, they have to be continued for a prolonged period of time and they are all potentially toxic drugs. The decision to treat epilepsy is dependent on the evidence of effect of AEDS on the risk of recurrence and prognosis of the disease.

The results of recent studies and clinical trials suggest that in most cases treatment should probably start after the first recurrence of seizures. The overall risk of recurrent seizure at 2 years following initial seizure was 42% across all the first seizure studies.[1]

After a second unprovoked seizure, the chances of a third unprovoked seizure are 80–90% within 2 years, if not treated. Therefore, treatment after the second (rather than the first) unprovoked seizure is recommended.[2] Moreover, delaying treatment until a second seizure can increase diagnostic certainty and prevent unnecessary treatment of nonepileptic events.

The risk of seizure relapse varies among patients depending on the presence or absence of specific prognostic factors. The major medical factors that influence the risk of recurrence after the first seizure include children with pre-existing neurologic deficits, partial seizures, definite epileptiform activity on electroencephalogram (EEG), and siblings with seizures.[3,4]

Presently the available data do not suggest that prior neonatal or febrile seizures are associated with increased risk of recurrence after a first attack.[5,6] Similarly family history of seizures and age and sex of the patients do not affect the recurrence rate after the first episode.[5,7,8]

Antiepileptic drugs in patients presenting with a first tonic-clonic seizure reduce the risk of relapse. However, 50% of patients who are not treated will never experience a second seizure. Moreover the probability of long-term remission is not influenced by treatment of the first seizure.[2,9]

The above findings are of considerable practical interest because it has been estimated that up to 30% of patients treated with AEDs experience moderate to severe adverse effects, which may cause drug withdrawal in up to 20% of patients.[10] The actual decision whether or not to treat patients who present with an initial seizure must be individualized. It depends on both the probability of having a recurrence and on the perceived risk/benefit ratio of treatment.

WHICH DRUG TO CHOOSE?

The selection of the antiepileptic drug is decided by various factors, which may be patient-specific and/or AED specific factors. Patient-specific factors include the child's nature of epilepsy (seizure type or the epilepsy syndrome), age, gender along with their comorbidities and comedications.[11] Affordability is also an important patient specific factor deciding the choice of AED. AED specific factors include efficacy and tolerability of the drug.

Principles of Starting Antiepileptic Drug

Patients should be started on small dose of one of the first line AEDs recommended for their type of seizure. It is usually the least toxic drug available. In children under the age of 10 or 12 years, dosages are usually based on mg/kg/body; this is important in view of the marked age range and different metabolic rates of children. Neonates, infants, and children under the age of 2 years frequently require relatively higher doses than older children because of a higher rate of drug metabolism. If the seizures are controlled with this small dose and there are no serious side effects, no further changes are necessary. If the seizures are not controlled with this dosage, and there is no serious toxicity the dosage should be systematically increased until the seizures are controlled or side effects preclude further dosage increase. If unacceptable side effects occur before control is reached, or where control is suboptimal, the patient will require either a different AED (substitute drug) or an additional AED (polytherapy). If there has been some initial control with the first drug, it would be reasonable to add the next most appropriate AED, without withdrawing the first drug. If complete seizure control is then achieved, consideration could be given for withdrawing the first drug after a seizure-free period of between 2 months and 3 months. If the initial AED has been wholly ineffective, it would seem logical to simultaneously replace the first drug with the second, to maintain mono therapy.

Here one should be aware of certain pharmacokinetic principles. One should not judge the efficacy of a drug and increase or decrease the dose of a drug until steady state of the drug is reached. Steady state refers to the time taken for a stable drug level to reach after each dose administration.

In order to achieve a new steady state serum concentration, five half-lives must elapse after the initiation of drug therapy. Therapeutic efficacy of a drug can be assessed only after this state has been reached. Too often, an AED is discarded as ineffective because inadequate time has been allowed to build up a steady state concentration. Similarly the dosage of a drug is sometimes increased too rapidly seeing no response. This may result in the accumulation of toxic concentration of the drug.

The half-life and the time taken for the steady state to reach are given in the following (**Table 18.1**).[12]

WHICH DRUG FOR INITIAL TREATMENT?

Clinicians may decide not to treat a patient who has a single, unprovoked, afebrile seizure because the chance of not having another seizure may be as high as 70%. For patients who have recurrent seizures, the accurate classifications of seizure type(s) and epilepsy syndrome are probably the most important determinants of the likelihood of seizure recurrence and of AED selection. Thus, certain benign epilepsies like benign rolandic epilepsy may not require any treatment or mono therapy with a low-toxicity-profile AED be started. In contrast, a diagnosis of infantile spasms, symptomatic, or localization-related epilepsy calls for aggressive use of potentially effective drugs.

As already told, the choice of the drug is mainly based on the efficacy of the drug for that particular type of epilepsy/epileptic syndrome. It is clear that choice of the best first AED is not a 'one size fits all' scenario.

The first step is to diagnose the epilepsy syndrome. If this is difficult, then at least try to ensure that the patient does not have juvenile myoclonic epilepsy, which can be exacerbated by carbamazepine and phenytoin, or absence seizures, which are likely to be worsened by carbamazepine, tiagabine, vigabatrin or phenytoin. **Table 18.2** provides a general recommendation for the choice of drugs for specific epileptic syndromes.[13]

If one cannot diagnose an epileptic syndrome, try to find out whether it is a partial or generalized seizure from the history (obtained from the patient and the eye witness) and EEG (if necessary video EEG). There is no hard and fast rules as to which drug should be used first. **Table 18.3** provides a general recommendation for the choice of drugs for specific seizure types.[13]

It is generally accepted that monotherapy is the best therapeutic option when a diagnosis of epilepsy has been made. Carbamazepine, phenytoin, valproic acid (sodium valproate), phenobarbital (phenobarbitone) and primidone are all effective for the treatment of partial and/or generalized tonic-clonic seizures. Within these seizure types, however, there are no hard and fast rules about the choice of the first-line drug.

Carbamazepine is generally regarded as the drug of choice for patients with partial seizures (with or without secondary generalization),

Table 18.1 Half–lives and time to achieve steady state for various AEDs

Drug	Half-life	Time to reach steady state
Phenytoin	15–30 hours	5–15 days
Phenobarbitone	46–136 hours	14–21 days
Carbamazepine	11–17 hours	3–10 days
Valproate	6–15 hours	1–2 days
Primidone	6–18 hours	4–7 days
Lamotrigine	10–15 hours	5–15 days
Oxcarbazepine	8–10 hours	3–4 days
Levetiracetam	7–8 hours	2–3 days
Topiramate	20–24 hours	5 days

Table 18.2 Antiepileptic drug choice based on epileptic syndrome

Epileptic syndrome	First choice drug	Other options
Neonatal seizures	Phenobarbitone	Phenytoin, topiramate, lamotrigine
Infantile spasms	Corticotropin	Topiramate, lamotrigine, valproic acid, zonisamide, felbamate
Lennox-Gastaut syndrome	Valproate	Topiramate, lamotrigine, zonisamide, felbamate
Childhood absence epilepsy	Valproate, ethosuximide	Lamotrigine
Juvenile absence epilepsy	Valproate	Lamotrigine, topiramate, zonisamide
Juvenile myoclonic epilepsy	Valproate	Lamotrigine, topirimate, zonisamide
Benign rolandic epilepsy	Carbamazepine	Gabapentin, topiramate, lamotrigine

Table 18.3 Antiepileptic drug choice based on seizure type

Epilepsy type	Most appropriate	Second preference
Idiopathic GTCs	Valproate	Lamotrigine, topiramate, phenytoin, zonisamide phenobarbitone
Absences	Valproate/ethosuximide	Lamotrigine, zonisamide
Tonic/atonic/myoclonic	Valproate	Topiramate, lamotrigine, phenytoin, phenobarbital, zonisamide, felbamate
Partial seizures (with/without generalization)	Carbamazepine	Oxcarbazepine, lamotrigine, topiramate, phenytoin, levetiracetam, zonisamide, gabapentin, valproic acid, phenobarbital

whereas valproic acid is usually recommended for initial treatment of most forms of generalized epilepsies. For partial seizures and secondarily generalized tonic-clonic seizures, the drugs effective are carbamazepine (CBZ), diphenyl hydantoin (DPH), phenobarbitone and primidone. The treatment success was highest with CBZ and DPH: CBZ is thought to be more advantageous considering dysmorphic and cognitive side effects of DPH. But DPH offers the advantage of the availability of an I/V preparation. If it is desirable to rapidly achieve therapeutic levels in a patient, DPH would seem to be the drug of choice.

As far as newer AEDs are concerned, the efficacy of lamotrigine, oxcarbazepine, gabapentin and TPM (topiramate) is same as that of carbamazepine or phenytoin. Carbamazepine, phenytoin, valproic acid, phenobarbital, lamotrigine, gabapentin, oxcarbazepine and topiramate can be used as first line treatment of new onset partial seizure. There is no clear superiority of one over other. Oxcarbazepine (OXC) is as effective as CBZ, LTG (lamotrigine), DPH or VPA (valproic acid): however, tolerability is better with OXC. Similarly LTG is as effective as PHT or gabapentin. But vigabatrin, tiagabine and gabapentin are less effective than CBZ in monotherapy studies.

Valproate is the first choice for the treatment of primary generalized epilepsies with onset in adolescence. Other classic antiepileptic drugs such as phenytoin, phenobarbital, or carbamazepine generally do poorly in terms of controlling these epileptic syndromes. Absence and myoclonic seizures not only fail to respond to these classic drugs but also may even be exacerbated.

For the treatment of absence seizures, both valproate and ethosuximide can be tried and there are of equal efficacy. However, if any one of the two is ineffective, then the combination of the two can be tried. If the combination also fails, the next drug to be tried is clonazepam. Lamotrigine is a newer AED found to be effective for this type of seizure.

Of the newer drugs lamotrigine, topiramate, zonisamide, and levetiracetam have shown promise in terms of being effective alternatives in the treatment of the idiopathic generalized epilepsies. Lamotrigine and topiramate are now licensed for this indication.

Lamotrigine is very effective in controlling generalized tonic-clonic and absence seizures. It is an ideal agent for patients with juvenile absence epilepsy or grand mal seizures on awakening. Topiramate has also shown excellent efficacy in idiopathic generalized epilepsies. It is particularly effective in generalized tonic-clonic and myoclonic seizures but shows limited efficacy in absence seizures. The rather high incidence of cognitive dysfunction limits the use of topiramate as a first-choice agent. In children topiramate can be effective in various generalized epilepsy syndromes when other anticonvulsants have failed. Levetiracetam (LEV) is another new AED with a wide spectrum of action that includes generalized tonic-clonic, absence, and myoclonic seizures. Behavioral changes, mostly irritability and mood swings, appear to be the main limitation with the use of levetiracetam.

Drugs effective for both generalized and partial include valproate, LTG, topiramate, and Zonisamide.

Usually the first choice is a standard AED because head-to-head trials have not shown superior efficacy for any of the new AEDs compared to the older drugs. An important factor in AED selection is the toxicity profile of each medication. What one patient tolerates may be unacceptable to another. The other deciding factor in choosing the AED is the presence of a comorbid medical condition. For example, choice in child with hepatic dysfunction may be gabapentin, topiramate or levetiracetam, which are cleared primarily by the kidney.[13] However, these AEDs should be used carefully in children with renal failure.

If it is not possible to classify the epilepsy, one may have to choose a broad spectrum AED like valproate, lamotrigine, topiramate or levetiracetum. All of these are effective across a wide range of seizures.

Studies[14] have shown that seizure freedom can be obtained in 46% of patients with the first AED: with second AED, it is 10%, and with the third AED, it is only 2.3%. Generally, about 60% of patients can be controlled with monotherapy.[14]

In the drug selection, it is very important to remember that wrong selection of AEDs can worsen seizure.

- CBZ may increase atypical absence, absence or even sometimes convulsive seizure especially among patients who have the Lennox-Gastaut syndrome.
- If ethosuximide is inappropriately prescribed to a patient with complex partial seizure, patient may remain vulnerable to continuing seizure activity.
- Phenobarbitone may increase absence, atonic and myoclonic seizures.
- CBZ may exacerbate myoclonic, atonic and absence seizures.
- Concurrent use of clonazepam with valproate may exacerbate absence status epilepticus.

One may also note that sudden withdrawal of phenobarbitone from epileptic patient may lead to exacerbation of seizures and sometimes develop into status epilepticus.

Polytherapy

In some children, polytherapy with two AEDs is justified; However, this may result in a significant control only in an additional 5–10% of children. The problems of using multiple AEDs ('polytherapy') include pharmacokinetic interactions (thereby potentially reducing the effectiveness of each of the drugs), difficulties in interpreting the effect of each drug, cumulative toxicity, and increasing the risk of idiosyncratic drug interactions. Choice of the second drug is dependent upon the seizure type/epilepsy syndrome and safety profile. Consideration must also be given to whether the two AEDs act synergistically or antagonistically, in terms of both effectiveness and safety.

Other Drug Treatments

Numerous other drugs have been used in pediatric epilepsy, usually in a desperate attempt to control multiple and refractory seizure types. Acetazolamide is a useful add-on drug (usually in combination with CBZ) in treating simple, and complex, partial seizures. Pyridoxine (vitamin B_6) is clearly the treatment of choice in the rare inherited disorder of pyridoxine-dependent seizures, but it also has been used in West syndrome (infantile spasms). Intravenous immune globulins have been used with varying success in intractable epilepsies, including children with both the West and Lennox-Gastaut syndromes.

DRUG INTERACTIONS

Older AEDs are the primary source of pharmacokinetic interactions with each other and with other drugs. Carbamazepine, phenytoin and phenobarbital reduce the levels of many AEDs and other drugs such as antiretroviral drugs, major immune suppressants, antineoplastic agents and oral anticoagulants.[15] Valproic acid is a broad spectrum enzyme inhibitor and will have the opposite effect. If administered without adjusting the dose of other drugs, it can lead to overdose and toxicity (particularly important when combined with lamotrigine, some antineoplastics and anticoagulants).

The interaction profile is generally much more favorable for most newer AEDs. Drugs such as gabapentin, levetiracetam, will not cause important interactions and therefore they are recommended for polytherapy in epileptic patients and in particular groups such as patients with cancer, transplants, anticoagulant treatments or HIV infection.[15] Lamotrigine has little potential for interactions except when combined with valproate.

Oxcarbazepine and topiramate are AEDs with an average potential for interactions with other AEDs according to the dose. **Table 18.4** gives the interaction potential of various commonly used AEDs.[15] **Table 18.5** gives the effect of older AEDs on the new AEDs.

There are certain important pharmacokinetic interactions by other commonly used drugs with AEDs. Drugs like certain macrolides, ritonavir, antifungals and verapamil grossly increase the blood level of carbamazepine leading to toxicity.[15] Antifungals also elevate the level of phenytoin. Similarly, carbapenem antibiotics block the intestinal absorption of valproic acid.

Newer AEDs (GBP, TGB (tiagabine), ZON (Zonisamide), LEV, LTG, TPM, OXC) have no significant effect on the blood level of phenytoin, carbamazepine, phenobarbitone or primidone. However, valproate level is decreased by 25%.

Pharmacokinetics in Children

Valproate and phenobarbitone have favorable kinetics, whereas carbamazepine and phenytoin have unfavorable kinetics. Carbamazepine daily dosages in infants need to be increased up to 30–50 mg/kg compared with 15–25 mg/kg for older children, and is to be given in tid dosage. The adequate dose of phenytoin is difficult to determine in infants in view of nonlinear pharmacokinetics. Infants and young children show increased clearance of lamotrigine and topiramate.

Tolerability of AEDs in children is different from adults. Valproate hepatotoxicity is increased below the age of 2 years, with polytherapy and with the presence of associated psychomotor delay. One-third of the children will demonstrate phenobarbitone induced behavioral side effects in the form of hyperexcitability/insomnia. Benzodiazepines can induce paradoxical hyperexcitation in children. Bronchorrhea and dysphagia can be seen with clonazepam and topiramate induced metabolic acidosis is more common in children.

WHEN TO STOP THE TREATMENT?

The primary risk of stopping AED treatment is the risk of seizure recurrence. Generally, the likelihood of seizure recurrence is about 30% for patients who have been seizure-free for at least 2 years.[16] Longer periods of seizure freedom before the tapering of AED treatment is associated with a lower risk of relapse. The factors predicting higher relapse after stopping AEDs include presence of cognitive or motor handicap, an abnormal EEG at the time of discontinuation and partial seizures. However, even for children with cerebral palsy, AED therapy withdrawal may not always be associated with a greatly increased risk of seizure relapse. In a recent study, the overall seizure relapse risk in children with cerebral palsy and seizures was only 40% after AED therapy withdrawal following a 2-year period without seizures.[17] Children with spastic diplegia had only a 14.3% relapse rate after AED therapy withdrawal.[17] Children with the onset of seizures before age 2 years or in adolescence also

Table 18.4 Antiepileptic drugs that do and do not induce hepatic enzyme

Enzyme inducing AEDs	Nonenzyme inducing AEDs
Carbamazepine	Lamotrigine
Oxcarbazepine	Levetiracetam
Phenobarbital	Benzodiazepines
Phenytoin	Valproate
Primidone	Gabapentin
Topiramate	Vigabatrin

Table 18.5 Effect of older AEDs on new AEDs

	Drug interaction						
	Gabapentin	Lamotrigine	Topiramate	Tiagabine	Levetiracetam	Zonisamide	Oxcarbazepine
DPH CBZ Pheno PRM	None	↓	↓	↓	None	↓	↓
VPA	None	↑	None	None	None	None	Slight ↓

have a higher likelihood of relapse. This is probably due to the fact that the onset of epilepsy before age 2 years may be associated with structural or metabolic disorders that have strong epileptogenic effects. Probably, the best predictor of relapse is the type of the epileptic syndrome. Eventually, all patients with benign rolandic epilepsy will have seizure remission. Conversely, nearly all patients with juvenile myoclonic epilepsy will have seizure recurrence if AED therapy is discontinued. Patients with the greatest number of risk factors have the highest rate of relapse.[18,19]

When a decision is made to discontinue AED treatment, medications are slowly tapered. Barbiturates and benzodiazepines may provoke seizures when abruptly withdrawn, and hence these drugs are be tapered more slowly. However, some of the studies have shown that the probability of seizure recurrence after a relatively short, 6-week tapering of medication is equivalent to the risk after a longer, 9-month-period of medication tapering.[20]

REFERENCES

1. Hauser WA, Rich SS, Jacobs MP, Anderson VE. Patterns of seizure occurrence and recurrence risks in patients with newly diagnosed epilepsy. Epilepsia. 1983;24:516-7.
2. Musicco M, Beghi E, Solari A, Viani F. Treatment of first tonic clonic seizure does not improve the prognosis of epilepsy. First Seizure Trial Group (FIRST Group). Neurology. 1997;49(4):991-8.
3. Hauser WA, Rich SS, Annegers JF, Anderson VE. Seizure recurrence after a 1st unprovoked seizure: an extended follow-up. Neurology. 1990;40:1163-70.
4. Berg AT, Shinnar S. Relapse following discontinuation of antiepileptic drugs: a meta-analysis. Neurology. 1994;44:601-8.
5. Shinnar S, Berg AT, Moshe SL, et al. The risk of recurrence following a first unprovoked seizure in childhood: a prospective study. Pediatrics. 1990;85:1076-85.
6. Camfield PR, Camfield CS, Dooley JM, Tibbles JAR, Fung T, Garner B. Epilepsy after a first unprovoked seizure in childhood. Neurology. 1985;35:1657-60.
7. Boulloche I, Leloup P, Mallet E, Parain D, Tron P. Risk of recurrence after a single unprovoked generalized tonic-clonic seizure. Dev Med Child Neurol. 1989;31:626-32.
8. Saunders M, Marshal C. Isolated seizures: an EEG and clinical assessment: Epilepsia. 1975; 16:731-3.
9. Stroink H, Brouwer OF, Arts WF, Geerts AT, Peters AC, van Donselaar CA. The first unprovoked, untreated seizure in childhood: a hospital based study of the accuracy of the diagnosis, rate of recurrence, and long term follow out come after recurrence. Dutch study of epilepsy in childhood. J Neurol Neurosurg Psychiatry. 1998;64(5):595-600.
10. Collaborative group for epidemiolgy of epilepsy. Adverse reactions to antiepileptic drugs: a multicenter survey of clinical practice. Epilepsia. 1986;27:323-30.
11. Glauser TA, Loddenkemper T. Management of childhood epilepsy. Continuum (Minneap Minn). 2013;19(3):656-81.
12. Schachter SC, Seizure disorders. Med Clin N Am. 2009;93:343-51.
13. Jarrar RG, Buchhalter JR. Therapeutics in pediatric epilepsy, Part 1: The new antiepileptic drugs and the ketogenic diet. Mayo Clin Proc. 2003;78:359-70.
14. Kwan P, Brodie MJ. Early identification of refractory epilepsy. NEJM. 2000;342:314-9.
15. Diaz RAS, Sancho J, Serratosa J. Antiepileptic drug interactions. The Neurologist. 2008;14: S55–65.
16. Berg AT, Shinnar S. Relapse following discontinuation of antiepileptic drugs: a meta-analysis. Neurology. 1994;44:601-8.
17. Delgado MR, Riela AR, Mills J, Pitt A, Browne R. Discontinuation of antiepileptic drug treatment after two seizure-free years in children with cerebral palsy. Pediatrics. 1996;97:192-7.
18. Medial Research Council antiepileptic drug withdrawal study group. Prognostic index for recurrence of seizures after remission of epilepsy. BMJ. 1993;306:1374-8.
19. Camfield C, Camfield P, Gordon K, Smith B, Dooley J. Outcome of childhood epilepsy: a population-based study with a simple predictive scoring system for those treated with medication. J Pediatr. 1993;122:861-8.
20. Tennison M, Greenwood R, Lewis D, Thorn M. Discontinuing antiepileptic drugs in children with epilepsy: a comparison of a 6-week and a 9-month taper period. N Engl J Med. 1994;330:1407-10.

CHAPTER **19**

Newer Antiepileptic Drugs in Treatment of Childhood Epilepsy

Kavita Srivastava

OBJECTIVES

- Introduction and overview of newer anti-epileptic drugs (AEDs)
- *Pharmacology of individual drugs*: Indications, efficacy and tolerability
- Practical considerations in use of newer AEDs
- Summary of formulations available, doses and adverse effects.

INTRODUCTION

Antiepileptic drugs form the most important part of the treatment of a child with epilepsy, even though other therapies like special diets, surgery, vagal nerve stimulation (VNS), etc. may be required in a proportion of cases. The clinician has to choose the first and if required, subsequent add-on or substitute drugs from the AED arsenal available.

Classically, the *older generation* AEDs include those marketed before 1980—phenobarbitone (1912), phenytoin (1938), carbamazepine (1974), primidone, clonazepam and valproate (1967). Most of these 'traditional' drugs were not intended to be used primarily as antiepileptics (e.g. phenobarbitone as hypnotic and carbamazepine as antidepressant) and hence, with the exception of valproate, these drugs shared the common problems of sedation and cognitive side effects. They also exhibit a high degree of plasma protein binding and significant drug interactions via hepatic metabolism.[1,2]

In last 25 years, about 17 new AEDs have been marketed, which are classified as *Newer generation AEDs*. These drugs offer the advantage of fewer drug interactions, unique mechanisms of action and a broader spectrum of activity. This has expanded the choices but has also become challenging for the clinicians to choose the drugs wisely for a given patient.[3]

These drugs include (in order of USFDA approval)—felbamate (1993), gabapentin (1993), lamotrigine (1994), topiramate (1996), tiagabine (1997), levetiracetam (1999), oxcarbazepine (2000), zonisamide (2000). Some authors classify the drugs marketed after 2010 as 3rd generation AEDs lacosamide (2007), retigabine (2010), perampanel (2012), stiripentol, rufinamide (2008), clobazam (2013) and eslicarbazepine (2013). Brivaracetam is in the pipeline for approval.[4]

INDIVIDUAL DRUGS: PHARMACOLOGY, INDICATIONS, EFFICACY AND TOLERABILITY

Oxcarbazepine

Pharmacology

Carbamazepine used to be the first line drug for children with partial epilepsy, but had problems of autoinduction (causing decrease in serum levels over a period of time) and drug interactions as it was oxidized by the CYP enzymes in liver to an active epoxide derivative, which are susceptible to stimulation or inhibition by many other drugs. The epoxide derivative was also responsible for many of the side effects like drowsiness, ataxia and rash.

Oxcarbazepine (OXC) is a keto-derivative of carbamazepine, it is completely absorbed after oral administration, with no effect of food. It does not have autoinduction or clinically significant drug interactions as it is not metabolized by CYP enzymes as well has only 38% binding to plasma proteins. It undergoes reduction in liver to 10 monohydroxy metabolite (MHD) which also has anticonvulsant activity and has a half-life of 8-9 hours, while the parent drug has half-life of 2 hours. There is no need for monitoring of drug levels, MHD is further conjugated and then excreted in urine as glucuronide. Dose adjustments are indicated in renal impairment.

It produces blockade of voltage sensitive sodium channels, increased potassium conductance and modulates high voltage activated calcium channels hence should not be combined with drugs acting similarly, e.g. carbamazepine, phenytoin and lamotrigine.

Adverse Effects

Common side effects include nausea, vomiting, dizziness, sleepiness, ataxia and cognitive slowing. Clinically significant hyponatremia (serum sodium less than 125 mmol/L) is seen in 2.5%, it is rare below the age of 17 years. Hyponatremia is mild and can be corrected with fluid restriction. Usually seen in first 3 months of treatment, sodium monitoring is needed only if additional risk factors of hyponatremia are present, e.g. SIADH, polytherapy, diuretics, elderly etc. or patient is symptomatic with headache, lethargy, increased seizure frequency, etc.[5]

Rash is seen in 4-7%, including serious reactions like Steven Johnson syndrome (SJS) and toxic epidermal necrolysis (TEN), with 3-10 fold higher risk as compared to general population. The median time of onset for reported cases was 19 days. The patient should be counseled to discontinue the drug immediately if a rash is seen.

Another serious hypersensitivity (median time to onset 13 days) reaction called DRESS (**D**rug induced **R**ash, **E**osinophilia with **S**ystemic **S**ymptoms) with multiorgan dysfunction in the form of hepatitis, lymphadenopathy, neutropenia and thrombocytopenia warrants immediate discontinuation of the drug, as these may be life-threatening. 30% of patients with hypersensitivity to carbamazepine may develop hypersensitivity on OXC and hence, it should not be substituted if possible.

Steven Johnson syndrome (SJS) and TEN are reported to be 2-3 times more common in Hans Chinese with underlying HLA B *1502 mutation. It has been proposed that this allele codes for a molecule that is displayed on the surface of antigen presenting cells. Oxcarbazepine and carbamazepine, or their metabolites bind to this molecule and activate CD8+ lymphocytes which proliferate to cause SJS.

The HLA B1502 gene mutation frequency among Indian castes and tribal population ranges from 1.1% to 33%. A 9-year-old Indian boy was reported to be positive for this allele after developing rash on OXC, within 1 hour of administration on two occasions.[6]

In a small percentage of patients, OXC may cause paradoxical worsening of seizures and/or EEG, hence EEG monitoring is indicated if patients show increase in seizure frequency, new type of seizures, e.g. myoclonic, behavioral abnormalities and deterioration of school performance. These abnormalities including EEG are reversible on discontinuation of OXC. One of the postulated mechanisms for this worsening is dysregulation of sodium channels leading to inhibition of inhibitory neurons.[7] It may also exacerbate myoclonic or absence seizures if used in generalized epilepsy.

Indications and Efficacy

Oxcarboxepine (OXC) is equivalent to carbamazeine and phenytoin in efficacy, but superior in dose-related tolerability, 75% of patients who had side effects on carbamazepine improved when switched to OXC without loss of seizure control.[8] It is available in the form of oral suspension which makes it easier to titrate the doses as well as improves acceptance by patients and parents.[9] The suspension is efficacious and well tolerated as monotherapy in children with partial seizures with no difference in effectiveness between intellectually normal and impaired children.[10] A Cochrane review found OXC and cabamazepine to be similar in efficacy and tolerability for partial onset seizures.[11]

Lamotrigine

Pharmacology

Lamotrigine (LTG) is an antifolate agent, blocks voltage-gated sodium channels and inhibits release of glutamate. It is rapidly and completely absorbed, with no interference by food. Peak levels are achieved in 1–3 hours. It is 55% bound to plasma proteins. It is mainly metabolized by glucuronic acid conjugation into an inactive metabolite. It's half-life when used alone is 30 hours, while it is 15 hours with concomitant enzyme inducers. With valproate which is an enzyme inhibitor, the half-life may be prolonged up to 60 hours.

Adverse Effects

Lamotrigine (LTG) is metabolized to an epoxide which is responsible for side effects like rash. The incidence of rash, including Steven Johnson syndrome is 8 per 1000 patients and this rash mostly develops in the first two to eight weeks of initiating treatment. There is no way to reliably predict which rash will prove to be serious; but usually life-threatening ones have vesiculobullous lesions like in Steven Johnson syndrome, toxic epidermal necrolysis, etc.[12]

Another type of hypersensitivity reaction, drug reaction with eosinophilia and systemic symptoms (DRESS) (like fever, multiorgan dysfunction, lymphadenopathy) is associated with maculopapular rash and is mediated through CD4+ T cells. Both types of reactions can be life-threatening and even fatal and warrant immediate withdrawal of drug.

A meta-analysis showed the incidence of rash is significantly higher than nonaromatic AEDs.[13] The risk of serious rash is higher in younger children, with concomitant valproate therapy and if the starting dose is high or rapid escalation of dose is done. Hence, the starting and titration dose of LTG is at one fourth the dose, when used as add on in a child on valproate therapy. Other side effects include aseptic meningitis, suicidal behavior in adolescents and blood dyscrasias are seen in a minority of patients.

Indications and Efficacy

A 2 year follow-up of 204 infants aged 1 month to 24 months on LTG as monotherapy or add on, showed reduction in seizure frequency in 74% with only 2% children showing side effect of irritability.[14] A Cochrane review compared LTG to carbamazepine as monotherapy and concluded that LTG was significantly less likely to be withdrawn but results for time to first seizure suggested that carbamazepine may be superior in terms of seizure control.[15]

The SANAD trial arm comparing newer drugs with carbamazepine for partial epilepsy concluded that LTG was superior in tolerability and quality of life, although efficacy was not different.[16] It is relatively safe in pregnancy hence can be prescribed to adolescent females with idiopathic generalized epilepsy as against valproate which has considerable risks of teratogenicity.

Lamotrigine (LTG) is an important option in children with mental retardation with refractory epilepsy and contribute to seizure reduction as well as significant improvements in behavior due to direct mood stabilizing properties.[17]

Levetiracetam

Pharmacology

Levetiracetam (LEV) is chemically unrelated to existing AEDs. It's unique mechanism of action is mediated through binding to synaptic vesicle protein SV2A, thus altering vesicle exocytosis. It is rapidly and almost completely absorbed, with plasma half-life of 6–8 hours. It has minimal plasma protein binding (<10%) and excreted mainly through renal route (66% as unchanged and rest as inactive metabolite). Its dose should be reduced in renal impairment.

Adverse Effects

These two properties contribute to its inert nature when used with other drugs. A study done in children with epilepsy did not show any significant interactions with other AED viz. carbamazepine, valproate, topiramate and lamotrigine.[18] It is, therefore, preferred as add on therapy to existing regimen although more neurologists are using it as first line in epilepsy.

It was hailed as the perfect drug but was noted to have significant side effects like somnolence and dizziness in up to 14% children. It is also shown to cause an increase in behavioral abnormalities like hyperactivity, hyperkinesias, aggression, etc.[19] It can increase the risk of suicidal thoughts, observed as early as one week after treatment.

It should be used with caution in patients with mental retardation as they are at increased risk of paradoxical seizure worsening in up to 14%, irrespective of the epilepsy syndrome.[20] It has been suggested that this adverse reaction can be partially avoided with slow titration.[21]

A small study found significant decrease in lymphocyte counts after 3-6 months of therapy which could explain increased incidence of nasopharyngeal infections in these children.[22] A recent study has found no correlation between efficacy and adverse effects of LEV with serum levels.[23] A meta-analysis suggested that these adverse effects may be less common in children than adults.[24]

A study of 82 cases with accidental overdose showed no significant side effects.[25] A recent review of 1213 patients confirmed the fetal safety of LEV monotherapy with overall risk of fetal malformation after first trimester exposure was within population baseline risk of 1-3% with no adverse effects on long-term child development.[26]

Indications and Efficacy

In a Cochrane review, children were better responders as add on for partial epilepsy than adults with no significant adverse events except certain behavior changes.[27] Young children in the age group of 1 month to 5 years showed shorter half-life and rapid clearance with good tolerance suggesting that higher doses may be required in this age group.[28] Children and adolescents with weight up to 60 kg need a higher weight-related dose of at least 10 mg/kg followed by titration to 20 mg/kg/day as compared to adults who will need 500 mg for 70 kg weight to achieve equivalent levels.[29]

Adjunctive LEV is an efficacious and well tolerated treatment for inadequately controlled partial onset seizures in age group of 1 month to 4 years.[30] In very young patients from the age of 2 weeks to 2 years, it was well tolerated and showed highest efficacy in generalized epilepsy.[31] It has shown considerable efficacy in up to 45% cases even when given after failure of 3 drugs with good retention rates.[32]

Levetiracetam (LEV) is also a preferred treatment of adolescent girls and women with idiopathic generalized epilepsy (IGE) for whom valproate is unsuitable due to adverse effects like weight gain, hair loss and teratogenicity. LEV does not interact with oral contraceptives thus having an advantage over LTG in this age group.[33]

Levetiracetam (LEV) is slowly gaining popularity in neonatal seizures with limited studies showing efficacy and good tolerability in newborns.[34] Doses tried were 16 mg/kg/day to 45 mg/kg/day which reduced seizures by more than 50% in 35% of treated patients.[35] LEV does not enhance neuronal apoptosis unlike phenobarbitone and phenytoin and in fact, may have neuroprotective and antiepileptogenic properties.[36]

There is anecdotal evidence that it may be effective in improvement in EEG and behavior in CSWS.[37] Intravenous LEV is particularly useful in treatment of status epilepticus as well as high dose IV LEV (150 mg/kg/day or more) has been used for acute seizure exacerbation leading to repetitive seizures in children with intractable epilepsy.[38]

A meta-analysis comparing LEV with other newer drugs in refractory partial epilepsy found that add on therapy with LEV has a favorable responder and withdrawal rate compared to LTG, OXC, TPM and ZNS.[39]

Topiramate

Pharmacology

Topiramate (TPM) is a sulfamate and exerts its action through blockage of voltage dependent sodium channels, increase in activity of GABA at GABA-A receptor, antagonism of AMPA/kainite subtype of glutamate receptor as well as inhibition of carbonic anhydrase.

It is rapidly absorbed without any interference by food. It has a half-life of 21 hours and 15-41% of drug is bound to plasma proteins. It is not metabolized much and is excreted unchanged in urine and has significant tubular reabsorption hence it is recommended to use one half of the usual starting and maintenance doses in patients with moderate-to-severe renal impairment.

Adverse Effects

Side effects are seen in up to 58% of children on TPM. It causes certain unique side effects like acute myopia with secondary angle closure glaucoma with symptoms of acute onset of decreased visual acuity with ocular pain with or without redness. These symptoms warrant immediate discontinuation of TPM or else may lead to permanent vision loss.

Another side effect that needs close monitoring is hypohidrosis (decreased sweating) and fever especially in hot weather may lead to hyperthermia, especially if the child is on anticholinergic drugs (e.g. pacitane) or carbonic anydrase inhibitors (e.g. acetazolamide).

The children may also develop metabolic acidosis of hyperchloremic non anion gap type, exacerbated in presence of renal disease, diarrhea, ketogenic diet or severe respiratory disorders. Bicarbonate levels lower than 17 mEq/L are seen in up to 67% of patients on doses more than 5 mg/kg/day. The symptoms of chronic metabolic acidosis include hyperventilation, anorexia, reduced growth rates and predisposes to arrhythmia, osteomalacia and nephrocalcinosis.

It promotes nephrolithiasis by inhibiting carbonic anhydrase thereby reducing urinary citrate excretion and increasing urinary pH. This complication may increase in the presence of ketogenic diet. Increase of fluid intake prevents formation of stones. Either the dose of topiramate should be reduced or alkali supplementation should be started. However, a recent population based cohort study suggests that topiramate use is not associated with nephrolithiasis.[40]

With concomitant valproate therapy, hyperammonemia should be suspected if there is unexplained vomiting or lethargy. This condition is associated with normal serum valproate levels and is reversible on cessation of either drug.[41] The other side effects include psychomotor slowing, word finding difficulties and increase in suicidal thoughts. The cognitive impairment may be severe enough to lead to drug discontinuation in up to 54% of patients on TPM (versus 39% on LEV).[42]

Anorexia can be significant enough to cause weight loss. A Cochrane review reported that the relative risk of treatment withdrawal due to side effects was 2.44 as compared to placebo and the risk of weight loss was 3.47 (1.55–7.79) along with other side effects.[43] However, a large multicenter study of TPM as add on in 284 infants less than 2 years old showed fever and respiratory infections in about 50% and anorexia, acidosis in about 30%.[44]

Indications and Efficacy

It is a broad spectrum drug and has been extensively used in children as add on in refractory partial epilepsy and catastrophic epilepsies like West syndrome, Dravet syndrome, Doose syndrome, Lennox Gastaut syndrome, Angelman syndrome, Rett syndrome and CSWS. It is also a useful adjuvant drug for refractory status epilepticus. The efficacy is more sustained in patients with localization related epilepsy as compared to the catastrophic epilepsies which may show initial reduction in seizure frequency in up to 48%.[45] In a retrospective review of 100 cases of West syndrome treated with topiramate, 64% patients showed reduction in spasms.[46]

Topiramate (TPM) was found to be effective in 50% of partial and 44% of generalized epilepsy and is particularly well tolerated in children below 4 years.[47] The probability of maintaining seizure freedom was higher on higher doses, up to 400 mg/day with minor side effects seen in 145 patients.[48]

Vigabatrin

Pharmacology

Vigabatrin (VGB) is a structural analog of GABA, which irreversibly binds to GABA transaminase which degrades GABA, the enzyme that degrades GABA thus allowing GABA to accumulate in brain. It can be taken with or without food, does not bind to plasma proteins and not significantly metabolized. It is excreted primarily through renal excretion, hence needs dose adjustment in renal impairment. The half-life is about 6 hours in infants and 9 hours in adolescents.

Adverse Effects

Up to 32% of infants on VGB may show symmetric T2 hyperintensities with restricted diffusion in centrencephalic structures—thalamus, basal ganglia, brainstem, cerebellum, etc. The postulated mechanisms include edema of myelin due to raised GABA levels or myelin vacuolization. These changes are mostly reversible, more common in infants <1 year and cryptogenic spasms but do not depend on the duration of treatment.[49] Relatively higher dose was also associated with more risk of these changes.[50]

The use of VGB is limited by the evidence of causing visual field loss in at least 20–40% of patients. This warrants monitoring of vision by an ophthalmologist with expertise in indirect ophthalmoscopy of retina. Peripheral visual field assessment is difficult in children below 9 years and cognitively impaired, nonetheless visual assessment should be performed at baseline, on therapy and up to 3–6 months after cessation of therapy. The onset and progression of vision loss is unpredictable, hence the drug should be immediately discontinued if vision loss is detected. Once detected, the loss is irreversible.[51]

In an observational cohort study, 146 infants in age group of 3–35 months were followed up with serial ERG (Electroretinogram) and VGB-induced retinal damage was picked up in 5.3% at 6 months and 13.3% at 12 months of treatment. It is suggested to minimize the duration of treatment to 6 months to reduce the chances of retinal damage.[52]

Patients may be left with tunnel vision to within 10 degrees of visual fixation resulting in severe disability. There may also be damage to central retina leading to decreased visual acuity. Informed consent should be taken from the caregivers about adequate explanation of the risks and benefits of VGB therapy. In symptomatic spasms, the potential benefit of reducing the risk of vision loss with shorter treatment should be weighed against the risk of seizure relapse and increased risk of mental deficiency. Few studies have suggested that avoiding light exposure and taurine supplementation may reduce the retinal damage. Some authors suggest ERG in a sedated infant is the only option appropriate for monitoring in infants and younger children.[53]

Indications and Efficacy

It is indicated in the treatment of infantile spasms from the age of 1 month to 2 years and for refractory partial epilepsy after the age of 10 years. The dose for infants with West syndrome is 50 mg/kg/day in two divided doses, further doses can be titrated by 25–50 mg/kg/day every 3 days to maximum of 150 mg/kg/day. A large randomized trial showed high doses (100–150 mg/kg/day) to be more effective than low dose (18–36 mg/kg/day) in controlling spasms.[54]

It is not freely available in India. If there is no clinical benefit seen by 2–4 weeks, it should be withdrawn. Usually, the duration of treatment of 6 months is sufficient. A retrospective review showed that spasms were controlled in 73% of patients with tuberous sclerosis while in 27% if other etiologies. Shorter time from spasm onset to VGB treatment and total duration of treatment were significantly associated with better neurodevelopmental outcome.[55] In another study of children with tuberous sclerosis and infantile spasms, VGB was highly effective in controlling spasms but had no effect on intellectual disability.[56]

However, for cryptogenic infantile spasms not associated with tuberous sclerosis, low dose ACTH started early is associated with better outcome as compared to VGB.[57] A Cochrane review for VGB in partial epilepsy showed that frequency of seizures was reduced on VGB but also more likely to be withdrawn due to side effects.[58] Amongst the other drugs used for spasms, VGB interacts significantly with clonazepam and valproate.

Clobazam

Pharmacology

Clobazam (CLB) is a benzodiazepine and acts through potentiation of GABA resulting from binding to benzodiazepine site of the GABA A receptor. It is rapidly absorbed after oral administration, unaffected by food, has 70–90% plasma protein binding. It is metabolized in liver to N-desmethyl clobazam which has 1/5 of activity but has 3–5 times higher levels as compared to the parent compound. It may increase the levels of other AED. It has a long half-life of 36–42 hours. Excretion is mainly through urine. Doses need to be adjusted in hepatic impairment.

Adverse Effects

Common side effects include sedation, behavioral abnormalities like aggression, irritability and serious skin reactions like Steven Johnson syndrome especially in first 8 weeks of treatment.

Indications and Efficacy

In India, it is commonly used in children as add on therapy, either during slow titration of other newly added drugs like LTG, TPM, or as add on after failure of 1-2 drugs. In doses of 0.2-0.3 mg/kg/day, seizure reduction is noted in 75% patients. At low doses, it is well tolerated with good retention rates suggesting good tolerability.[59]

It is recommended for children above 2 years with Lennox Gastaut syndrome (LGS) or as add on drug for refractory partial epilepsy. Initial dose is 0.25 mg/kg/day in 2 divided or single dose at night. In LGS, it was associated with more than seizure 50% reduction in more than half of patients with 10% achieving freedom from drop attacks without developing tolerance.[60] Clobazam has a sustained effectiveness over the first 3 years of use in LGS and other intractable epilepsy syndromes which makes it a viable long-term treatment option.[61] Clobazam has shown efficacy against a wide spectrum of seizure types and etiologies. An early, low dose response is a favorable indicator of sustained response.[62]

It has demonstrated efficacy as monotherapy as well. A Cochrane review found no advantage of clobazam over carbamazepine for retention at 12 months in drug naïve children and a slight advantage over phenytoin for retention at 6 months in adolescents.[63]

Zonisamide

Pharmacology

Zonisamide (ZNS) is a sulfonamide, acts through blockade of sodium and calcium channels and also has weak carbonic anhydrase inhibitor activity. It is 40% bound to plasma proteins, with a long half-life of 63 hours. It is metabolized by acetylation and glucoronide formation. It needs dose adjustment in renal impairment.

Adverse Effects

Being a sulfonamide, there is a risk of causing Stevens Johnson syndrome in 2%, with rash appearing early in treatment, 85-90% occurred within 2-14 weeks of initiation. It can also cause oligohydrosis, hyperthermia and nephrolithiasis.

A Cochrane review concluded that in adults, zonisamide is effective as add on treatment of people with drug resistant partial epilepsy but showed significant side effects like ataxia, somnolence, agitation and anorexia.[64] However, it appears to be better tolerated by children, being effective in up to 62% irrespective of seizure type, it was uncommon to discontinue due to side effects.[65]

Indications and Efficacy

Another study in children aged more than 8 months with intractable epilepsy, the efficacy of ZNS was independent of cognitive status and there was no correlation between adverse events and dose.[66] A multicenter review of children aged 1-18 years, showed good response in 35% patients who had been refractory to at least 3 drugs. Side effects were seen in 43% but warranted withdrawal in 17% patients only.[67]

A meta-analysis of 398 children below the age of 16 years treated with ZNS reported no significant ECG abnormalities and acceptable safety profile when used as adjunctive treatment.[68] ZNS has been widely used in Japan for West syndrome. In a Japanese institute-based survey, vitamin B6 was used most frequently followed by valproic acid, ZNS and ACTH.[69]

Lacosamide

Lacosamide is a novel antiepileptic approved for adjunctive treatment of refractory partial epilepsy in patients more than 17 years. It has 100% oral absorption, limited hepatic metabolism, low protein binding and no known drug interactions. It selectively enhances the slow inactivation of voltage-gated sodium channels. It also modulates a phosphoprotein CRMP-2, involved in neuronal growth and differentiation, raising concern regarding its use in younger children.

In a study of 40 children with refractory epilepsy with age from 1.4 years onwards, with multiple seizure types, had tried 5–6 antiepileptic drugs, some of them failed VNS and ketogenic diet, 42.5% children showed reduction of seizures by 50% and 15% became seizure free. The doses used ranged from 2 mg/kg/day to 7 mg/kg/day. Side effects were seen in 37%—mainly lethargy, tremor, weight loss, etc.[70]

In a study of young children with refractory focal epilepsy, LCM was found to be effective and well tolerated but loss of efficacy was reported in significant proportion of initial responders.[71] IV LCM is available and is slowly emerging as one of the drugs for refractory status epilepticus.

Rufinamide

Rufinamide (RFN) is indicated for children with Lennox Gastaut syndrome aged 4 years or older, initial dose is 10 mg/kg/day, increased slowly to 45 mg/kg/day. It is contraindicated in long QT syndrome.

It has been found to be especially effective in tonic-atonic seizures in Lennox–Gastaut syndrome as well as has been proven effective and in many other types of seizures as well. The common adverse events noted were somnolence, dizziness etc.[72] It is likely to be a cost-effective alternative to TPM as adjunctive therapy for children with LGS.[73]

Amongst other newer drugs not available in India, stiripentol is a useful drug for Dravet syndrome and retigabine which modulates the KCNQ potassium channels, and is a potential agent for benign familial neonatal seizures.

Other newer drugs like brivaracetam, carisbamate, marijuana, ganaxolone, perampanel and eslicarbazepine have limited experience in children and will not be discussed further.

PRACTICAL CONSIDERATIONS: PLACE OF NEWER DRUGS IN MANAGEMENT OF PEDIATRIC EPILEPSY

When choosing an AED for a given patient, the following patient-related variables need to be considered—type of seizures, epilepsy syndrome, age, gender, comorbidities, comedications, genetic background, affordability, ability to swallow, etc. The AED characteristics to be considered include suitability for the epilepsy type, adverse effects, idiosyncratic reactions, interaction potential, teratogenicity, cost and availability.[74]

For partial and secondarily generalized seizures, carbamazepine, valproate, lamotrigine and oxcarbazepine are all efficacious as first line agents. As second line, vigabatrin, lamotrigine, topiramate, levetiracetam are equally efficacious and well-tolerated except vigabatrin which should be the last choice due to the risk of visual field defects.

For primary generalized seizures, valproate and lamotrigine are drugs of choice. These are also the first choice if unclassified seizures. As second line for generalized epilepsy—lamotrigine, topiramate, levetiracetam can be used. Lamotrigine may worsen myoclonic seizures. Clonazepam can be used for refractory myoclonic seizures.[75]

As vitamin D deficiency is endemic in our population, and antiepileptics can worsen the same, it is recommended to supplement it, irrespective of the antiepileptic given.[76]

There is no indication for routine monitoring of AED levels, except in limited situations.[77] The first drug is effective in 60% patients, adding the second drug may control in 40% of the remainder patients. The odds of further success with subsequent drug attempts are far lower. In view of the law of diminishing returns, the diagnosis should be reviewed carefully and other suitable options like surgery (for lesional epilepsy) or ketogenic diet (and vagal nerve stimulation) for non-lesional epilepsy should be considered.[78]

When adding another drug, consideration should be given to the mechanism of action. Drugs with action on same receptors (e.g. carbamazepine, oxcarbazepine, lamotrigine) should be avoided. Similarly, drugs with similar adverse risk profile (e.g. topiramate and zonisamide) should be avoided. Caution needs to be exercised when starting and titrating lamotrigine to a patient on valproate.[79]

Adolescents need to be educated regarding lot of lifestyle issues like adequate sleep, avoiding flickering lights if photosensitive, driving, etc. In adolescent females with idiopathic epilepsy, lamotrigine or levetiracetam should be considered as the drug of first choice, in view of adverse endocrine effects of valproate as well as the risk of teratogenicity.[80]

Table 19.1 Newer antiepileptic drugs (AEDs) ready reckoner

Drug name	Formulations available, dose	Indications	Side effects	Comments
Oxcarbazepine	Syrup: 300 mg/5 mL Tablets: 150/300/600 mg Start at 5 mg/kg/day, increase weekly to 15–20 mg/kg/day. Max dose: 60 mg/kg/day	As monotherapy in partial epilepsy, as adjunctive therapy. Syrup can be given BD, has been tested >1 month	Rash, including SJS, TEN. Initial sedation. Paradoxical worsening of seizures and EEG in 15–20% cases. Hyponatremia	Less chances of drug interactions, autoinduction than carbamazepine. Rash in 25–30% of those who had rash on carbamazepine
Levetiracetam (IV available)	Syrup: 500 mg/5 mL Tablets: 250/500/750/1000 mg Start 10 mg/kg/day Maintenance 20–30, maximum 60–80 mg/kg/day	Broad spectrum drug for partial and generalized epilepsy, first line for females with IGE	Hyperactivity, behavioral disturbances, depression, suicidal ideation in adolescents	Novel mechanism of action, least interactions, considered safe during pregnancy, newborn
Topiramate	Tablets: 25/50/100 mg Tablets are enteric coated Start 1–3 mg/kg/day Maximum 5–9 mg/kg/day	Broad spectrum drug for partial and generalized epilepsy, West syndrome Concomitant Migraine	Anorexia, urolithiasis, oligohydrosis, myopia, glaucoma, hyperthermia, word finding difficulties	Ensure good hydration, dose adjustment with renal failure
Lamotrigine	Tablets: 5/25/50/100/200 mg Start: 0.6 mg/kg/day, increase slowly to 3–5 mg/kg/day, maximum—7.5 mg/kg/day	Broad spectrum drug for partial and generalized epilepsy, may worsen myoclonic seizures	Rash/Steven Johnson syndrome, may be fatal especially if used with valproate. No significant drug interactions	If child on valproate, start dose: 0.15 mg/kg/day, increase by 0.3 mg/kg/day every 1–2 weeks, max. 1–3 mg/kg/day (200 mg/day)
Zonisamide	Capsules: 25/50/100 mg Initial dose: 100 mg/day, increase 2 weekly to maximum 400 mg/day	Adjunctive therapy for partial seizures, anecdotal reports in West syndrome	Rash/Steven Johnson syndrome, Hypohidrosis, hyperthermia, arrhythmia	Has been used extensively in Japan for infants with West syndrome
Vigabatrin	Tablets: 500 mg 50 mg/kg/day, can increase to maximum of 150 mg/kg/day	1 month to 2 years: West syndrome, especially with tuberous sclerosis More than 10 years: Add on for partial epilepsy	Dose and duration dependent bilateral progressive irreversible peripheral visual field constriction	Periodic visual assessment, use limited to 3–6 months. Taper gradually. MRI may show nonspecific white matter changes
Clobazam	Tablets: 5/10 mg Start with 5 mg/day, can titrate to 20 mg daily for weight <30 kg and 40 mg daily for weight >30 kg	Above 2 years: As adjunctive therapy for Lennox Gastaut syndrome, partial epilepsy	Rash/Steven Johnsons, sedation, hyperactivity, behavioral abnormalities	Not approved by USFDA for intermittent febrile seizure prophylaxis

In epileptic encephalopthies like West syndrome, first line drugs include ACTH and vigabatrin (if secondary to tuberous sclerosis). Second line drugs include topiramate, valproate, zonisamide, levetiracetam, lamotrigine and vitamin B6.[81]

However, the cost of these drugs increases the cost of therapy and limits their use in less affording patients.[82] The average cost of carbamazepine Syrup is ₹ 24/- while syrup oxcarbazepine is ₹ 137. For 10 tablets: carbamazepine plain, chrono 200, 300 mg cost ₹ 15, 23 and 38, respectively, while the corresponding cost for tablet oxcarbazepine 150 mg is ₹ 64 per 10 tablets. Levetiracetam was very costly when introduced (₹ 1200 per bottle) gradually the cost has been brought down to ₹ 300–400. Tablets of topiramate 25 mg, lamotrigine 25 mg, clobazam 5 mg are in the range of ₹ 50–70 per 10 tablets.

There is enough evidence that many newer AEDs are effective in status epilepticus and refractory status epilepticus, e.g. IV levetiracetam, IV lacosamide, topiramate through nasogastric tube, etc.

Please see **Table 19.1** *summarizing details regarding preparations available, dosing and side effects of commonly used newer antiepileptic drugs.*

CONCLUSION

Even with all these developments in the past two decades, none of the newer AEDs are 100% effective, devoid of side effects and prevent relapse when withdrawn. For a given patient, balance has to be achieved between efficacy and side effects. The goal should be to choose the most suitable drug in minimum doses to control seizures and minimize the side effects. The newer drugs may not score in efficacy over the older drugs, but has better tolerability which translates to better quality of life on chronic treatment.

As yet, there is no perfect antiepileptic drug. The search for that perfect AED continues…

ACKNOWLEDGMENTS

Sincere thanks to Profs S Rajadhyaksha, J Oswal and R Jahagirdar, Department of Pediatrics, for critical review of the manuscript.

REFERENCES

1. Brodie MJ. Review: Antiepileptic drug therapy the story so far. Seizure. 2010;(19):650-5.
2. Vajda FJE, Eadie MJ. The clinical pharmacology of traditional antiepileptic drugs. Seminars in Epileptology. Epileptic Disord. 2014;16(4):395-408.
3. LaRoche SM, Helmers SL. The new antiepileptic drugs-Scientific Review. JAMA. 2004;291:605-14.
4. Arzimanoglou A, Ben-Menachem E, Cramer J, et al. The evolution of antiepileptic drug development and regulation. Epileptic Disord. 2010;12(1):3-15.
5. Kim YS, Kim DW, Jung KH, et al. Frequency of and risk factors for oxcarbazepine-induced severe and symptomatic hyponatremia. 2014;23(3):208-12.
6. Shankarkumar U, Shah KN, Ghosh K. HLA B* 1502 allele association with oxcarbazepine induced skin reactions in epilepsy patient from India. Epilepsia. 2009;50(7):1833-9.
7. Vendrame M, Khurana DS, Cruz M, et al. Aggravation of seizures and/or EEG features in children treated with Oxcarbazepine monotherapy. Epilepsia. 2007;48(11):2116-20.
8. French JA, Kanner AM, Bautista J, et al. Special report: Practice parameters. Efficacy and tolerability of the new antiepileptic drugs: I: Treatment of new onset Epilepsy: Report of the TTA and the QSS subcommittees of the American Academy of Neurology and American Epilepsy Society. Epilepsia. 2004;45(5):401-9.
9. Rufo-Campos M, Casas-Fernandes C, Marrtinez-Bermejo A. Long term use of Oxcarbazepine oral suspension in childhood epilepsy: Open label study. J Child Neurol. 2006;21:480-5.
10. Eun SH, Kim HD, Chung HJ, et al. A multicentre trial of oxcarbazepine oral suspension monotherapy in children newly diagnosed with partial seizures: a clinical and cognitive evaluation. 2012;21(9):679-84.
11. Koch MW, Polman SK. Oxcarbazepine versus carbamazepine monotherapy for partial onset seizures. Cochrane Database Rev. 2009.
12. French JA, Gazzola DM. Review: New generation antiepileptic drugs: what do they offer in terms of improved tolerability and safety? Ther Adv Drug Saf. 2011;2(4):141-58.
13. Wang XG, Xiong J, Xu WH, et al. Risk of a lamotrigine-related skin rash: current meta-

analysis and post marketing cohort analysis. Seizure. 2015;25:52-61.
14. Pina-Garza JE, Elterman RD, Ayala R, et al. Long-term tolerability and efficacy of Lamotrigine in infants 1 to 24 months old. J Child Neurol. 2008; 23:853-61.
15. Gamble CL, Williamson PR, Marson AG. Lamotrigine versus carbamazepine monotherapy for epilepsy. Cochrane Database Syst Rev. 2006.
16. Chadwick D, Marson T. Choosing first drug treatment for epilepsy after SANAD: Randomized controlled trials, systematic reviews, guidelines and treating patients. Epilepsia. 2007;48(7):1259-63.
17. McKee JR, Sunder TR, Vuong A, et al. Adjunctive Lamotrigine for refractory epilepsy in adolescents with mental retardation. J Child Neurol. 2006;21:372-9.
18. Otoul C, Smedt HD, Stockis A. Lack of pharmacokinetic interaction of Levetiracetam on Carbamazepine, Valproic acid, Topiramate, and lamotrigine in children with epilepsy. Epilepsia. 2007;48(11):2111-5.
19. Halma E, de Louw AJA, Klikenberg S, et al. Behavioral side effects of levetiracetam in children with epilepsy: A systematic review. Seizure. 2014;23(9):685-91.
20. Szucs A, Clemens Z, Jakus R, et al. The risk of paradoxical Levetiracetam effect is increased in mentally retarded patients. Epilepsia. 2008;49 (97):1174-9.
21. Vigevano F. Topical review: Levetiracetam in Pediatrics. J Child Neurol. 2005;20:87-93.
22. Dinopoulos A, Attilakos A, Paschalidou M, et al. Short-term effect of levetiracetam monotherapy on hematological parameters in children with epilepsy: A prospective study. Epilepsy Research. 2014;108(4):820-3.
23. Sheinberg R, Heyman E, Dagan Z, et al. Correlation between efficacy of levetiracetam and serum levels among 50 children with refractory epilepsy. Pediatr Neurol. 2015.
24. Mbizvo GK, Dixon P, Hutton JL, et al. The adverse effect profile of levetiracetam in epilepsy: a more detailed look. Int J Neurosci. 2014;124(9):627-34.
25. Lewis JC, Albertson TE, Walsh MJ. An 11-year review of levetiracetam ingestions in children less than 6 years of age. Clin Toxicol. 2014;52(9):964-8.
26. Chaudhry SA, Jong G, Koren G. The fetal safety of Levetiracetam: a systematic review. Reprod Toxicol. 2014;46:40-5.

27. Mbizvo GK, Dixon P, Hutton JL, et al. Levetiracetam add on for drug-resistant epilepsy: an updated Cochrane review. Cochrane Database Syst Rev. 2012.
28. Glauser TA, Mitchell WG, Weinstock A, et al. Pharmacokinetics of Levetiracetam in infants and young children with epilepsy. Epilepsia. 2007;48(6):1117-22.
29. Chhun S, Jullien V, Rey E, et al. Population pharmacokinetics of levetiracetam and dosing recommendation in children with epilepsy. Epilepsia. 2009;50(5):1150-7.
30. Pina-Garza E, Nordli Jr DR, Rating D, et al. Adjunctive Levetiracetam in infants and young children with refractory partial onset seizures. Epilepsia. 2009;50(95):1141-9.
31. Krief P, Kan L, Maytal J. Efficacy of levetiracetam in children with epilepsy younger than 2 years of age. J Child Neurol. 2008;23:582-4.
32. Goldberg-Stem H, Feldman L, Eidlitz-Markus T, et al. Levetiracetam in children, adolescents and young adults with intractable epilepsy: Efficacy, tolerability and effect on EEG—a pilot study. 2013;17(3):248-53.
33. Grunewald R. Levetiracetam in the treatment of idiopathic generalized Epilepsies. Epilepsia. 2005;46(9):154-60.
34. Furwentsches A, Bussmann C, Ramantani G, et al. Levetiracetam in the treatment of neonatal seizures: A pilot study. Seizure. 2010;19:185-9.
35. Abend NS, Gutierrez-Colina AM, Monk HM, et al. Levetiracetam for treatment of neonatal seizures. J Child Neurol. 2011;26(4):465-70.
36. Glass HC. Neonatal seizures: Advances in mechanisms and management. Clin Perinatol. 2014;41(1):177-90.
37. Abey A, Poznanski N, Verheulpen D, et al. Levetiracetam efficacy in epileptic syndromes with continuous spike waves during slow sleep. Epilepsia. 2005;46(12):1937-42.
38. Depositario-Cabacar D, Peters JM, Pong AW, et al. High dose intravenous levetiracetam for acute seizure exacerbation in children with intractable epilepsy. Epilepsia. 2010;51(7):1319-22.
39. Otoul C, Arrigo C, van Riickevorsel K, et al. Meta-analysis and indirect comparisons of levetiracetam with other second generation antiepileptic drugs in partial epilepsy. Clin Neuropharmacol. 2005;28(2):72-8.
40. Shen A-L, Lin H-L, Tseng Y-F, et al. Topiramate may not increase risk of urolithiasis: A nationwide population-based cohort study. Seizure. 2015;29:86-9.

41. Cheung E, Wong V, Fung C-W. Topiramate-valproate-induced hyperammonemic encephalopathy: Case report. J Child Neurol. 2004; 19:157-60.
42. Bootsma HPR, Aldenkamp AP, Diepman L, et al. The effect of antiepileptic drugs on cognition: Patient perceived cognitive problems of topiramate versus levetiracetam in clinical practice. Epilepsia. 2006;47(S2):24-7.
43. Pulman J, Jette N, Dykeman J, et al. Topiramate add on for drug resistant partial epilepsy. Cochrane Database Syst Rev. 2014.
44. Puri V, Seth N, Jayalakshmi S, et al. Long term Open label study of adjunctive topiramate in infants with refractory partial onset seizures. J Child Neurol. 2011; 26(10):1271-83.
45. Grosso S, Franzoni E, Lannetti P, et al. Efficacy and safety of topiramate in refractory epilepsy of childhood. J Child Neurol. 2005;20:893-7.
46. Korinthenberg R, Schreiner A. Topiramate in children with West syndrome: A retrospective multicenter evaluation of 100 patients. J Child Neurol. 2009;24(94):400-5.
47. Mikaeloff Y, de Saint-Martin A, Mancini J, et al. Topiramate: efficacy and tolerability in children according to epilepsy syndrome. Epilepsy Research. 2003;53(3):225-32.
48. Glauser T, Dlugos DJ, Dodson WE, et al. Topiramate monotherapy in newly diagnosed epilepsy in children and adolescents. J Child Neurol. 2007;22:693-9.
49. Dracopoulos A, Widjaja E, Raybaud C, et al. Vigabatrin associated reversible MRI signal changes in patients with infantile spasms. Epilepsia. 2010;41(7):1297-304.
50. Pearl PL, Vezina LG, Saneto RP, et al. Cerebral MRI abnormalities associated with vigabatrin therapy. Epilepsia. 2009;50(2):184-94.
51. Gaily E, Jonsson H, Lappi M. Visual fields at school age in children treated with vigabatrin in infancy. Epilepsia. 2009;50(2):206-16.
52. Westall CA, Wright T, Cortese F, et al. Vigabatrin retinal toxicity in children with infantile spasms: An observational cohort study. Neurology. 2014;83:2262-8.
53. Willmore LJ, Abelson MB, Ben-Minachem E, et al. Vigabatrin: 2008 update. Critical review and commentary. Epilepsia. 2009;50(2):163-73.
54. Elterman RD, Shields WD, Bittman RM, et al. Vigabatrin for the treatment of infantile spasms: Final report of a randomized trial. J Child Neurol. 2010;25:1340-7.
55. Camposano SE, Major P, Halpern E, et al. Vigabatrin in the treatment of childhood epilepsy: A retrospective chart review of efficacy and safety profile. Epilepsia. 2008;49(7):1186-91.
56. Yum M-S, Lee E-H, Ko T-S. Vigabatrin and mental retardation in Tuberous sclerosis: infantile spasms versus focal seizures. J Child Neurol. 2013;28:308-13.
57. Go CY, Mackay MT, Weiss SK, et al. Evidence-based guidelines update: Medical treatment of infantile spasms: report of the guideline development subcommittee of the American Academy of Neurology and the Practice committee of the Child Neurology. Neurology. 2012;78:1974-80.
58. Hemming K, Maguire MJ, Hutton JL, et al. Vigabatrin for refractory partial epilepsy. Cochrane Database Syst Rev. 2013.
59. Joshi R, Tripathi M, Gupta P, et al. Effect of Clobazam as add on antiepileptic drug in patients with epilepsy. Indian J Med Res. 2014; 140:209-14.
60. Wheless JW, Phelps SJ. Clobazam: A newly approved but well-established drug for the treatment of intractable epilepsy syndromes. J Child Neurol. 2013;28:218-29.
61. Purcarin G, Ng Y-T. Experience in the use of clobazam in the treatment of Lennox Gastaut syndrome. Therapeutic Advances in Neurol Disord. 2014;7:169-76.
62. Perry MS, Bailey L, Malik S, et al. Clobazam for the treatment of intractable epilepsy in children. J Child Neurol. 2013;28:34-9.
63. Arya R, Anand V, Garg SK, et al. Clobazam monotherapy for partial-onset or generalized onset seizures. Cochrane Database Syst Rev. 2014.
64. Carmichael K, Pulman J, Lakhan SE, et al. Zonisamide add on for drug resistant partial epilepsy. Cochrane Database Syst Rev. 2013.
65. Kim HL, Aldridge J, Rho JM. Clinical experience with zonisamide monotherapy and adjunctive therapy in children with epilepsy at a tertiary care referral centre. J Child Neurol. 2005;20: 212-9.
66. Mandelbaum DE, Bunch M, Kugler SL, et al. Broad spectrum efficacy of Zonisamide at 12 months in children with intractable epilepsy. J Child Neurol. 2005;20:594-7.
67. Tan HJ, Martland TR, Appleton R, et al. Effectiveness and tolerability of zonisamide in children with epilepsy. Seizure. 2010;19(1):31-5.

68. Cross JH, Auvin S, Patten A, et al. Safety and tolerability of zonisamide in pediatric patients with epilepsy. 2014;18(6):747-58.
69. Okumura A, Ozawa H, Ito M, et al. Current treatment of West syndrome in Japan. J Child Neurol. 2007;22:560-4.
70. Yorns Jr WR, Khurana DS, Carvalho KS, et al. Efficcay of Lacosamide as adjunctive therapy in children with refractory epilepsy. J Child Neurol. 2014;29(1):23-7.
71. Grosso S, Parisi P, Spalice A, et al. Efficacy and safety of lacosamide in infants and young children with refractory focal epilepsy. European J Pediatr Neurol. 2013.
72. Hsieh DT, Thiele EA. Efficacy and safety of rufinamide in pediatric epilepsy.Therapeutic Adv Neurol Disord. 2013;6:189-96.
73. Verdian L, Yi Y. Cost utility analysis of rufinamide verus topiramate and lamotrigine for the treatment of children with Lennox Gastaut Syndrome in the United Kingdom. Seizure. 2010;19(1):1-11.
74. Glauser T, Ben-Menachem E, Buurgeois B, et al. ILAE treatment Guidelines: Evidence based analysis of antiepilptic drug efficacy and effectiveness as initial monotherapy for epileptic seizures and syndromes. Epilepsia. 2006;47(7):1094-120.
75. Glauser T, Ben-Menachem E, Bourgeois B, et al. Updated ILAE evidence review of antiepileptic drug efficacy and effectiveness as initial monotherapy for epileptic seizures and syndromes. Epilepsia. 2013.
76. Menon B, Harinarayan CV. The effect of antiepileptic drug therapy on serum 25 hydroxy vitamin D and parameters of calcium and bone metabolism—A longitudinal study. Seizure. 2010;19:153-8.
77. Patsalos PN, Berry DJ, Bourgeois BFD, et al. Antiepileptic drugs—best practice guidelines for therapeutic drug monitoring: A position paper by the subcommission on therapeutic drug monitoring, ILAE Commission on Therapeutic Strategies. Epilepsia. 2008;49(97):1239-76.
78. Kenney D, Wirrell E. Patient considerations in the management of focal seizures in children and adolescents. Adolescent Health, Medicine and Therapeutics. 2014;5:49-65.
79. Lee JW, Dworetzky B. Review: Rational polytherapy with antiepileptic drugs. Pharmaceuticals. 2010;3:2362-79.
80. Montouris G, Bassel AK. The first line of therapy in a girl with juvenile myoclonic epilepsy: Should it be valproate or a new agent? Epilepsia. 2009;50(8):16-20.
81. Riikonen R. Recent advances in the management of infantile spasms. CNS drugs. 2014.
82. Aneja S, Sharma S. Review article: Newer antiepileptic drugs. Indian Pediatrics. 2013;50: 1033-40.

CHAPTER 20

Practical Management of Status Epilepticus

Yeeshu Singh Sudan, Vinayan KP

INTRODUCTION

Status epilepticus (SE) is a medical emergency and is associated with high morbidity and mortality. The best outcome of status epilepticus depends upon an early diagnosis and an aggressive treatment. Management of status epilepticus requires a team approach which should at least include epileptologist or neurologist, critical care expert, and electrophysiologist.

DEFINITION

Status epilepticus is described as two or more sequential seizures without full recovery of consciousness between seizures, or more than 30 minutes of continuous seizure activity.[1]

Recently for clinical management of seizures operational definition has gained importance. It has shown that once a seizure lasts for more than 5 minutes it is unlikely to stop spontaneously within the next few minutes, therefore the time duration for generalized status epilepticus has reduced from 30 minutes to 5 minutes of continuous seizure activity.[2]

Refractory status is a condition in which minimum duration of status is 60 minutes (by history or on observation) despite the administration of two appropriate anticonvulsants at acceptable doses. Sometimes the term super-refractory status epilepticus is used in which seizures continue for 24 hours or more after the onset of anesthesia, including those cases in which the status epilepticus recurs on the reduction or withdrawal of anesthesia.[3]

CLASSIFICATION OF STATUS EPILEPTICUS

Broadly divided into:
- Generalized status epilepticus—types (tonic-clonic, myoclonic, absence, atonic, akinetic)
- Focal status epilepticus—which includes the older terminologies of simple or complex partial status epilepticus. Epilepsia partialis continua is another term commonly used for the focal motor status.

Another approach is to classify as generalized convulsive status epilepticus and nonconvulsive status epilepticus (simple partial, complex partial, absence).

Status epilepticus of partial onset followed by secondarily generalized status epilepticus accounts for the majority of episodes.

Incidence

There is significant lack of epidemiological data on status epilepticus especially from pediatric population. Data from all over the world has shown that majority of childhood SE occurred in previously neurologically healthy children.

One study from India has shown that 53% had SE as their first seizure and only 60% had received any treatment prior to coming to the pediatric intensive care unit (PICU).[4]

Infants younger than 12 months have the highest incidence and frequency of status epilepticus with more than 40 % cases of childhood cases occurring in those younger than 2 years.[5] Etiologies are highly age-dependent, with more than 80% of children under the age of two having febrile or acute symptomatic origin. Cryptogenic and remote symptomatic causes are more common in older children. The common causes are infection/fever (52%) and decreased antiepileptic drug levels (21%).[6]

There is significant mortality and morbidity associated with status epilepticus in children. However, it is less as compared to adult population.[6] The primary determinants of mortality in children with status epilepticus are duration of seizures, age at onset, and etiology.[7,8]

Nonconvulsive Status Epilepticus

Nonconvulsive status epilepticus (NCSE) is defined as an epileptic state lasting more than 30 minutes with some clinically evident change in mental status or behavior from baseline along with ictal activity on electroencephalogram (EEG). Clinically patient can present with agitation, lethargy or aggressive behavior, confusion, decreased speech, mutism, verbal perseveration or echolalia, confusion or delirium, staring, blinking, chewing or picking, tremulousness and subtle periorbital, facial or limb myoclonus.[9] It could be generalized or focal based on the EEG findings. EEG is a diagnostic tool in this scenario especially when the cause of acute confusional state is not clinically apparent. Etiology of NCSE could be due to various causes including hypoxic injury, infective causes, metabolic disturbances and after convulsive seizures.

MANAGEMENT

Treatment of seizure needs to be initiated possibly at home by caregiver. Pre-hospital management includes both first-aid during seizures, and pharmacotherapy.

Benzodiazepines like diazepam and midazolam can be used by a caregiver. Pre-hospital treatment with benzodiazepines has been shown to reduce seizure activity significantly compared with seizures that remain untreated until the patient reaches the emergency department.[10] The various routes employed include per-rectal (diazepam, lorazepam, paraldehyde), intranasal (midazolam), buccal (midazolam, lorazepam) and intramuscular (midazolam).[3] Nowadays buccal or intranasal midazolam is commercially available which is as effective as rectal diazepam and socially more acceptable.

The first step in managing status epilepticus is assessing the patient's airway and oxygenation. Cervical spine should be immobilized if trauma is suspected. Use an oral airway to prevent tongue from falling back. Children should be preferably admitted to pediatric intensive care unit (PICU) with continuous monitoring of pulse, blood pressure and good venous access with two intravenous lines should be done. Oxygen should be given in patients with SE to avoid desaturation. The airway compromise can occur at any stage due to ongoing seizures or to respiratory depressant effect of medications, therefore oral airway and intubation should be kept ready. Intravenous fluids should be initiated to maintain hydration and blood pressure preferably dextrose normal saline (DNS) or normal saline (NS). If the airway is clear and intubation is not immediately required, blood pressure and pulse should be checked and oxygen administered. In patients with a history of epilepsy, check the medicine the child is taking with any history of drug default. Always check sugar and send calcium levels immediately especially in newborn and infants and glucose and calcium infusion may be initiated depending on the clinical suspicion.

During the initial phase, there may be acidosis, hyperpyrexia, and hypertension need not be treated, because these are common findings in early status epilepticus and should resolve on their own with prompt and successful general treatment but in case if SE is prolonged it results in cerebral dysregulation resulting in hypoxia, cerebral ischemia, hypoglycemia, along with lactic acidosis **(Table 20.1 and Flow chart 20.1)**.

Table 20.1 Systemic complications of generalized convulsive status epilepticus[11]

Cardiovascular system	Cardiac arrhythmia, cardiac arrest, congestive heart failure
Respiratory system	Hypoventilation, apnea, hypoxia, hypercarbia, aspiration pneumonia, pulmonary edema
Metabolic	Lactic acidosis, hypercapnia, hypoglycemia
Renal system	Acute renal failure, myoglobinuria, tubular necrosis, cortical necrosis
Central nervous system	Cerebral edema, CSF pleocytosis, hypoxic ischemic encephalopathy
Endocrine system	Hyperglycemia, hypoglycemia, altered cortisol, pituitary failure
Autonomic system	Vomiting, urine/stool incontinence, tachycardia, bradycardia, hypertension, hypotension, hyperthermia, sweating

INVESTIGATIONS

Blood investigations depend on whether it is the first episode of SE in a normal child, or SE in a child with pre-existing epilepsy and already receiving antiepileptic drugs (AEDs). Early identification of the etiology can result in aggressive specific management of cause.[3] The investigations may include complete blood count, serum electrolyte, blood urea nitrogen, glucose, and antiepileptic drug levels, as well as a toxic drug screen. AED levels should be done receiving AED and presenting with SE, as it has both etiologic (non-compliance/low drug-level as a cause) and therapeutic (loading dose of the previously effective drug for management) implications.[3]

Imaging with computed tomography or magnetic resonance imaging (MRI) is recommended after stabilization of the airway and circulation. MRI is more sensitive and specific than CT scanning, but CT is more widely available and quicker in an emergency setting. If imaging is negative, lumbar puncture is required to rule out infectious etiologies.

If the routine blood test and imaging finding are normal, rare causes like inborn errors of metabolism, genetic causes and autoimmune encephalopathy should be ruled out by appropriate investigations.

Electroencephalography

EEG monitoring is helpful in management of status epilepticus especially in ICU setting. It can be done for short period or as continuous monitoring to rule out electrographic seizures. Sometimes video EEG can be utilized in deciding whether the ongoing clinical activity is epileptic or non-epileptic. After convulsive SE, one-third of children who undergo EEG monitoring are reported to have electrographic seizures, and among these, one-third experience entirely electrographic-only seizures.[12] An EEG should also be done if there is suspicion of non-convulsive SE (child not returning to the pre-SE state or remaining persistently encephalopathic even after the control of convulsive SE).[3] EEG is also important in differentiating focal or generalized seizure discharges and in deciding chronic AED therapy for the patient.

PHARMACOLOGIC MANAGEMENT

Rapid treatment of status epilepticus is crucial to prevent neurologic and systemic complications **(Flow chart 20.1)**. The goal of treatment always should be immediate diagnosis and termination of seizures. For an anti-seizure drug to be effective in status epilepticus, the drug must be administered intravenously to provide quick access to the brain without the risk of serious systemic and neurologic adverse effects **(Table 20.2)**.

Benzodiazepines

The benzodiazepines are some of the most effective drugs in the treatment of acute seizures and status epilepticus. The benzodiazepines most commonly used to treat status epilepticus are diazepam, lorazepam and midazolam. All three compounds work by enhancing the inhibition of γ-aminobutyric acid (GABA) by binding to the benzodiazepine-GABA and barbiturate-receptor complex.

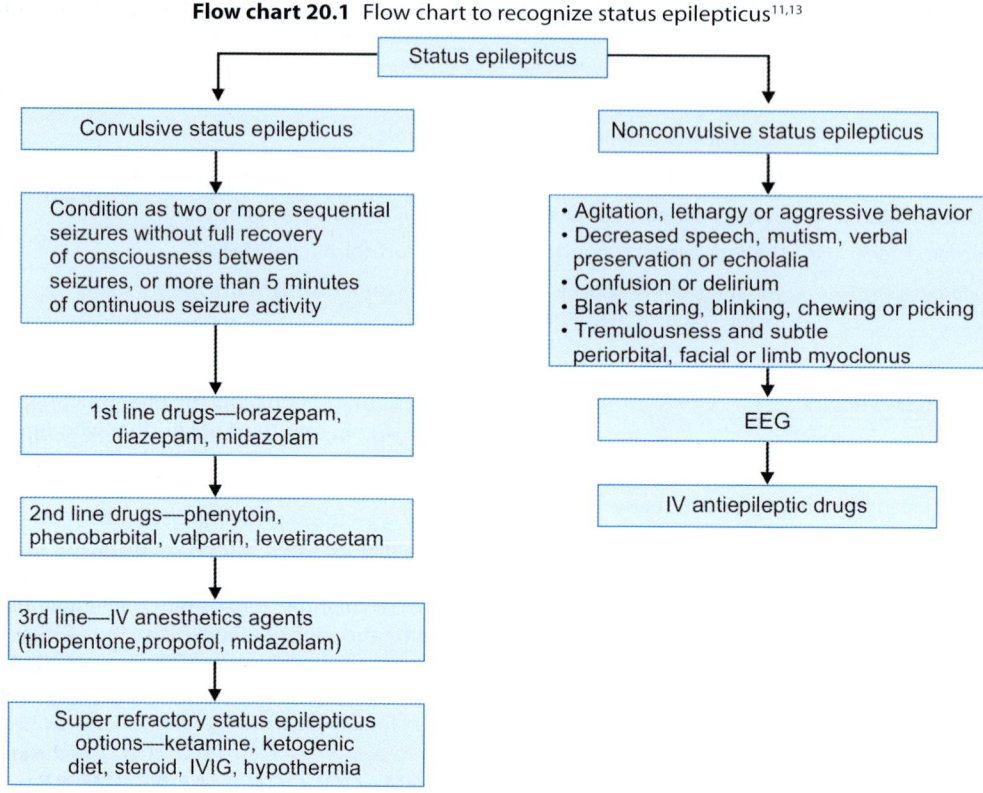

Flow chart 20.1 Flow chart to recognize status epilepticus[11,13]

Diazepam

Diazepam is cheap and easily available benzodiazepine. It is one of the drugs of choice for first-line management of status epilepticus because of its rapid action.[14] It acts within minutes because of its high lipid solubility it redistributes to other areas of the body quickly reducing its clinical effect.[15] The elimination half-life is around 24 hours, thus sedative effects potentially could accumulate with repeated administration. Adverse effects include respiratory suppression, hypotension, sedation, and local tissue irritation. The advantage with diazepam is that it can be stored at room temperature.

Lorazepam

Lorazepam is now regarded as drug of choice for acute management of status epilepticus.[16] It is less lipid-soluble than diazepam, with a distribution half-life of 2-3 hours versus 15 minutes for diazepam. Therefore, it should have a longer duration of clinical effect. The anticonvulsant effects of lorazepam last 6–12 hours.

Midazolam

Midazolam is another benzodiazepine which can be used but the effect is short lasting as compared to lorazepam. Advantage of midazolam is that it can be used as a continuous infusion therapy with a loading dose of 0.2 mg/kg followed by a maintenance infusion of 0.1–2.0 mg/kg/h. As it can cause hypotension and respiratory depression infusion therapy is recommended only under ICU setting.

Phenytoin

Phenytoin is one of the most effective drugs for treating acute seizures and status epilepticus.

The loading dose of the drug offers long-duration seizure—suppression. In addition, it is effective in the management of chronic epilepsy, particularly in patients with partial and secondarily generalized seizures. The main advantage of phenytoin is the lack of a sedating effect. Side effects including arrhythmias and hypotension, local irritation, phlebitis, and dizziness may accompany intravenous administration.

Fosphenytoin

Fosphenytoin is a water-soluble prodrug of phenytoin that completely converts to phenytoin following parenteral administration. Thus, the adverse events that are related to propylene glycol are avoided. It is useful in treating acute partial and generalized tonic-clonic seizures. 1.5 mg of fosphenytoin is equivalent to 1 mg of phenytoin and a rate of infusion that is three times faster than that of intravenous phenytoin. It is metabolized by the liver and has a half-life of 14 hours. Intramuscular doses also can be given, but the drug does not reach a therapeutic level for 30 minutes. Unlike phenytoin, fosphenytoin does not cause local irritation. Intravenous therapy has been associated with hypotension, so continuous cardiac and blood pressure monitoring are recommended.

Phenobarbitone

Phenobarbital typically is used after a benzodiazepine or phenytoin has failed to control status epilepticus. The loading dose is 20 mg/kg and maintenance dose is between 3-5 mg/kg/day in two divided doses. It is particularly effective in newborn and infants. Major side effects are sedation, respiratory depression and hypotension, therefore airway protection and mechanical ventilation should be available. A full therapeutic dose may take 30 minutes to infuse. It is diluted in 60–80 percent propylene glycol, which is associated with a number of complications, including renal failure, myocardial depression, and seizures.[15,17]

Valproate

Recent studies have shown good efficacy of valproic acid in management of status epilepticus similar or superior efficacy to phenytoin and phenobarbitone with fewer side effects.[18,19] The major advantage of valproic acid is the relative lack of sedation, respiratory depression or adverse hemodynamic events. It should be avoided in children with liver disease and suspected metabolic disorders. It has a broad spectrum of efficacy and may be useful in patients with absence or myoclonic status epilepticus.

Levetiracetam

This is the one of the most promising newer anti-epileptic drugs because of fewer side effects, broad spectrum of action and minimal drug interaction. It is particularly suitable in children with liver disease, bleeding diasthesis or metabolic disease. It lacks sedation and respiratory depression.

MANAGEMENT PROTOCOL

First line of drugs are rapidly acting benzodiazepines because of their rapid action and termination of seizures. Lorazepam has few advantages but diazepam is cheap and freely available. Midazolam can also be given but it has short duration of action. These drugs can be repeated twice or thrice but repeated doses are avoided to prevent respiratory depression and sedation.

Second line drugs are usually given in loading dose form. Phenytoin or fosphenytoin is usually the drug of choice but in newborn and infants phenobarbitone is a good option. Recent studies have shown that valproic acid can be loaded with good response.[18] Newer AEDs like levetiracetam and lacosamide are available in parentral preparation.

In case of refractory seizure not controlled with above mentioned drugs, next step is to repeat one of the above mentioned drugs or directly go to infusion therapy with anesthetic agents, if the ICU facilities are available. Anesthetic agents are better option as they are more effective but patient usually requires intubation and ventilatory support. Aim is to achieve burst suppression pattern (BSP) on EEG in which there is a burst of activity followed by a suppression period of at least 10 seconds to make an effective control in seizure activity. Once a good BSP is achieved, it should be maintained for at least 24–48 hours and then only consider tapering

Table 20.2 Management of status epilepticus[13,20]

Timeline 0 to 10 min		
Drugs	Dosage	Comments/precautions/side effects
Diazepam	0.2–0.3 mg/kg IV Max dose—10 mg	*Side effects:* Respiratory depression, sedation
Lorazepam	0.05–0.1 mg/kg/IV Max dose—4 mg	Longer acting then diazepam
Midazolam	0.15–0.2 mg/kg;/IV Max dose 5 mg	Can be given by IM route
If seizure persist at this stage, the above doses can be repeated once or twice		
Timeline 10 to 30/60 min		
Phenytoin or Fosphenytoin	20 mg/kg IV slowly at 1 mg/kg/min in NS *Max:* 1000 mg 30 mg/kg IV at 3 mg/kg/min	Side effects—cardiac arrhythmias, hypotension, 'purple glove syndrome'. Lesser side effects compared with phenytoin. Can be given IM if IV route not available. The maximum rate to infusion is 3 times greater than for phenytoin
Phenobarbitone	20 mg/kg in NS at 1.5 mg/kg/min	*Side effects:* Sedation, respiratory depression, and hypotension
Valproate	IV infusion 25 mg/kg at 3–6 mg/kg/min followed by infusion of 1–2 mg/kg/h	Should be avoided presence in of liver disease, suspected metabolic disease, and in newborn and infants
Levetiracetam	20 mg/kg over 15 min	Minimal interaction with other AEDs. Can be given safely in metabolic diseases, liver disease or coagulopathy
If seizure persist at this stage—repeat half dose of any of the above mentioned AEDs if intubation is not possible.		
Timeline 30/60 min onwards		
Midazolam infusion	*Loading:* 0.2 mg/kg by slow IV bolus *maintenance cIV dose:* 0.1–0.4 mg/kg/h, *maximum cIV dose:* 2.0–3.0 mg/kg/h	*Side effects:* Respiratory depression, sedation
Thiopental sodium	Loading 3 to 5 mg/kg at 0.2–0.4 mg/kg/min *maintenance cIV dose:* 3.0–5.0 mg/kg/h *maximum cIV dose:* 5.0 mg/kg/h	*Side effects:* Respiratory depression, hypotension, heart failure and increased risk of nosocomial infections
Propofol infusion	*Loading dose:* 1–5 mg/kg at 10 mg/min maintenance cIV dose: 2–10 mg/kg/h maximum cIV dose: 15 mg/kg/h	*Side effects:* Lactic acidosis, rhabdomyolysis, hypotension, and hypothermia *Advantage:* Less sedation, shorter time to extubation after discontinuation of the drug
Super- refractory status epilepticus		
Immunotherapy	IVMP 1 g/day × 5 days IVIG 0.4 g/kg/day × 5 days	Limited data available

Contd...

Practical Management of Status Epilepticus

Contd...

Magnesium infusion	Loading: 2-6 g/h to attain a level of 3.5 mmol/L	Limited data available
Ketogenic diet	1:1 or 1:4 ketogenic diet with initial complete avoidance of glucose	Close monitoring of urinary ketones and blood glucose is required
Surgery		Consider surgery in lesional cases
Other therapies		Topiramate, ketamine, inhalational anesthetics, hypothermia, electroconvulsive therapy

Abbreviations: NS, normal saline; cIV, continuous intravenous infusion; IVMP, intravenous methylprednisolone; IVIG, intravenous immunoglobulin; AEDs, antiepiliptic drugs

anesthetic agents. In case of recurrence of seizures during tapering of anesthetic agents, these drugs should be given again for another 12–24 hours, and then tapering of drugs should be attempted again. This cycle may need to be repeated every 24 hours until seizure control is achieved. Ideally continuous EEG monitoring should be done during the IV infusion to look for electrographic seizures and relapse. In a scenario where seizures are controlled but sensorium is not improved a possibility of nonconvulsive status should be considered and a continuous EEG monitoring should be started.

If the seizures are still persisting despite adequate loading with AEDs and anesthetic agents, this condition is termed as super refractory status epilepticus. This condition is difficult to treat. Pulse dose methylprednisolone, IVIg, ketamine, ketogenic diet can be tried with limited success. Recent data have shown that ketogenic diet is effective in controlling seizures in refractory status epilepticus in both adult and pediatric population.[21,22]

Practical Tips

- Treat fever aggressively as it can precipitate seizure recurrences.
- In case of difficult IV access phenobarbital, midazolam and fosphenytoin can be given intramuscularly.
- CSF pleocytosis can occur with repeated seizures.
- AED level monitoring during SE is useful to determine optimal doses.
- Oral AEDs the patient already taking should be continued during the management of SE. Oral route can be changed to IV if drug is available
- Always look for hypoglycemia and correct it.
- Avoid phenytoin in patient with primary generalized epilepsy or idiopathic epilepsy.
- In patients with chronic liver disease levetiracetam is a safe option.

REFERENCES

1. Bone Rc. Treatment of convulsive status epilepticus. Recommendations of the Epilepsy Foundation of America's Working Group on Status Epilepticus. JAMA. 1993;270:854-9.
2. Shinnar S, Berg AT, Moshe SL, Shinnar R. How long do new-onset seizures in children last? Ann Neurol. 2001;49:659-64.
3. Devendra Mishra, Suvasini Sharma, Naveen Sankhyan. Consensus Guidelines on Management of Childhood Convulsive Status Epilepticus. Indian Pediatrics. 51:975-90.
4. Gulati S, Kalra V, Sridhar MR. Status epilepticus in Indian children in a tertiary care center. Indian J Pediatr. 2005;72:105-8.
5. DeLorenzo RJ, Hauser WA, Towne AR, Boggs JG, Pellock JM, PenberthyL, et al. A prospective, population-based epidemiologic study of status epilepticus in Richmond, Virginia. Neurology. 1996;46:1029-35.
6. Shinnar S, Pellock JM, Moshe SL, Maytal J, O'Dell C, Driscoll SM, Al et al. In whom does status epilepticus occur: Age-related differences in children. Epilepsia. 1997;38(8):907-14.
7. DeLorenzo RJ, Ko D, Towne AR, Garnett LK, Boggs JG, Water house EJ, et al. Prediction

of outcome in status epilepticus. Epilepsia. 1997;38(suppl 8):210-5.
8. Towne AR, Pellock JM, Ko D, DeLorenzo RJ. Determinants of mortality in status epilepticus. Epilepsia. 1994;35:27-34.
9. Kaplan PW. Nonconvulsive status epilepticus. Seminars in Neurology. 1996;16:33-40.
10. Alldredge BK, Gelb AM, Isaacs SM, Corry MD, Allen F, Ulrich S, et al. A comparison of lorazepam, diazepam, and placebo for the treatment of out-of-hospital status epilepticus. N Engl J Med. 2001;345:631-7.
11. Sirven JI, Waterhouse E. Management of status epilepticus. American Family Physician. 2003;68(3).
12. Sánchez Fernández I, Abend NS, Arndt DH, Carpenter JL, Chapman KE, Cornett KM, et al. Electrographic seizures after convulsive status epilepticus in children and young adults: a retrospective multicenter study. J Pediatr. 2014; 164:339-46.
13. Guidelines for diagnosis and management of childhood epilepsy. Indian Pedaitrics. 2009:46.
14. Lowenstein DH, Alldredge BK. Status epilepticus. N Engl J Med. 1998;338:970-6.
15. Ramsay RE, Hammond EJ, Perchalski RJ, Wilder BJ. Brain uptake of phenytoin, phenobarbital, and diazepam. Arch Neurol. 1979;36:535-9.
16. Alldredge BK, Gelb AM, Isaacs SM, Corry MD, Allen F, Ulrich S, et al. A comparison of lorazepam, diazepam, and placebo for the treatment of out-of-hospital status epilepticus. N Engl J Med. 2001;345:631-7.
17. Shaner DM, McCurdy SA, Herring MO, Gabor AJ. Treatment of status epilepticus: a prospective comparison of diazepam and phenytoin versus phenobarbital and optional phenytoin. Neurology. 1988;38:202-7.
18. Misra UK, Kalita J, Patel R. Sodium valproate vs phenytoin in status epilepticus: a pilot study. Neurology. 2006;67:340-2.
19. Malamiri RA, Ghaempanah M, Khosroshahi N, Nikkhah A, Bavarian B, Ashrafi MR. Efficacy and safety of intravenous sodium valproate versus phenobarbital in controlling convulsive status epilepticus and acute prolonged convulsive seizures in children: A randomised trial. Eur J Paediatr Neurol. 2012;16:536-41.
20. Appleton R, Choonara I, Martland T, Phillips B, Scott R, Whitehouse W. The treatment of convulsive status epilepticus in children. The Status Epilepticus Working Party, Members of the Status Epilepticus Working Party. Arch Dis Child 2000;83:415-9.
21. Thakur KT, Probasco JC, Hocker SE, et al. Ketogenic diet for adults in super-refractory status epilepticus. Neurology. 2014;82(8):665-70. doi: 10.1212.
22. Nam SH, Lee BL, Lee CG, et al. The role of ketogenic diet in the treatment of refractory status epilepticus. Epilepsia. 2011;52(11): e181-4.

CHAPTER 21

Role of Ketogenic Diet in Management of Pediatric Epilepsy

Kavita Srivastava

OBJECTIVES

- Overview of ketogenic diet.
- *Mechanism of action*: How does it work?
- Efficacy, indications and contraindications of ketogenic diet.
- *The diet protocol*: Prerequisites, initiation, monitoring.
- Adverse effects of ketogenic diet in children.
- Other diets in management of pediatric epilepsy.

OVERVIEW OF KETOGENIC DIET

As early as 500 BC, fasting was recognized as a treatment for many ailments, including seizures and many dietary cures for epilepsy were advocated in the past. The term 'ketogenic diet' (KD) was coined and designed in 1924 by Dr Russell Wilder at the Mayo Clinic, as a means to attain the ketonemia associated with starvation as this could be given for prolonged periods. It seemed to be quite effective in controlling seizures[1] but fell out of fashion due to the surge of antiepileptic drugs (AED) in 1940s.

In 1994, Charlie Abraham, a 2-year-old child of a Hollywood director was featured in a television program, who had intractable seizures, had failed multiple AED as well as a surgery. After starting ketogenic diet, the child rapidly became seizure free and improved cognitively as well. The child went on to become a college graduate. His father founded the Charlie foundation which disseminates information to patients and doctors regarding this effective therapy. Following this, there was a renewed interest in KD, which is now available in 45 countries.[2] The classical ketogenic diet is high in fat (mainly long chain fatty acids) and supplies adequate proteins with minimal carbohydrates. The ratio of fats to (protein plus carbohydrates) is 4:1.

Almost 30% of children with epilepsy are drug resistant, i.e. fail trial of 2 AED. The KD plays an important role in such children, especially if nonlesional epilepsy. The diet is more successful in children as they are dependent on adults for their nutrition and KD has an important place in catastrophic epilepsy syndromes like Dravet, West and Lennox-Gastaut syndromes. Recently, its potential is being tapped for many other neurological disorders including brain tumors. Due to unpalatability of classical ketogenic diet with 4:1 ratio, various modifications like medium chain triglyceride (MCT) diet, Modified Atkins, low glycemic index diets, etc. have evolved to improve the chances of sustaining the diet.

MECHANISM OF ACTION: HOW DOES IT WORK?

Although decades of research have gone into the mechanisms of the diet in epilepsy, they are largely unknown. The saturated fat is converted to mainly long chain fatty acids, high rate of fatty acid oxidation generates large amounts of acetyl–CoA, which exceed the capacity of tricarboxylic acid cycle (TCA), leading to synthesis of ketone bodies (beta hydroxybutyrate, acetoacetate and acetone) in the liver mitochondria. The ketone bodies are elevated 2–4 times, contribute to ketosis and these readily cross the blood brain barrier. The extra hepatic tissues including brain utilize the ketone bodies for energy production: the ketones are oxidized, releasing acetyl-CoA which re-enters the TCA cycle.[3]

Ketone bodies are utilized efficiently and can provide 65% of the brain energy requirements during starvation. Some of the proposed mechanisms include:

The ketone bodies have structural similarity to inhibitory neurotransmitter GABA and may have anticonvulsant action.[4] Ketone bodies are thermodynamically more efficient fuels than glucose because they avoid the less efficient glycolytic pathway. This contributes to higher energy reserves in the brain. This may contribute to increased resistance to seizures as well as cognitive improvement seen in these patients.

Ketogenic diet may be neuroprotective by diminishing reactive oxygen species production through activation of mitochondrial uncoupling proteins. Independently, neither beta hydroxybutyrate nor acetoacetate have proven to have anticonvulsant action. But acetone showed clearly anticonvulsant properties in mice, comparable to phenytoin and valproate—suggesting a possibility that there may be a separate receptor for its action.[5]

As it usually takes about 2 weeks to be effective, it is possible that the effect is mediated through mitochondrial proliferation, upregulation of receptors/transporters, gene expression, etc. thus adaptation to the diet playing a major role in anticonvulsant action. The number of mitochondria was shown to increase by 46% in neurons after KD, the enhanced energy metabolism makes neurons more resistant to metabolic stress in epileptic foci, as well as compensates for transient failures of GABAergic inhibition, thus limiting seizure activity and propagation. Carbohydrate restriction may reduce energy production through glycolysis, limiting the neuronal ability to reach seizure threshold. Glucose restriction causes reduced adenosine diphosphate/adenosine triphosphate (ATP/ADP) ratios, leading to opening of K_{ATP} channels causing hyperpolarization of neurons.[6]

Calorie restriction, glucose deprivation activate an adenosine monophosphate (AMP) kinase, which is a ubiquitous protein that serves as energy sensor in cells. AMP kinase activates tuberous sclerosis complex which reduces the mTOR (mammalian target of rapamycin) pathway thereby reducing protein synthesis and cell growth and proliferation.[7] The ketotic brain astrocyte is more active, converting glutamate (most important excitatory neurotransmitter) to glutamine which is then converted to gamma-aminobutyric acid (GABA), the major inhibitory neurotransmitter.[8]

EFFICACY OF KETOGENIC DIET

The largest single intention to treat prospective study of 150 patients demonstrated at 3 months, 31% had more than 90% reduction in seizures, 26% had 50–90% reduction. After 12 months, 20% had more than 90% reduction while 23% had 50–90% reduction in seizures.[9]

A randomized control trial involving 145 children aged 2–16 years with daily seizures and failed 2 or more antiepileptic drugs showed that 38% in the diet group had more than 50% reduction in seizures.[10]

A meta-analysis of 38 studies to look at therapeutic success rate (>50% reduction in seizures) on KD showed success rates of 58.4% at 3 months, 42.8% at 6 months and 30.1% at 1 year. The reduction in success rates was attributed to reduced compliance. The corresponding figures for prospective studies were 53.9%, 53.2% and 55%. The diet was found to have higher success rates in younger children mainly due to compliance issues.[11] A Cochrane review (2012) showed that KD results in short to medium term benefits in seizure control, the effects of which are comparable to modern antiepileptic drugs.[12]

INDICATIONS AND CONTRAINDICATIONS

The indications and contraindications for ketogenic diet are summarized in **Table 21.1**. Ketogenic diet is the therapy of choice for glucose transporter type 1 deficiency syndrome (GLUT1DS) which is caused by impaired glucose transport into brain and

Role of Ketogenic Diet in Management of Pediatric Epilepsy

Table 21.1 Indications and contraindications are summarized as follows[13]

Indications	Contraindications
Definitely beneficial • Glucose transporter deficiency (Glut 1 DS), • Pyruvate dehydrogenase deficiency (PDHD) • Myoclonic astatic epilepsy (Doose syndrome) • Severe myoclonic epilepsy of infancy (Dravet) • Lennox gastaut syndrome	*Absolute* • Carnitine deficiency, carnitine translocase deficiency, pyruvate carboxylase deficiency, carnitine pamitoyl transferase (I and II) deficiency Beta oxidation defects (MCAD, SCAD, LCAD), Porphyria
Suggestion of benefit • Rett syndrome • Tuberous sclerosis complex • Selected mitochondrial disorders • Glycogenosis type V • Landau-kleffner syndrome • Lafora body disease • Sub-acute sclerosing panencephalitis	*Relative* • Hyperlipidemia • Inability to maintain nutrition • Surgical focus • Parent or child noncompliance

Novel indications (anecdotal evidence)[14]
Alzheimer's disease, parkinsonism, migraine, autism, traumatic brain injury, amyotrophic lateral sclerosis, stroke, CSWS (Continuous spike wave in sleep), refractory and super-refractory status epilepticus, FIRES—Febrile infection related refractory status epilepticus, neonates with catastrophic epilepsies, brain tumors: especially malignant glioma, etc.

manifests with early onset epilepsy, developmental delay and a complex movement disorder. The diet provides ketones as an alternative fuel to the brain. It should be introduced early to meet the demands of the developing brain and continued till puberty. Seizures are effectively controlled but the effect on movement disorder and neurodevelopment are less impressive.[15]

In children with intractable epilepsy, KD also improves the sleep quality and thereby the quality of life.[16] In such children, it has also shown significant improvement in epileptiform abnormalities in EEG, especially during sleep which correlated with improved seizure outcome and attention.[17] In another study, 24 hours EEG was done before and after 3 months of diet. The EEG showed significant reduction in interictal discharges in both responders as well as non-responders although it did not always correlate with reduction in seizures.[18] Serial EEGs can be helpful in predicting positive therapeutic outcomes on the diet.[19]

All patients with intractable epilepsy who have failed a reasonable dose of correctly chosen two antiepileptic drugs and nonresectable focus on MRI should be considered for a trial of ketogenic diet. There are very few centers offering ketogenic diet in India due to low level of awareness and lack of trained dieticians. Dr Janak Nathan, Mumbai has pioneered the Indianization of the ketogenic recipes (e.g. Dhokla, Idli, etc.) to suit Indian tastes and has contributed largely to the cultural acceptance of the diet among patients and spreading awareness regarding dietary therapies for epilepsy amongst neurologists in India.

PREDIET EVALUATION

If there is a clinical suspicion of inborn error of fat metabolism (e.g. developmental delay, cardiomyopathy, hypotonia, etc.), testing should be done to rule them out before initiation of the diet. Typically, 2–3 visits are scheduled before the actual initiation of the diet. Evaluation to rule out any metabolic disorders as well as complicating factors like dyslipidemia, gastroesophageal reflux, liver disease, kidney stones, constipation, etc. is done prior to start of diet in a suitable candidate. The parent is counseled to shift the child's medications from any liquid (syrup) to tablet forms, without sugar. It is important for them to realize that even a small amount of sugar (as in toothpaste/cough syrups, etc.) can interfere with ketosis.

The importance of strict adherence to the diet, restriction of carbohydrates and potential side effects are explained in detail. Any psycho-behavioral issues which may interfere with compliance should be identified. The parents should be given realistic expectations regarding seizure control, reduction of concomitant medications, etc. The weighing of meals, substitutions, managing sick days, nutritional supplementation, etc. is discussed.

The evaluation prior to diet and on follow-up is summarized in **Table 21.2**.

INITIATION OF DIET

Staple Indian diet consists of 65% carbohydrates, 12% proteins and 25% as fats, while ketogenic diet consists of 66% fats, 20% proteins and 14% carbohydrates. The classic KD is calculated in a ratio of grams of fat to grams of protein plus carbohydrate. Most common ratio being 4:1 (i.e. 4 g of fat to 1 g of protein plus carbohydrate). There is some evidence that 4:1 ratio may be more advantageous in the first 3 months.[13]

CLASSICAL/JOHNS HOPKINS HOSPITAL PROTOCOL[20]

Day 1: This consisted of admitting the child with strict fasting period of 2–3 days. No solid foods are given, fluids are restricted to 70 cc/kg body weight and consist of sugar free beverage, water etc. During the fasting period, glucose is monitored 6 hourly or earlier if lower values. If sugar falls below 40, orange juice is given. The urine is monitored for ketones.

Day 2: Fasting continues till the child is ketotic with 4+ ketones in urine, then feeds are introduced. The first 3 meals are 1/3 of calculated diet, meals 4th–6th are 2/3rd, followed by full meals from 7th meal onwards. This gradual progression helps the child to get accustomed to the diet. Also, the ratio can be adjusted early if intolerance is seen.

Day 3: The typical diet will consist of three meals and two snacks in 24 hours. Once the child is tolerating the diet well and ketosis is maintained, the child is discharged, usually by day 4. Family is taught to monitor urinary ketones at home.

MODIFICATIONS TO JOHNS HOPKINS HOSPITAL PROTOCOL

It was established later that there was no need for hospitalization to initiate diet and it could be started on outpatient basis.[9] Also, the need for fasting was questioned as studies have shown that slow initiation (1:1 ratio followed by gradual buildup to 4:1) is as good as fast initiation and children as far as efficacy is concerned while improving the tolerability. It was shown that children in non-fasting group had less hypoglycemia, acidosis and dehydration while time to ketonuria was not different.[21]

Table 21.2 Recommendations for evaluation at initiation and follow-up visits on ketogenic diet[13]

At initiation	During follow-up visits
Nutritional Baseline weight, height, body mass index Diet recall, food preferences, calorie requirement, protein: Fat ratio according to diet chosen	*Nutritional:* Same as initiation Check vitamin supplementation: B complex, vitamin D, calcium, zinc, trace minerals: selenium, magnesium, phosphorus *Optional:* Citrate, carnitine (*all as tablets*)
Lab evaluation Complete blood count, fasting lipid profile, serum acylcarnitine profile, urine analysis, serum sodium, potassium, bicarbonate, calcium, magnesium serum amino acids, urine organic acids SGOT, SGPT, serum urea, creatinine renal ultrasound (if family history of urolithiasis)	*Lab evaluation* Complete blood count, fasting lipid profile, serum electrolytes, urea, creatinine, SGOT, SGPT Urine analysis, serum acylcarnitine profile *Optional:* Anticonvulsant drug levels, renal ultrasound, bone mineral density EEG if desired by neurologist
Counseling Nature of diet, compliance, ketone monitoring, preparation of meals, anticonvulsant formulation	*Other issues:* Efficacy, compliance, side effects, whether any of the anticonvulsants can be tapered, adjust therapy to balance efficacy and tolerability

Although higher ketogenic ratio (4:1) contributed to better efficacy, the tolerability was poor. It was shown later that KD was effective in controlling seizures even at lower ratios of 3:1. There was also no evidence to support fluid restriction, and given the higher risk of nephrolithiasis, adequate fluid intake is encouraged.[22]

A typical meal consists of eggnog (egg with whipped cream), fats (oils, butter, *ghee*, margarine), proteins (vegetarian-cheese, paneer or nonvegetarian—eggs, chicken, fish, mutton) etc. Carbohydrates are allowed only as fruits or vegetables. For vegetarians, the major source of proteins are soya products. The diet control required is very strict and even an occasional 'cookie' can break the ketosis and cause breakthrough seizures. Vitamin and mineral supplements should be prescribed.

The algorithm to determine the meals require extensive calculations by an experienced dietician. Presently, a web based tool called keto-calculator is available.[23] Monitoring on the diet is listed in the **Table 21.2**. A trial of reduction or omission of one or more of anticonvulsants may be given if there is a good control for at least 3 months. Certain drugs like topiramate, zonisamide may add to the side effects of nephrolithiasis, acidosis while valproate may worsen the secondary carnitine deficiency. The diet is adjusted to maintain proper growth and follow-up is planned at least every 3 monthly. When effective, usually improvement is noted within 7–14 days. The time to improvement was quicker in fasted children but the long-term outcomes did not differ.[24]

ADVERSE EFFECTS OF THE KETOGENIC DIET

Most complications of the KD are transient and can be managed easily. The early and late onset complications are summarized in **Tables 21.3** and **21.4**. Gastrointestinal discomfort, though not usually life threatening, is the most important factor contributing to tolerability. Despite a long list of possible complications, only a small number of patients are known to stop the diet due to complications.[25]

The long-term complications of the diet are summarized in **Table 21.4**. It is recommended to keep a protein to energy ratio of 1.5 g/100 calories

Table 21.3 Early onset complications of ketogenic diet		
Early onset complications	Measures to avoid	Remedy
Dehydration (common if fasting protocol)	No fasting at KD initiation	Oral/IV fluids @ 75%
Gastrointestinal discomfort: Nausea, vomiting, diarrhea. These are mainly due to intolerance of fat, prolonged gastric emptying time. Constipation may also be seen due to low fiber/volume of the diet	Modification of menu, frequent intake of smaller amounts, treatment of concomitant GERD, gastritis (if on steroids)	Antiemetics, antacids, GI motility modifying agents, antidiarrheals Laxatives for constipation
Metabolic: Transient hypoglycemia (asymptomatic)	Step wise increase in calories	Orange juice (no sugar)
Lipids Hypertriglyceridemia, Hypercholesterolemia, low HDL values	Usually do not need treatment as no long-term risk of cardiovascular events	Combination of oils and ghee is used. Soya products and fiber help to reduce cholesterol
Secondary hypocarotenemia	Avoid valproate if possible	Carnitine supplementation
Hypoproteinemia, hyperuricemia, hyponatremia, acidosis, hypomagnesemia	Diet adjustments for salt, protein, minerals	Vitamin and mineral supplementation
Life threatening complications: Lipoid pneumonia (uncontrolled vomiting may require fundoplication), *Acute hepatitis and pancreatitis* (hypertriglyceridemia and valproate), *Severe sepsis* (immunologic dysfunction in severely retarded children due to protein imbalance), *Severe prolonged hypoglycemia* (seen if underlying metabolic defect has been missed)		

Table 21.4 Late onset complications of ketogenic diet

Complications	Measures to avoid	Remedy
Osteopenia: Can cause fractures	Monitoring with bone densitometry, exposure to sunlight, weight bearing exercises	Vitamin D and calcium supplementation
Urolithiasis: Usually formed in 5–14 months: uric acid, calcium oxalate, mixed stones may be formed, mostly due to chronic acidosis and dehydration)	Hydration with larger amounts of water, citrate supplement, avoid carbonic anhydrase inhibitors like topiramate, zonisamide	Stop offending drugs, rarely hydrochlorothiazide, extra-corporeal shock wave lithotripsy (ESWL) may be required for obstructive/symptomatic stones
Cardiac: Cardiomyopathy due to selenium and carnitine deficiency, acidosis, etc.	Periodic ECG for bradycardia, prolonged QT, reduced QRS voltage. May be fatal	Selenium and carnitine supplementation, rule out metabolic disorders
Growth: Conflicting reports whether growth retardation	Periodic growth monitoring	Adequate calorie, proteins and vitamin-mineral supplements

to prevent growth retardation.[26] There is some concern regarding increased arterial stiffness which may be an early marker of vascular damage, and such children may warrant aggressive treatment of hyperlipidemia with statins or conversion to less fat versions.[27]

DISCONTINUATION OF KETOGENIC DIET

If the seizures worsen for more than a few days after starting of KD, the diet can be immediately discontinued. In children with >50% seizure response, the KD can be discontinued after 2 years. If seizures were controlled by > 90%, with no significant side effects, it can be given for longer periods, especially if GLUT1 deficiency, tuberous sclerosis, etc.

If the diet has been effective, 80% of children will remain seizure free after the diet has been discontinued. If seizures worsen, it can be increased to a previously effective formulation. Gradual weaning over 2-3 months is advisable, similar to antiepileptic withdrawal. Abnormal EEG, abnormal MRI predict a higher risk of recurrence on withdrawal.[13] Long-term study after discontinuation showed that most subjects were doing well and had normal lipid profiles and body mass indices even if they were abnormal while on diet.[28]

Like all therapies, KD also has potential adverse effects. Overall, the risk of serious adverse events is low and the KD does not need to be discontinued for these reasons in most children. However, the treating physician should be aware of the complications to monitor and prevent if possible.

RECENT ADVANCES IN KETOGENIC DIET

Recently, ketogenic diet has been recognized for its neuroprotective and anti-inflammatory properties.[29,30] KD not only improves seizure control but also has significant effects on sleep and EEG. It is becoming an important supplement to antiepileptics, including general anesthesia in children with refractory and super-refractory status epilepticus, especially FIRES (febrile infection induced refractory epilepsy syndrome).[31] Intravenous ketogenic diet was found to be successful in attaining fast ketosis resulting in successful control of super refractory status epilepticus.[32]

MORE LIBERAL KETOGENIC DIETS

In view of poor tolerability of the classical ketogenic diet, several less strict diets with high fats and low carbohydrates were developed and found to be effective. These are *modified Atkin's diet* (MAD), *low glycemic index diet* (LGID), and *medium chain triglyceride* (MCT) diet. Some important features of these are summarized in **Table 21.5**.

Table 21.5 Comparison of ketogenic diet with other diets[33]

Parameter	Ketogenic diet	MCT oil diet	Low glycemic index diet	Modified Atkins diet
Design of the diet	Highly structured diet with fat: protein ratio of 3-4:1. Carbohydrates are allowed only as vegetables and fruits. Fats are mainly LCT (Long chain triglycerides)	Structured diet, MCT oils produce more ketones, hence allows more carbohydrate and proteins to be given. Avoid on valproate MCT proportion decided according to tolerance	Less structured, based on exchange lists with complex, low glycemic carbohydrates. Leads to steady glucose levels with no ketosis	High fat diet with low carbohydrates, proteins not limited. Meal plans given accordingly
Fat to protein and carb ratio	4:1 (Classic) To 1:1 (modified)	1:1	1:1	0.9:1
Carbohydrates allowed/1000 Kcal	8 g (4:1) to 50 g (1:1)	40–60 g	40–60 g	10 g for 1 month, then 20 g
How are foods measured?	Weighed	Weighed or measured	Measured or estimated	Estimated
Are calories controlled?	Strictly controlled	Yes	Yes	No
Vitamin and mineral supplements	Required	Essential fatty acids also supplemented	Required	Required
Efficacy	Well established in literature	Equivalent to KD for elimination of seizures, but more expensive	Efficacy comparable to KD, simpler to implement	Efficacy good, gaining popularity in adults

Medium chain triglyceride diet has been studied in children and found to be effective as well as better tolerated, compared to KD. It is especially suited for children who have large appetites, or cannot accept the restrictions of classic KD.[34] As more variety is allowed, less chances of growth failure and fewer supplements are required. There are also fewer side effects of calculi, acidosis, hypoglycemia, etc. It should not be combined with valproate as there are case reports of liver failure.[35]

The LGID restricts carbohydrates to those with low glycemic index (GI). The glycemic index is a measure of a food's tendency to elevate blood glucose. Foods are classified according to glucose generating potential from 0 to 100. Foods with high glycemic index like watermelon, potatoes, etc. are avoided and those of less than 50 (apple, cucumber, whole grain breads, etc.) are used. The factors affecting the GI of a diet include particle size, type of starch, presence of fiber, fats and acidity. It provides comparable efficacy to KD but better tolerability due to flexibility and simpler implementation.[36]

The MAD has less fat than KD but still has three times fat of the normal diet. There is no restriction on type of carbohydrate, unlike LGIT, but the quantity is restricted to 10 g/day for the first month. It is more popular among adults where acceptability of KD is very poor. One more advantage is that the family members can also be on diet to improve compliance, as it leads to health benefits like weight loss. It is slowly becoming popular as step down diet if KD has been found effective in seizure control but is difficult to continue due to side effects.[37] In a study of intractable childhood epilepsy, liquid ketogenic supplement was added to MAD in the initial one month with beneficial effects.[38]

KEY MESSAGES

Traditionally, KD has been reserved as a last treatment option after failure of three or more anticonvulsants. Given its efficacy, it should be offered early, after two anticonvulsant drugs have failed. It is particularly useful for certain devastating epilepsy syndromes like Glut 1 transporter deficiency, Dravet, Doose, West, Lennox Gastaut syndrome, etc. The contraindications should be kept in mind, viz. mitochondrial disorders, disorders of fatty acid metabolism, etc.

Families are often interested in nonmedicinal avenues of treatment and knowledge of these options can empower a pediatrician to help families make choices that have scientific validity.[39] It should be initiated in consultation with a dietician trained in this field with periodic follow-up and monitoring for seizure reduction and complications. The more liberal options like MCT, LGID and MAD are slowly gaining favor due to increased tolerability.

In the coming years, as more centers across India offer ketogenic diets, and more neurologists become aware of this efficacious option, it should find its rightful place in management of pediatric patients with nonlesional intractable epilepsy who otherwise are condemned to indefinite trials of multiple AEDs. Recent (June 2015) recommendations published by the International league Against Epilepsy Task Force for dietary therapy provide excellent and practical guidance for minimum requirements for establishment of a new ketogenic diet center in resource limited settings.[40]

ACKNOWLEDGMENTS

Professor S Rajadhyaksha, Vijay Kalrao and Jitendra Oswal (Department of Pediatrics, Bharati Vidyapeeth Medical College, Pune, Maharashtra, India) for critical review of the manuscript

REFERENCES

1. Freeman JM, Vining EPG, Pillas DJ, et al. The efficacy of the ketogenic diet: a prospective evaluation of intervention in 150 children. Pediatrics. 1998;102:1358-63.
2. Wheless JW. History of the ketogenic diet. Epilepsia. 2009;49(S8):3-5.
3. Kosoff EH, Vining EPG. The Ketogenic diet. In: Shorvon S (Ed) Treatment of epilepsy. Oxford Press. 2004.pp.262-8.
4. Nordli Jr DR, De Vivo DC. The ketogenic diet. In: Pellock JM, Bourgeois BFD, Dodson WE (Eds). Pediatric Epilepsy. 3rd edn. Demos Medical Publishing. 2008.pp.739-50.
5. Likhodii S, Nylen K, Burham WM. Acetone as an anticonvulsant. Epilepsia. 2008:49(S8):83-6.
6. Bough KJ, Rho JM. Anticonvulsant mechanisms of the ketogenic diet. 2007;48(1):43-58.
7. Yamada KA. Calorie restriction and glucose regulation. Epilepsia. 2008;49(S8):94-6.
8. Yudkoff M, Daikhin Y, Horyn O, et al. Ketosis and brain handling of glutamate, glutamine and GABA. Epilepsia. 2008;49(8):73-5.
9. Hartman AL, Vining EPG. Critical reviews: Clinical aspects of the ketogenic diet. Epilepsia. 2007;48(1):31-42.
10. Neal EG, Chaffe H, Schwartz RH, et al. The ketogenic diet for the treatment of childhood epilepsy: a randomized control trial. Lancet Neurol. 2008;7(6):500-6.
11. Li H-F, Zou Y, Ding G. Therapeutic success of the ketogenic diet as a treatment option for epilepsy: a meta-analysis. Iran J Pediatr. 2013;23 (6):613-20.
12. Levy RG, Cooper PN, Giri P, et al. Ketogenic diet and other dietary treatments for epilepsy. Cochrane Database of Systematic Reviews, Issue 3, 2012.
13. Kossoff EH, Zupec-Kania BA, Amark PE, et al. Optimal clinical management of children receiving the ketogenic diet: Recommendations of the International Ketogenic diet Study group. Epilepsia, 2008.
14. Special supplement on Ketogenic diet. Journal of Child Neurology: August, 2013.
15. Klepper J. Glucose transporter deficiency syndrome (GLUT1DS) and the ketogenic diet. Epilepsia. 2008; 49(8):46-9.
16. Hallbook T, Lundgren J, Rosen I. Ketogenic diet improves sleep quality in children with therapy resistant epilepsy. Epilepsia. 2007;48(1):59-65.
17. Hallbook T, Kohler S, Rosen I. Effects of ketogenic diet on epileptiform activity in children with therapy resistant epilepsy. Epilepsy Res. 2007;77(2-3):134-40.
18. Remahl S, Dahlin MG, Amark PE. Influence of the ketogenic diet on 24 hour EEG in children with epilepsy. Pediatr Neurol. 2008;38(1):38-43.

19. Walker I, Said RR. Predictors of ketogenic diet efficacy in children based on the EEG. J Child Neurol, 2014.
20. Swink TD, Vining EPG, Freeman JM. The Ketogenic diet: Mosby Year Book, Advances in Pediatrics. 1997;44:297-329.
21. Bergquist AGC, Schall JI, Gallagher PR, et al. Fasting versus gradual initiation of the ketogenic diet: A prospective, randomized clinical trial of efficacy. Epilepsia. 2005;46(11):1810-9.
22. Wirrell EC. Ketogenic ratio, calories, and fluids: Do they matter? Epilepsia. 2008;49(8):17-9.
23. Zupec-Kania B. Ketocalculator: A web based calculator for the ketogenic diet. Epilepsia. 2008; 49(8):14-6.
24. Kossoff EH, Laux LC, Blackford R, et al. When do seizures usually improve with the ketogenic diet? Epilepsia. 2008;49(2):329-33.
25. Kang HC, Chung DE, Kim DW, et al. Early and Late onset complications of the ketogenic diet for intractable epilepsy. Epilepsia. 2004;45(99): 1116-23.
26. Nation J, Humphrey M, Mackay M, et al. Linear growth of children on a ketogenic diet : Does the protein to calorie ratio matter? J Child Neurol. 2014;29:1496-501.
27. Coppola G, Natale F, Torino A, et al. The impact of the ketogenic diet on arterial morphology and endothelial function in children and young adults with epilepsy: A case-control study. Seizure. 2013;23:260-5.
28. Patel A, Pyzik PL, Turner Z, et al. Long term outcomes of children treated with the ketogenic diet in the past. Epilepsia. 2010;51(7):1277-82.
29. Gasior M, Rogawski MA, Hartman AL, et al. Neuroprotective and disease modifying effects of the ketogenic diet. Behav Pharmacol. 2006; 17(5-6):431-9.
30. Duplus N, Curatolo N, Benoist JF, et al. Ketogenic diet exhibits anti-inflammatory properties. Epilepsia, 2015, ahead of publication.
31. Kossoff E. The fat is in the fire: Ketogenic diet for refractory status epilepticus. Epilepsy Currents 2011;11(3): 88-89.
32. Lin JJ, Lin KL, Chan OW, et al. Intravenous ketogenic diet therapy for the treatment of the acute stage of super-refractory status epilepticus in a pediatric patient. Pediatr neurol. 2015;52(4): 442-5.
33. Zupec-Kania B. The Charlie Foundation Position statement on the diet therapies for epilepsy. Available on *http://www.charliefoundation.org* (accessed on 14th March 2015).
34. Liu YC. Medium chain triglyceride (MCT) ketogenic therapy. Epilepsia. 2008;49(8):33-6.
35. Liu YC, Wang HS. Medium chain triglyceride ketogenic diet, an effective treatment for drug resistant epilepsy and a comparison with other ketogenic diets. Biomed J. 2013;36:9-15.
36. Pfeifer HH, Lyczkowski DA, Thiele EA. Low glycemic index treatment: Implementation and new insights into efficacy. Epilepsia. 2008;49(8): 42-5.
37. Kossoff EH, Dorward JL. The modified Atkins diet. Epilepsia. 2008;49(8):37-41.
38. Kossoff EH, Dorward JL, Turner Z, et al. Prospective study of the modified atkins diet in combination with a ketogenic liquid supplement during the initial month. J Child Neurol. 2011;26(92):147-51.
39. Sharp GB, Smanta D, Willis E. Options for pharmacoresistant epilepsy in children: when medications don't work. Pediatr Ann. 2015;44 (2):43-8.
40. Kossoff EH, Al-Macki N, Cervenka MC, et al. What are the minimum requirements for keto-genic diet services in resource limited regions? Recommendations from the International League Against Epilepsy Task Force for dietary therapy. Epilepsia, 2015, ahead of print.

CHAPTER **22**

Neurological Dysfunctions in Iron Deficiency Anemia

TM Ananda Kesavan

OBJECTIVES

- To know about magnitude of iron deficiency anemia in India
- Role of iron in brain function
- To know neurologic sequelae of iron deficiency in children.

INTRODUCTION

Iron is the one of the most abundant element in the earth. But iron deficiency (ID) is the most common micronutrient deficiency in the world! Nutritional anemia is a major public health problem in India and is primarily due to iron deficiency. The National Family Health Survey-3 (NFHS-3) data suggests that anemia is widely prevalent among all age groups, and is particularly high among the most vulnerable—nearly 58% among pregnant women, 50% among nonpregnant nonlactating women, 56% among adolescent girls (15–19 years), 30% among adolescent boys and around 80% among children under 3 years of age.[1]

Seven out of every 10 children aged 6–59 months in India are anemic—3% are severely anemic, 40% are moderately anemic, and 26% are mildly anemic. The prevalence of anemia ranges from 38% in Goa to 78% in Bihar. More than half of young children in 24 states have anemia, including 11 states where more than two thirds of children are anemic. It is very sad to notice that the prevalence of anemia has actually increased from NFHS-2 to NFHS-3. The percentage of children with any anemia increased from 74.3% in NFHS-2 to 78.9% in NFHS-3. In the period between the two surveys, there was an increase in the prevalence of mild anemia (from 23% to 26%) and moderate anemia (from 46% to 49%).

Although the most common manifestation of ID is anemia, it is frequently associated with neurologic disorders presenting to general pediatric neurologic practices. These disorders include developmental delay, stroke, breath-holding episodes, attention deficit hyperactive disorder, etc. The identification of iron deficiency as part of the differential diagnosis in these disorders is uncommon and frequently goes untreated. The purpose of the current review is to highlight what is understood regarding ID and it's underlying pathophysiology as it relates to the brain and the association of ID with common neurologic pediatric disease.

PATHOPHYSIOLOGY

The blood-brain barrier provides an effective regulatory point for iron movement from the plasma pool to the cerebral spinal fluid. The choroids plexus is also a likely source of iron movement into and out of the brain. Not all brain regions contain the same amount of iron.

Iron, transported by transferrin, enters brain endothelial cells via receptor-mediated endocytosis.[2] Once in the brain, the transportation of iron is poorly understood. Iron uptake during early postnatal development is rapid, leading to brain iron concentrations that are one-half that of the adult rat (most investigations of brain iron have been performed in the rat model) by as early as the third week of life.[3] Iron uptake subsequently decreases with age. The iron attained by the developing brain becomes sequestered.

The distribution of brain iron changes with age, presumably as a result of the altering brain region requirements of iron at different neuro developmental stages.[4] Iron is distributed unevenly and is present in both gray and white matter.[5] It is most commonly located in oligodendrocytes of rat and human brains.[3] Iron-rich areas in the mature rat include the circumventricular regions and regions in which iron is associated with oligodendrocytes and the neuropil network **(Table 22.1)**.

Iron-binding capability diminishes with age, suggesting that aged animals are unable to remove free iron that can lead to free radical production and cell death.[6] Free iron has been implicated in the pathophysiology of several brain diseases, including Parkinson's disease, Alzheimer's disease and multiple sclerosis.[7]

The biological basis of the behavioral and cognitive developmental delays observed in iron-deficient infants is not completely understood but possibilities include:
- Decreased myelin formation
- Alterations in brain energy metabolism
- Abnormalities in neurotransmitter metabolism.

Iron and myelin formation: Oligodendrocytes are the myelin-producing cells in the brain. Iron is required for myelin production, in that it is a cofactor for cholesterol and lipid bio-synthesis.[2] Also oligodendrocytes have a high level of oxidative metabolism and therefore require iron for metabolic processes. In addition to myelin production, oligodendrocytes have the additional function of storing and mobilizing iron in the central nervous system.[2,8] Early exposure to ID during critical periods of brain development is believed to result in "irreversible" damage, resulting in clinical sequelae such as developmental delay.

Delayed myelination and hypomyelination have been demonstrated in rats with prenatal and lactational ID.[9] The synthesis of nervonic acid is decreased and the ratio between sphingolipids and nervonic acid is abnormal in IDA. The direct effect of decreased nervonic acid synthesis is the postulated mechanism by which ID delays myelination.

Alteration in brain energy metabolism: Iron is directly or indirectly involved in various metabolic process in brain. A large number of enzymes are known to contain iron or require iron as a co-factor, including cytochrome oxidase, succinate dehydrogenase, aconitase, catalase, myelo peroxidase, cytochrome C reductase, ribonucleotide reductase, tyrosine hydroxylase, and xanthine oxidase. Consequently in ID, there are changes in nucleic acid biosynthesis, oxidative respiration and mitochondrial function, detoxification of metabolic byproducts, and catecholamine metabolism.[3,4] Because iron is imperative to maintain normal organ function at a cellular level, it is not surprising that its deficiency results in a variety of clinical manifestations affecting most organ systems including nervous system **(Table 22.2)**.

Table 22.1 Iron-rich area in the brain[5]

- Globus pallidus
- Ventral pallidum
- Substantia nigra reticulata
- Interpeduncular nucleus
- Cerebellar nuclei
- Facial nucleus
- Superior olive

Table 22.2 Neurological manifestation of iron deficiency

• Fatigability	• Cognitive impairment
• Anorexia	• Sensorineural hearing loss
• Reduced attention span	• Restless leg syndrome
• Irritability	• Febrile seizure
• Growth retardation (weight > height)	• Stroke
• Behavioral changes	• Breath-holding episodes
• Developmental delay	• Pseudotumor cerebri
• Learning disability (writing, mathematics)	• Cranial nerve palsies
• Poor scholastic performance	

Table 22.3 Neurochemical effect of iron deficiency[10,11]

Neurochemical	Metabolic effect	Clinical effect	Reversibility
GABA	+/− GABA Decreased GAD, GABA-T	Impaired neurotransmitter regulation of hypothalamic-hypophyseal hormones	Irreversible in gestational iron deficiency
Dopamine	Decreased D2 receptor binding sites	Decreased motor activity and learning processes	Irreversible
Phenylalanine	Increased phenylalanine secondary to decreased phenylalanine like" effect hydroxylase activity	Decreased learning secondary to "PKU- like" effect	Reversible
Serotonin	Decreased 5-HT via decreased, tryptophan or tyrosine hydroxylase activity, Or Increased 5-HT via decreased degradation by aldehyde oxidase	Impairs neurodevelopment Or Increased drowsiness, decreased attention and learning due to serotonergic effect	Irreversible Or Reversible

Abbreviations: GABA, gamma aminobutyric acid; GAD, glutamate decarboxylase; D, dopamine; 5-HT, 5-hydroxy tryptophan; PKU, phenylketonuria

Neurochemical effects: In iron deficiency, there is decrease in neurotransmitter synthesis. The change in neurotransmitter activity has been a suggested mechanism resulting in the clinical abnormalities observed in ID **(Table 22.3)**.

NEUROLOGIC SEQUELAE OF IRON DEFICIENCY IN CHILDREN

Neurological problems postulated to be associated with ID is described below.

Poor Cognitive Development

Cognitive performance and school achievement scores are low in children with low Hb.[12] Children with ID in early life demonstrate lower academic performance during their school years even after the anemia had been treated. When comparing to nonanemic children, ID children showed poor performance on tests assessing development, cognitive performance and in subjects like mathematics.[13] It is not reversible with an iron-replete diet.

A Cochrane review examined the impact of iron therapy in children less than three years with IDA.[14] Improvement was observed in mental and motor development, cognitive performance and language skills. Studies in developing countries have found a beneficial effect of long-term treatment of anemic children.[15]

The children with moderately severe anemia in infancy had lower mental and motor scores in most areas compared with their nonanemic peers. It was suggested that prolonged severe iron deficiency in infancy is associated with poor developmental outcome at 5 years of age.[16] Unfortunately, no practice guidelines have been published on screening for ID or use of iron supplementation to prevent cognitive or behavioral defects.

Low iron exposure during lactational period results in irreversible brain ID despite adequate therapy. Early exposure to ID during critical periods of brain development is believed to result in "irreversible" damage, resulting in clinical sequelae such as delayed development.[17]

Walter, et al.[18] studied a cohort of 196 Chilean infants from infancy to 5 years of age. IDA infants had lower baseline mental and psychomotor scores that were not corrected after 3 months of iron therapy. Further analysis of the data suggested that prolonged iron deficiency and severe anemia in infancy result in irreversible developmental changes despite correction of anemia.

Lozoff has looked further at behavior of ID infants.[19] The study concluded that anemic infants are "functionally isolated" as a result of altered interaction with their physical and social environment. This in turn interferes with their natural development, resulting in motor and cognitive delay. Other authors have also noted similar observation.[20]

Pediatric Stroke

Pediatric stroke is uncommon, occurring in approximately 2–3/1L/year. Stroke in association with ID has been reported in the pediatric and adult literature in a number of case reports.[21] Several mechanisms have been proposed (**Table 22.4**).

Breath-holding Spells

Breath-holding spells (BHS) have been associated with ID and can occur in up to 27% of affected children.[24] Autonomic dysregulation resulting in vagally mediated cardiac arrest or bradycardia has been proposed, as have the effects of anemia on reducing oxygen carrying capacity. ID children also are known to be more irritable; presumably, this may increase the likelihood of an event. Treatment with iron supplementation has been shown to significantly reduce or eliminate the risk of recurrence.[24]

Benign Intracranial Hypertension

ID as a cause of benign intracranial hypertension has been recognized years back.[23] It is most commonly seen in young females. Although the underlying mechanism is unknown it has been proposed that the tissue hypoxia leads to increased capillary permeability and development of brain edema or abnormalities in cerebrovascular hemodynamics that increase the cerebral blood flow, leading to increased intracranial pressure. Depletion of iron containing enzymes also may contribute to the development of cerebral edema. Benign hypertension due to ID is reversible with iron supplementation.[25]

Cranial Nerve Palsy

Another neurologic abnormality observed with iron deficiency anemia (IDA) is bilateral 6th cranial nerve palsy. This is proposed to be a consequence of increased intracranial pressure or focal pontine ischemia.

Hearing Problem

Auditory evoked brain stem response is found to be prolonged in ID children. It may be due to impaired myelin synthesis.[26] ID has also been hypothesized to be a cause of sensorineural hearing loss in the rat model. It is proposed that decreased iron-dependent enzyme activity in the cochlea, decreased spiral ganglion cells, and changes in stereocilia function result in hearing loss. Sun AH, et al. demonstrated that 10% of ID rats had moderate to profound sensorineural hearing loss.[27]

In humans, auditory brainstem-evoked response was measured in 5.5–6-month-old infants of which 29 had marginal iron deficiency.[26]

Table 22.4 Proposed hypothesis to explain the association between iron deficiency and stroke[22,23]

- Thrombocytosis secondary to iron deficiency. Megakaryocytes and normoblasts are derived from a common committed progenitor cell, the CFU-GEMM. Thrombopoietin, the molecule that stimulates the growth of megakaryocytes and production of platelets, is structurally homologous to erythropoietin. The high levels of erythropoietin produced by iron deficiency anemia conceivably could cross react with megakaryocyte thrombopoietin receptors, modestly raising the platelet count
- Iron deficiency results in a hypercoagulable state. The microcytic poorly deformable red blood cells increase blood viscosity' and increase risk of venous thrombosis
- Some group of children also had cerebrovascular dilatation, which slows blood flow and further promotes thrombosis
- Anemic hypoxia may contribute to transient hemiplegia and cerebellar infarct. The anemic state is well tolerated until some infection (e.g. viral illness) increases metabolic demands that cannot be met in the face of anemia. Decreased iron-dependent enzymes necessary to metabolic processes may contribute to impaired energy metabolism and oxygen utilization

Central conduction was delayed in the ID group. Algarin demonstrated impaired visual evoked potential in ID children.[28]

Attention-deficit Hyperactivity Disorder

Attention-deficit hyperactivity disorder (ADHD) is associated with ID. Serum ferritin levels were inversely correlated with the severity of ADHD. The children with the most severe iron deficiency were the most inattentive, impulsive, and hyperactive. Low iron stores may explain as much as 30% of ADHD severity.[28] Iron supplementation has been reported incidentally to decrease the cognitive deficiency in children with ADHD, decreasing the need for psycho stimulants.

ADHD possibly modulated by the dopaminergic mesocortical pathways, and because patients with ADHD have increased dopamine transporter–binding potential and genetic polymorphisms in the dopamine receptor. It has been suggested that the symptoms of ADHD may be caused by dopamine dysfunction (children with ADHD benefit from dopamine stimulants). Because iron is a coenzyme of dopamine synthesis and iron deficiency alters dopamine receptor density and activity, brain iron stores may influence dopamine-dependent functions.

Restless Legs Syndrome

Iron deficiency in the central nervous system is known to cause motor impairment and periodic limb movement in the sleep. Restless legs syndrome (RLS) is frequently associated with low serum iron and a tendency toward low serum ferritin levels. Treatment with iron is associated with clinical improvement in most of these patients. Recent work shows that blood brain barrier epithelial cells in persons with RLS have decreased iron stores, suggesting that there is insufficient availability of iron to meet the dynamic circadian iron requirements.[29]

Abnormal dopamine metabolism is a possible link between ID and each of these pathological conditions—BHS, RLS, and ADHD. Iron is a cofactor in catecholamine metabolism and in dopamine synthesis through tyrosine hydroxylase, the rate-limiting enzyme for catecholamine neurotransmitter synthesis.[30] Therefore, deficiency of iron would reduce dopamine synthesis and could exacerbate a variety of common clinical states.

Febrile Seizure

Children with febrile seizures were almost twice as likely to be iron deficient as those with febrile illness alone. The screening for ID should be considered in children presenting with febrile seizure.[31] In a study conducted by Daoud, et al. also showed there is significant association between ID and febrile seizure.[32]

In a retrospective case control study of 361 children who presented to an emergency department with febrile seizures, compared to a control group of 390 children who presented with fever only, those with febrile seizures were almost twice as likely to be iron deficient.[33]

Reasons for this increased febrile seizure susceptibility are unclear. There is no established connection between dopaminergic systems and febrile seizures per se. Dopamine can modulate neuronal excitability in either direction—excitatory or inhibitory—depending on the specific neural circuit, cell type, and brain region.[34] The correlation between ID and febrile seizures might be secondary to a nonspecific alteration of cortical excitability, particularly in the setting of age-dependent fever, since there is no known predilection to seizures in iron deficient older individuals.

Other Neurological Manifestations

Iron is also critical for a many other biological functions including muscle metabolism, sleep regulation, heat production, catecholamine metabolism, immune function, pain perception, thermo regulation, circadian cycles, altered behavioral inhibition and abnormal responses to reward.[35,36]

CONCLUSION

Iron has important role in normal brain development, myelination, and neurotransmitter production. ID during gestation and lactation results in abnormalities in brain iron that are irreversible. So, we have to prevent iron deficiency in women of childbearing age, during gestation, and throughout infancy and childhood.

ID is rarely considered as a primary etiology infrequently observed pediatric neurologic disease, even though IDA is a very common problem in developing countries like India. The developmental sequelae and other neurologic abnormalities caused by iron deficiency, are costly to society and devastating to those affected. With appropriate recognition and treatment the neurologic sequelae of iron deficiency are entirely preventable and reversible.

REFERENCES

1. National Family Health survey 3, India: 2005-06.
2. Connor JR, Fine RE. Development of transferrin-positive oligodendrocytes in the rat central nervous system. J Neurosci Res. 1987;17:51-9.
3. Dwork AJ, Lawler G, Zybert PA, et al. An auto radiographic study of the uptake and distribution of iron by the brain of the young rat. Brain Res. 1990;518:31-9.
4. Beard JL. Iron deficiency and neural development: An update. Arch Latinosam Nutr. 1999;49:34S-9S.
5. Hill JM, Switzer RC. The regional distribution and cellular localization of iron in the rat brain. Neuroscience. 1984;11:595-603.
6. Barkai AI, Durkin M, Dwork AJ, Nelson HD. Autoradiographic study of iron-binding sites in the rat brain: Distribution and relationship to aging. J Neurosci Res. 1991;29:390-5.
7. Beard JL, Connor JD, Jones BC. Brain iron: Location and function. Prog Food Nutr Sci. 1993;17:183-221.
8. Gerber MR, Connor JR. Do oligodendrocytes mediate iron regulation in the human brain? Neurology. 1989;26:95-8.
9. Yu GSM, Steinkirchner TM, Rao GA, Larkin EC. Effect of prenatal iron deficiency on myelination in rat pups. Am J Pathol. 1986;125:620-4.
10. Taneja V, Mishra K, Agarwal KN. Effect of early iron deficiency in rat on the gamma-aminobutyric acid shunt in brain. J Neurochem. 1986;46:1670-4.
11. Taneja V, Mishra KP, Agarwal KN. Effect of maternal iron deficiency on GABA shunt pathway of developing rat brain. Ind J Exp Bio. 1990;28:466-9.
12. Sungthong R, Mo-suwan L, Chongsuvivatwong V. Effects of haemoglobin and serum ferritin on cognitive function in school children. Asia Pac J Clin Nutr. 2002;11:117.
13. Halterman JS, Kaczorowski JM, Aligne CA, Auinger P, Szilagyi PG. Iron deficiency and cognitive achievement among school aged children and adolescents in the United States. Pediatrics. 2001;107:1381-6.
14. Logan S, Martins S, Gilbert R. Iron therapy for improving psychomotor development and cognitive function in children under the age of three with iron deficiency anaemia. Cochrane Database Syst Rev. 2001;CD001444.
15. Stoltzfus RJ, Kvalsvig JD, Chwaya HM, et al. Effects of iron supplementation and anti-helmintic treatment on motor and language development of preschool children in Zanzibar: Double blind placebo controlled study. BMJ. 2001;323:1389.
16. Lozoff B, Jimenez E, Wolf AW. Long-term developmental outcome of infants with iron deficiency. N Engl J Med. 1991;325:687-94.
17. Lozoff B, Wolf AW, Jimenez E. Iron-deficiency anemia and infant development: Effects of extended oral iron therapy. J Pediatr. 1996;129:382-9.
18. Walter T, De Andraca I, Chadud P, Perales CG. Iron deficiency anemia: Adverse effects on infant psychomotor development. Pediatrics. 1989;84:7-17.
19. Lozoff B, Klein NK, Nelson EC, McClish DK, Manel M, Chacon ME. Behavior of infants with iron-deficiency anemia. Child Dev. 1998;69:24-36.
20. Deinard AS, List A, Lindgren B, Hunt JV, Chang PN. Cognitive deficits in iron-deficient and iron-deficient anemic children. J Pediatr. 1986;108:681-9.
21. Belman AL, Rouque CT, Ancona R, et al. Cerebral venous thrombosis in a child with iron deficiency anemia and thrombocytosis. Stroke. 1990;21:488.
22. Bruggers CS, Ware R, Altman AJ, et al. Reversible focal neurological deficits in severe iron deficiency anemia. J Pediatr. 1990;117:430.
23. Yager JY, Hartfield DS. Neurologic manifestations of iron deficiency in childhood. Pediatr Neurol. 2002;27:85.
24. Daoud AS, Batieha A, Al-sheyyab M, et al. Effectiveness of iron therapy on breath-holding spells. J Pediatr. 1997;130:547.

25. Tugal O, Jacobson R, Berezin S, et al. Recurrent benign intracranial hypertension due to iron deficiency anemia: Case report and review of literature. Am J Pediatr Hematol Oncol. 1994;16:266.
26. Roncagliolo M, Garrido M, Walter, et al. Evidence of altered central nervous system development in infants with iron deficiency anemia at 6 mo; delayed maturation of auditory brainstem responses. Am J Clin Nutr. 1998;68:683.
27. Algarin C, Peirano P, Garrido M, et al. Iron deficiency anemia in infancy: Long-lasting effects on auditory and visual system functioning. Pediatr Res. 2003;53:217EE.
28. Eric K, Lecendreux M, Isabelle A, Marie CM. Iron deficiency in children with attention-deficit/hyperactivity disorder. Arch Pediatr Adolesc Med. 2004;158(12):1113.
29. Connor JR, Ponnuru P, Wang XS, Patton SM, Allen RP, Earley CJ. Profile of altered brain iron acquisition in restless legs syndrome. Brain. 2011;134:959-68.
30. Walter T. Effect of iron-deficiency anaemia on cognitive skills in infancy and childhood. Baillieres Clin Haem. 1994;7:815-27.
31. Alfredo, Renato S, Nicola I, Angelo C, Paolo R, Alfonso D, Ciro I, et al. Iron deficiency anaemia and febrile convulsions: case-control study in children under 2 years. BMJ. 1996;313:343.
32. Daoud AS, Batieha A, Abu-Ekteish F, Gharaibeh N, Ajlouni S. Iron status: a possible risk factor for the first febrile seizure. Epilepsia. 2002;43:740-3.
33. Hartfield DS, Tan J, Yager JY, et al. The association between iron deficiency and febrile seizures in childhood. Clin Pediatr (Phila). 2009;48:420-6.
34. Idjradinata P, Pollitt E. Reversal of developmental delays in iron-deficient anaemic infants treated with iron. Lancet. 1993;341:1-4.
35. Lozoff B, Beard J, Connor J, Felt B, Georgieff M, Schallert T. Long-lasting neural and behavioral effects of iron deficiency in infancy. Nutr Rev. 2006;64:34-43.
36. Beard JL. Iron biology in immune function, muscle metabolism and neuronal functioning. J Nutr. 2001;131:568-79.

CHAPTER 23

Cerebral Edema

S Mini

Cerebral edema is a fairly common accompaniment of many medical and surgical emergencies. Untreated cerebral edema can lead to elevated intracranial pressure (ICP), which can have lethal consequences due to secondary cerebral ischemia and herniation syndromes. Hence prompt management of cerebral edema and associated elevation of intracranial pressure (ICP) have become corner stone in neurocritical care.

BASIC PHYSIOLOGY

The cranial vault is a box like structure with fixed volume. The intracranial vault is constituted by three compartments—the brain (1200–1600 mL), cerebrospinal fluid (CSF) (100–150 mL) and blood (100–150 mL). Intracranial pressure is the pressure exerted by these three constituents. According to Monroe-Kellie Doctrine,[1,2] the volume of brain, CSF and intracranial blood is a constant and any increase in the volume of one compartment is compensated by reduction of the other two. The infant's cranium has the potential for growth due to open fontanels and sutures, therefore it has there greater total compliance than that of adult. Hence, it is likely that infants and young children have advanced cranial pathology at the time of clinical presentation with little reserve left.

The intracranial pressure in an adult is normally in the range of 5–15 mm Hg. Normal CSF opening pressure on LP in children ranges from 11.5 cm to 28 cm of water or 9–21 mm Hg.[3] Normal values of CSF pressure in newborns are usually less than these values, at 3–8 cm of H_2O or 2–6 mm Hg. Even though the exact upper limit of intracranial pressure is not well defined, a pressure above 20 mm Hg can be considered as raised ICP for all practical purposes.

Intracranial pressure (ICP) is determined by cerebral blood flow (CBF) and CSF circulation. Cerebral blood volume (CBV) is determined by cerebral blood flow (CBF) and the diameter of capacitance vessels, i.e. small veins and venules. CBV increases with vasodilatation and decreases with vasoconstriction. The cerebral blood flow is autoregulated as long as the cerebral perfusion pressure is 60–160 mm Hg. Beyond this reserve, autoregulation fails. Although CBF frequently changes in the same direction as CBV, these variables are inversely related under normal situations due to auto regulation.

Cerebral perfusion pressure (CPP) is the difference between mean arterial pressure (MAP) and intracranial pressure (ICP).

CPP = MAP–ICP

where MAP = (1/3 systolic BP) + (2/3 Diastolic BP).

DEFINITION

Cerebral edema is defined as the swelling of brain due to the excess accumulation of water in the intra and/or extracellular spaces of the brain.[4] Volumetric enlargement due to cerebral engorgement which results from an increase in blood volume either due to vasodilatation secondary to hypercapnia or impairment of venous flow secondary to obstruction of the cerebral veins and venous sinuses are excluded from this definition. Cerebral edema may or may not be associated with increased intracranial pressure.

TYPES OF CEREBRAL EDEMA

The following subtypes of cerebral edema are mentioned below.

Cytotoxic/Cellular Edema

This is due to fluid accumulation within cellular elements, i.e. neurons, glia or endothelial cells. It can result from almost any injury to brain due to predominantly due to hypoxic—ischemic injury, traumatic brain injury, infections and inflammation of CNS, toxic and metabolic perturbations affecting brain. Cellular edema is primarily due to dysregulation of osmotic gradient across the cell membrane.

Vasogenic Edema

This is due to the influx of fluid and solutes into the extracellular space of brain parenchyma through an incompetent blood brain-barrier (BBB).[4] This is the most common type of brain edema and results from increased permeability of the capillary endothelial cells. Breakdown in the blood-brain barrier allows movement of albumin and other plasma proteins from the intravascular space through the capillary wall into the extracellular space. It primarily affects the white matter. Vasogenic edema is predominantly encountered in primary and metastatic tumors of CNS, abscess, infections and intracranial hemorrhage. This type of edema is sensitive to steroid therapy.

Interstitial/Hydrocephalic Edema

This is best characterized in noncommunicating hydrocephalus where there is obstruction to flow of CSF within the ventricular system or communicating hydrocephalus where the obstruction is distal to the ventricles and results in decreased absorption of CSF into the subarachnoid space. In hydrocephalus, a rise in the intraventricular pressure causes CSF to migrate through the ependyma into the periventricular white matter, thus, increasing the extracellular fluid volume.[5,6]

Osmotic Edema

Normally CSF and extracellular fluid osmolality in the brain is slightly greater than that of plasma. In osmotic edema, an osmotic gradient is present between plasma and the ECF. The BBB is intact, otherwise an osmotic gradient cannot be maintained. This situation occurs with hypo osmolar conditions (dilutional hyponatremia) like SIADH, excessive hemodialysis of uremic patients and diabetic ketoacidosis. There is a decrease of serum osmolality due to reduction of serum Na^+ and when serum Na^+ drops below 120 mmol/L, water enters the brain and distributes evenly within the ECSs of the gray and white matter.[7,8] The formation of osmotic edema can lead to a significant increase in the rate of CSF formation[9] without any contribution of the choroid plexuses. Since osmotic edema is vented rapidly, the increase in brain volume tends to be modest. Osmotic brain edema can also occur when the plasma osmolality is normal but tissue osmolality is high in the core of the lesion as occurs following brain hemorrhage, infarcts or contusions.[10,11]

Hydrostatic Edema

This form of cerebral edema is seen in acute, malignant hypertension. It is thought to result from direct transmission of pressure to cerebral capillary with transudation of fluid into the ECF.

Even though different subtypes of edema are described, in clinical practice, these sub types often coexist, with one type predominating over the other, depending on the underlying cause of cerebral edema and stage of progression of disease.

PATHOPHYSIOLOGY

Cellular Edema

Pathophysiology of cerebral edema at cellular level is complex. Insults like ischemia, hypoxia, trauma or inflammation initiate a cascade of events which ultimately leads to damage of neuroglia and endothelial cells of blood vessels. The cascade begins with cellular depletion of ATP and release of excitatory neurotransmitters like glutamate into extracellular space. Glutamate can trigger or inhibit sodium and calcium entry channels on cell membrane. As glutamate opens the calcium channel on cell membrane calcium accumulates within cell. Membrane ATPase pumps extrude one calcium ion exchange for three sodium ions. Sodium builds up within the cell creating an osmotic gradient and this leads to increase in cellular volume due to subsequent entry of water into cell. There is also accumulation of other osmoles like H- and, HCO_3^- within the cell. As long as the cell membrane remains intact, in water causes dysfunction but not necessarily permanent damage. Excess intracellular calcium activates a cytotoxic cascade leading to cell death. Within six hours of initial injury, immediate early genes like *c-fos* and *c-jun* are activated. This in turn leads to activation of cytokines, chemokines and microglial cells leading to release of arachidonic acid, free radicals (oxygen species and nitric oxide) and proteases. Theses lead to disruption of cell membrane. Once the membranes are disrupted recovery of the cells is impossible.[12]

Recent research has shed light on the role of Aquaporin-4 water channels in the formation of cytotoxic edema and resolution of vasogenic and interstitial edema. AQP4, the principal AQP in mammalian brain, is expressed in glia at the borders between major water compartments and the brain parenchyma. It is expressed in the basolateral membrane of the ependymal cells lining the cerebral ventricles and subependymal astrocytes which are located at the ventricular CSF fluid-brain interface. Expression of AQP4 in astrocytic foot processes brings it in close proximity to intracerebral vessels, and thus, the blood–brain interface. Water molecules moving from the blood pass through the luminal and abluminal endothelial membranes by diffusion and across the astrocytic foot processes through the AQP4 channels. AQP4 is also expressed in the dense astrocytic processes that form the glia limitans which is at the subarachnoid—CSF fluid interface. Studies imply that AQP4 has a significant role in water transport and development of cellular edema following cerebral ischemia.[13]

Vasogenic Edema

This is primarily due to breakdown of blood brain barrier (BBB). Ultra structural studies have shown an increase in the number of endothelial caveolae in the vessels with breakdown of BBB within minutes after the onset of pathological states.[14,15] The enhanced caveolae appear to be the major route by which early passage of plasma proteins occurs in brain diseases associated with vasogenic edema. Caveolae allow protein passage across endothelium via fluid-phase transcytosis and transendothelial channels. The tight junctions remain intact during early phase. The junctional breakdown to proteins occurs late in the course of brain injury probably during end-stage disease and precedes endothelial cell breakdown. Recent evidence suggests that aquaporin 4 channels located in the ependyma and astrocytic foot processes have an important role in the clearance of the interstitial water in vasogenic and interstitial edema.[15]

Causes

Cerebral edema can occur encountered in almost many CNS disorders and extra-cerebral causes. Some of the well-known causes of cerebral edema are enlisted in **Table 23.1**.

CLINICAL FEATURES

Cerebral edema can occur due to wide range pathology of neurological or non-neurological nature. Cerebral edema alone may not be associated with specific clinical features of its own until elevation in ICP leads to focal or global cerebral ischemia and herniation syndromes. Headache in early morning worsened by recumbent posture, double vision, transient visual obscurations and, projectile vomiting are the usual symptoms when raised ICP evolves gradually. Cerebral edema may however add on to or complicate the clinical features of underlying pathological condition. As features of cerebral edema can be subclinical and difficult to detect, a high index of suspicion should be exercised. With elevations in intracranial pressure, cerebral edema can cause cerebral ischemia and various types of Herniation syndromes due to pressure gradients between various intracranial compartments.

Table 23.1 Etiology of cerebral edema	
Neurological causes	Non-neurological causes
• Traumatic brain injury • Meningitis and meningoencephalitis • Ischemic and hemorrhagic stroke • Brain tumors and other space occupying lesions like subdural hematoma (SDH), abscess, tuberculomas, etc.	• Diabetic ketoacidosis • Lactic acidosis and organic acidemia's like Maple syrup urine disease (MSUD) • Malignant hypertension and hypertensive encephalopathy • Hepatic encephalopathy, Reye's syndrome • Systemic poisoning (carbon monoxide and lead) • Hyponatremia, syndrome of inappropriate antidiuretic hormone secretion (SIADH) • Opioid drug abuse and dependence • Bites of certain reptiles and marine animals • High altitude cerebral edema

In an appropriate clinical scenario, alteration in level of consciousness, bradycardia, hypertension, abnormal breathing patterns, external ocular movement abnormalities, alteration and inequality of pupillary size and extensor plantar response on the side of the lesion should raise strong suspicion of cerebral edema. Cushing's triad (bradycardia, hypertension and irregular breathing patterns) however is a late manifestation of raised ICP. Papilledema may not be present in cases with acute elevation of ICP.

HERNIATION SYNDROMES

The pressure difference between various compartments within the cranial vault can lead to various types of Herniation syndrome. The signs and symptoms associated with various Herniation syndromes are due to compression or distortion of the reticular activating system causing altered level of consciousness, compression of brainstem structures leading to cranial nerve palsies, motor deficits, bradycardia, hypertension and abnormal patterns of respiration, compression of blood vessels leading to reduced cerebral perfusion pressure leading to ischemia and further elevation of ICP. The features of major herniation syndromes are shown in **Table 23.2**.

IMAGING FEATURES OF CEREBRAL EDEMA

The most feasible brain imaging modality in the setting of suspected elevated ICP is CT brain. It is less time consuming than MRI and gives a clue to underlying etiology in most cases. Apart from the features of underlying etiology, the evidence of elevated ICP in CT include effacement of cerebral sulci, poor gray—white differentiation, chincking of ventricles, effacement of perimesencephalic cisterns, midline shift in unilateral supratentorial lesions, etc. MRI is more helpful to detect the etiology of cerebral edema like early cerebral infarct. The diffusion weighted images (DWI) with corresponding absolute diffusion coefficient map (ADC map) is the MRI sequence which helps to differentiate cytotoxic edema and vasogenic edema. In cytotoxic edema, areas of hyperintense intense signals in DWI appear to be hypointense in ADC map due to restricted movement of water molecule (restricted diffusion in DWI) **(Figs 23.1 and 23.2)**. In vasogenic edema is the reverse is noted. **Figures 23.3 and 23.4** shows the CT and MRI findings described.

MONITORING OF INTRACRANIAL PRESSURE

The main rationales for measuring ICP are:
- Measurement of ICP can be accomplished using detection and treatment of fatal cerebral herniation events
- Detection of possible secondary insults related to either increased intracranial pressure or decreased brain perfusion.

Studies by Gopinath et al.[16] demonstrated that episodes of intracranial pressure greater than 20 mm Hg correlated with poor neurological outcome in adults after traumatic brain injury (TBI). This threshold value has been adopted in adult TBI and pediatric TBI. However, there is only sparse evidence to support this threshold for children with

Cerebral Edema

Table 23.2 The stages of reproductive aging workshop classification of reproductive aging woman

Herniation syndrome	Location	Clinical features
Uncal/lateral transtentorial	Medial part of temporal lobe (uncus and parahippocampal gyrus) gets displaced and forced into the free edge of tentorial opening (incisura) at the level of midbrain	• Ipsilateral third nerve palsy—ptosis, pupil fixed and dilated (Hutchison pupil), eye deviated down and out • Ipsilateral hemiparesis from compression of the contralateral cerebral peduncle against Kernohan's notch • Other signs of brainstem dysfunction from ischemia secondary to compression of posterior cerebral artery
Subfalcine (Cingulate) herniation	Increased pressure in one cerebral hemisphere leads to herniation of cingulate gyrus underneath falx cerebri	Compression of anterior cerebral arteries results in contralateral lower extremity paresis or paraparesis
Central tentorial herniation	Supratentorial mass lesions causing downward displacement of one or both cerebral hemispheres causing compression of diencephalon and midbrain through tentorial notch	Impaired consciousness and eye movements, decorticate and decerebrate posturing
Cerebellar-tonsillar herniation or trans foramen magnum herniation	Most commonly seen with mass lesion in the posterior fossa. Unilateral or bilateral downward and mesial displacement of cerebellar hemispheres/Magnum (ventral parafolliculi or tonsillae) though foramen magnum leading to medullary compression	Episodic tonic extension ("cerebellar fits"), arching of the back and neck, extension and internal rotation of limbs, loss of consciousness, cardiac arrhythmias, precipitous changes in BP, heart rate, small pupils, ataxic breathing, disturbance of conjugate gaze and quadriparesis

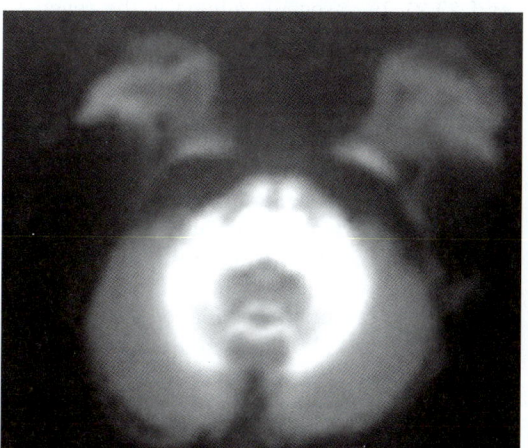

Figure 23.1 Diffusion weighted MRI (DWI) showing hyperintense signals of cerebellar peduncles and brainstem in a child with Maple syrup urine disease (MSUD)

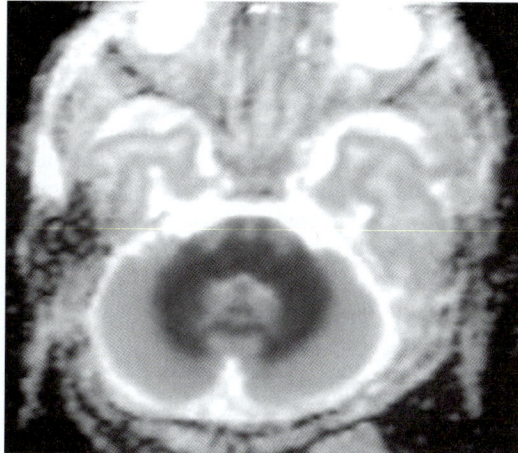

Figure 23.2 The apparent diffusion coefficient (ADC) map of same child showing hypointense signals due to cytotoxic edema

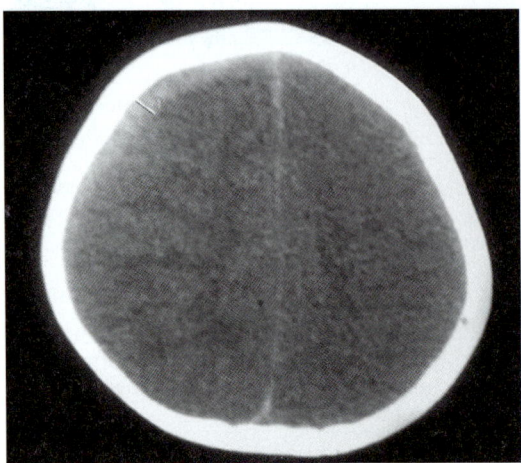

Figure 23.3 CT head (noncontrast) showing subdural hematoma overlying right frontal cortex. Note the effacement of sulci and poor gray white differentiation due to accompanying brain edema

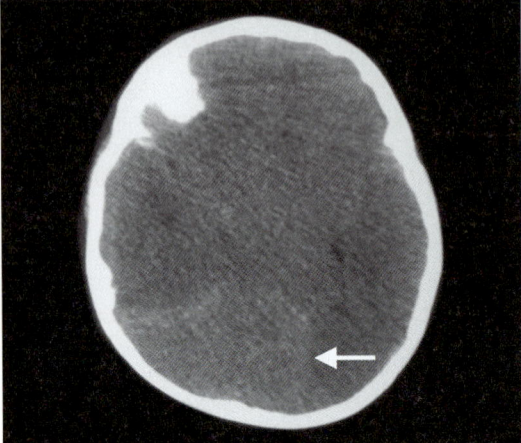

Figure 23.4 CT head of same patient showing effacement of cisterns around midbrain and white cerebella sign (Arrow) due to redistribution of cerebral blood volume (CBV) to posterior circulation secondary to brain edema. Also note the ventricles are not visualized properly

TBI. There is hardly any data on the threshold of ICP requiring intervention in other conditions such as meningitis, hydrocephalous or stroke, etc.

Currently ICP monitors are placed either in the brain parenchyma or in the ventricular space. Parenchymal monitors are easy to place (requiring only a reflection of the dura) and are believed to carry a decreased risk for infection. However, intraparenchymal monitors were found to have significant drift. Newer intraparenchymal monitors have corrected this problem. The advantages of intraventricular monitors are the ability to withdraw CSF as a therapy for increased ICP and the ease of recalibration. They are more technically challenging to place, especially when significant cerebral swelling has already occurred. They may carry increased risk of infection. In selecting monitor location, careful considerations should be given to locations based on individual risk/benefit profiles for each patient.

Waveforms Encountered During Intracranial Pressure Recording

Recording of ICP in normal individual two pressure wave forms. There is a rise with cardiac systole (due to distention of intracranial arteriolar tree) which follows a slower change in pressure with respiration, falling with each inspiration and rising with expiration. Normal intracranial pressure in adults is 8–18 mm Hg and in children it ranges from 10 mm to 20 mm. ICP is less when measured through a lumbar puncture. It is not a static state, but one that is influenced by several factors. Sustained increase of ICP > 20 mm Hg is considered pathological. Lundberg has described three types of wave forms. These are:

1. *A waves or plateau waves* have amplitudes of 50 mm Hg to 100 mm Hg, lasting 5–20 minutes. These waves are always pathological. During such waves, it is common to observe evidence or early herniation, including bradycardia and hypertension. It is postulated that as CPP becomes inadequate to meet metabolic demand, cerebral vasodilation ensues and cerebral blood volume increases. This leads to a vicious circle, with further CPP decrease, predisposing patients to other plateau waves. If low CPP is not corrected, global cerebralischemia ensues and eventually results in cerebrocirculatory arrest and brain death.
2. *B waves* oscillate up to 50 mm Hg in amplitude with a frequency 0.5–2/min and are thought due to vasomotor center instability when CPP

is unstable or at the lower limits of pressure autoregulation.
3. *C waves* oscillate up to 20 mm Hg in amplitude and have a frequency of 4–8/min. These waves have been documented in healthy individuals and are thought to occur because of interaction between cardiac and respiratory cycles.

Noninvasive Methods

Several noninvasive methods have been tried over many years to measure ICP, including transcranial Doppler (TCD), middle ear endolymph pressure estimation, visual evoked potentials and optic nerve sheath diameter. None of them are being used widely due to lack of reliability.

MANAGEMENT OF PATIENT WITH RAISED INTRACRANIAL PRESSURE

The treatment of intracranial hypertension depends upon the etiology and the clinical condition of the child. The best therapy for raised ICP is resolution of underlying cause.

Steps in Intracranial Pressure Management

- Initial stabilization
- Evaluation for etiology and monitoring of ICP and vital signs
- General measures to reduce ICP
- Special measures to reduce ICP.

Initial Stabilization

The initial management strategy is to stabilize the cardiopulmonary status according to standard PALS. If required child should be intubated and ventilated. The indications for intubation are shown in **Table 23.3**. Maintenance of adequate ventilation and blood pressure are the cornerstones of management of elevated intracranial pressure. Adequate ventilation prevents the vasodilation that occurs in response to hypercapnea. Attention should be paid to appropriate fluid and ionotropic supports to maintain adequate systemic blood pressure. Maintenance of normal blood pressure is of utmost importance in preventing fall in CPP which will otherwise lead to infarction of vital tissues and accentuate cerebral edema.

Table 23.3 Indications for endotracheal intubation in children with elevated intracranial pressure

- Refractory hypoxia
- Hypoventilation
- Glasgow coma score of ≤8
- Loss of airway protective reflexes
- Acute herniation requiring controlled hyperventilation
- Need for administration of resuscitation medications through endotracheal route
- Aspiration pneumonia
- ARDS

Rapid sequential intubation in cases with raised ICP

- Lidocaine may be used intravenously or locally to prevent ICP surges.
- Etomidate is the favored as a sedative because of its rapid onset of action and minimal side effects when patient hemodynamically unstable. Thiopental is classically recommended for patients with elevated ICP who are hemodynamically stable. It can cause cardiac suppression and vasodilatation, leading to decreased mean arterial pressure and should be used with caution for patients who may develop hemodynamic instability. Midazolam provides some cerebral protective effects, but it can also cause hypotension in the dose required for RSI. In addition, its onset of action is slower and less reliable than thiopental. Recent studies suggest use of ketamine is not associated with elevated ICP. Nondepolarizing muscle relaxants like Rocuronium are preferred for paralysis because succinyl choline may cause increases in ICP.
- Avoidance of hypoxemia and maintenance of PaO_2 at approximately 100 mm Hg are recommended. $PaCO_2$ should be maintained that support adequate regional CBF or CPP to the injured brain, and a value of approximately 35 mm Hg is a generally accepted target in the absence of ICP elevations or clinical herniation syndromes. Hyperventilation causes hypocapnia, which leads to cerebral vasoconstriction and reduced CBF. Decrease in CBF is accompanied by a decrease in cerebral blood volume, which in turn decreases ICP. Aggressive hyperventilation with $PaCO_2$ in the range of 25–30 mm Hg is indicated only if there are clinical signs of acute herniation. Its effects

are transient. This may prevent herniation by relieving the pressure differential in the intracranial compartments. There is associated risk of cerebral ischemia with excessive lowering of CBF if prolonged hypocapnia is maintained.
- Positive end-expiratory pressure can increase ICP in two ways; firstly through impedance of venous return, increasing cerebral venous pressure and ICP and secondly through decreased BP and reflex increase of CBV, increasing ICP. Therefore, delivery of PEEP more than 10 cm H_2O in patients with elevated ICP should be avoided.

Maintenance of blood pressure is necessary to prevent secondary cerebral ischemia due to reduction in cerebral perfusion pressure. Euvolemia should be maintained using isotonic saline to keep CPP above 60 mm Hg. Fluid should not be restricted unnecessarily as it may reduce BP and CPP. Hypovolemia should be treated promptly with hypertonic fluids with a goal of attaining a state of normal volume. Hypotonic solution and plain dextrose infusions should be avoided. However, excess intravascular volume may exacerbate the development of cerebral edema and hence should be avoided. Rigorous attention should be paid to daily fluid balance, body weight, and serum electrolyte monitoring.

Use of antihypertensives: Intracranial pressure can also be influenced by antihypertensive drugs. Vasodilator drugs like nitroprusside, nitroglycerin, and nifedipine can be expected to increase ICP and hence better avoided in patients with raised ICP. Conversely, nonvasodilator antihypertensive drugs, like the sympatholytic drugs such as beta-adrenergic blocking drugs, can be expected to have little or no effect on ICP.

Evaluation and Monitoring

Once the child is stable, head computed tomography (CT) scan without contrast should be performed. MRI is time consuming and may not be feasible in a critically ill child. LP should be avoided in patients with raised ICP. If intracranial infection is suspected, deferral of LP should not delay initiation of appropriate antibiotics or antiviral therapy. Early neurosurgical consultation should be taken to assist with management decisions like excision of intracranial tumor or hematoma, external ventricular drainage, implantation of ICP monitoring device etc. The indications for ICP monitoring are not well defined except in cases of traumatic brain injury.

> *The Brain Trauma Foundation guidelines for ICP monitoring in patients with TBI*
> - GCS score <9 and abnormal CT scans
> - In patients with a GCS score <9 and normal CT scans in the presence of two or more of the following:
>   – Age greater than 40 years
>   – Unilateral or bilateral motor posturing
>   – Systolic blood pressure greater than 90 mm Hg.

General Measures to Reduce Elevated Intracranial Pressure

- *Positioning:* If raised ICP is suspected, the head should be elevated to 30° to facilitate venous drainage through jugular veins and decrease hydrostatic pressure, thereby lowering ICP. Use of restricting devices and garments around the neck like devices for securing endotracheal tubes may impair cerebral venous outflow by compression of the internal jugular veins and should be avoided. Head elevation beyond 40 degrees can be detrimental due to lowering of CPP elevation of head position may be harmful in ischemic stroke, because it may further compromise perfusion to ischemic tissue.
- *Management of hyperpyrexia*: Hyperpyrexia can increase cerebral metabolism and cerebral blood flow and lead to further elevation of ICP. Fever should be promptly controlled with antipyretics and cooling blanket. Shivering associated with hyperpyrexia may be controlled with muscle relaxants. A mild hypothermia (32–36°C) has been shown to be protective.
- *Provision of analgesia and sedation:* Adequate analgesia and sedation should be maintained. These measures are used to avoid and treat increases in ICP, especially when this is associated with pain and increased cerebral metabolism. These agents also facilitate the general care of ventilated patients. Analgesia should be provided even in drowsy or unresponsive patients while procedures like ET suctioning, catheterization, insertion of IV

access, etc. are attempted. Administration of lidocaine before endotracheal tube suctioning to blunt the gag and cough responses. Little data is available for children. Although opioids are used commonly for analgesia, a recent systematic review of sedation for adults with severe traumatic brain injury highlighted the observation that high bolus doses of opioid sedation were associated with an increase in ICP and reduced brain perfusion pressure. Little data is available in children. Although ketamine was initially thought to increase ICP, a number of recent studies have demonstrated no increase in ICP in patients given ketamine infusions either together with other sedative agents. Etomidate may have some ICP-lowering effects; however there is a risk of adrenal suppression. Propofol is used as a long-term sedative in adult TBI, but not in the pediatric critical care unit because of the risks of propofol infusion syndrome. Neuromuscular blockade is recommended for patients if ICP remains elevated in spite of adequate sedation. It also prevents patient fighting the ventilator and ensures hyperventilation if required.

- *Maintenance of euglycemia*: Both hyperglycemia and hypoglycemia in children with head injuries have been associated with poor outcomes. Routine use of plain dextrose and hypotonic fluids should be avoided. Many centers aggressively treat hyperglycemia in patients with head injuries with insulin. Patients also should be monitored for hypoglycemia, which can adversely affect brain tissue, particularly in infants and small children who have smaller glycogen stores. The optimal target blood glucose level remains to be determined in patients with brain injury.
- *Anticonvulsant therapy*: There is no recommendation for use of prophylactic anticonvulsant therapy. However, many centers administer prophylactic phenytoin or phenobarbital to patients who are at high risk of developing seizures. Breakthrough seizures are best treated with benzodiazepines injections.
- *Nutritional support*: Unless contraindicated, enteral route of nutrition is preferred. Special attention should be given to the osmotic content of formulations, to avoid free water intake that may result in a hypo osmolar state and worsen cerebral edema.

Specific Measures to Reduce Elevated Intracranial Pressure

Controlled Hyperventilation

Controlled hyperventilation remains the most efficacious therapeutic intervention for cerebral edema, particularly when cerebral edema is associated with persistent elevations in ICP. A decrease in $PaCO_2$ to 30–35 mm Hg produces proportional decreases in regional CBF resulting in rapid and prompt reduction in ICP. Features of impending herniation in a patient warrants hyperventilation to lower $PaCO_2$ to 25–30 mm Hg. The vasoconstrictive effect of respiratory alkalosis on cerebral arterioles lasts only for 10–20 hours. Continuation hyperventilation beyond this time period may result in exacerbation of cerebral edema due vasodilatation and rebound elevations in ICP. Prolonged hyperventilation has been shown to result in worse outcomes in patients with TBI. Hence, controlled hyperventilation is to be used as a rescue or resuscitative measure for a short duration until more definitive therapies are instituted. Caution must be exercised while reversing hyperventilation over 6–24 hours to avoid cerebral hyperemia and rebound elevations in ICP.

Osmotherapy

The fundamental goal of osmotherapy is to create an osmotic gradient to cause egress of water from the brain extracellular and possibly intracellular compartment into the vasculature, thereby decreasing intracranial pressure. The target is to maintain euvolemic or a slightly hypervolemic state with a serum osmolality of 300–320 mOsm/L.

Concentrated urea was the first agent to be used clinical practice as an osmotic agent. Its use was short-lived due to its side effects such as nausea, vomiting, diarrhea, and coagulopathy. Currently used agents include mannitol, furosemide, hypertonic saline. Glycerol is still used by some clinicians.

Mannitol, an alcohol derivative of simple sugar mannose, was introduced in 1960 and has since remained the major osmotic agent of choice in clinical practice. It has rapid onset of action within 20–40 minutes and the effect lasts for 4–6 hours. Apart from its osmotic properties, mannitol seems to provide additional beneficial effects in brain injury by increasing deformability of RBCs, decreasing blood viscosity resulting in increases in rCBF and CPP and a resultant cerebral vasoconstriction leading to decreased CBV, increasing free radical scavenging, inhibition of apoptosis. It is administered as intravenous bolus injection of 20% solution at a dose of 0.25–1.5 g/kg by. Repeated dosing of Mannitol may be instituted every 6 hours and should be guided by serum osmolality to a recommended target value of approximately 320 mOsm/L; higher values result in renal tubular damage. T ½ increases from 0.25–1.7 hours to 6–36 hours in renal failure. Contraindications for using Mannitol are systemic hypotension, acute tubular necrosis, anuria, pulmonary edema, acute left ventricular failure, CHF. Excessive use of mannitol without adequate water replacement can result in severe dehydration, free water losses, and hypernatremia.

Administration of hypertonic saline lowers ICP and increases rCBF extra osmotic properties of hypertonic saline include modulation of CSF production and resorption, accentuation of tissue oxygen delivery, probable modulation of inflammatory and neurohumoral responses (arginine-vasopressin and atrial natriuretic peptide). It is especially useful in the setting of systemic hypotension, where Mannitol is contraindicated. Formulations include 2% NaCl, 3% NaCl (513 mEq/L of Na and Cl), 5% NaCl (856 mEq/L of Na and C), 7% (1200 mEq/L), 7.5%, 10% and 23.4% (approx 4000 mEq/L). Usual dose is 1–2 mL/kg/hour of 3% normal saline with a target to increase serum sodium concentration to a range of 145–155 mEq/L (serum osmolality approximately 300–320 mOsm/L). Bolus doses may also be used instead of continuous infusion. This level of serum sodium is maintained for 48–72 hours until patients demonstrate clinical improvement or there is a lack of response despite achieving the serum sodium target. During withdrawal of therapy, caution has to be exercised against possible rebound hyponatremia and cerebral edema. Serum sodium and potassium are monitored every 4–6 hours during both institution and withdrawal of therapy and other serum electrolytes (particularly calcium and magnesium) should be monitored daily. Myelinolysis (Osmotic demyelination), the most serious complication of hypertonic saline therapy, typically occurs when rapid corrections in serum sodium arise from a chronic hyponatremic state to a normonatremic or hypernatremic state. Intravenous bolus injections of 30 mL of 23.4% hypertonic saline have been used in cases of intracranial hypertension refractory to conventional ICP-lowering therapies.

Glycerol is another useful agent given in doses of 30 mL every 4–6 hours orally or daily IV 50 g in 500 mL of 2.5% saline solution. Its effectiveness appears to decrease after few days. It is used in a dose of 0.5–1.0 g/kg body weight. In unconscious or uncooperative patients it is given by nasogastric tube.

Use of Diuretics

Role of loop diuretics (commonly furosemide) for the treatment of cerebral edema, particularly when used alone, remains controversial. Furosemide (0.7 mg/kg) is found to prolong the reversal of blood brain osmotic gradient established with the osmotic agents by preferentially excreting water over solute. Combining furosemide with mannitol produces a profound diuresis; however, the efficacy and optimum duration of this treatment remain. If loop diuretics are used, rigorous attention to systemic hydration status is advised, as the risk of serious volume depletion is substantial and cerebral perfusion may be compromised. A common strategy used to raise serum sodium rapidly is to administer an intravenous bolus of furosemide (0.7–1 mg/kg) to enhance free water excretion and to replace it with intravenous bolus of 3% hypertonic saline.

Corticosteroids

Some clinicians still try corticosteroids. It tends to reduce vasogenic edema associated with brain tumors or accompanying brain irradiation and surgical manipulation. It decreases tight-junction permeability and stabilizes the disrupted blood brain barrier. Glucocorticoids, especially dexamethasone, are the preferred steroidal agents, due to their low mineralocorticoid activity. Steroids deleterious side effects are stress ulcers, hyperglycemia, impairment of wound healing, psychosis, and immunosuppression.

Pharmacological Coma

Barbiturates reduce ICP suppressing cerebral metabolism. In addition it is thought to have some neuroprotective effect. The goal of therapy is to achieve burst suppression on EEG, at which point its effects are maximal. Very few studies have evaluated barbiturates in children, all as cases series. There is no clear evidence till date that barbiturate therapy benefits patients. Pentobarbital and thiopental have been used with no clear evidence to choose between the twos. The major limitations of barbiturate therapy are their potential adverse effects—hypotension, decreased cardiac output, immune modulation, and prolonged sedation after terminating therapy. Patients on barbiturate therapy usually require inotropic support to avoid hypotension.

Therapeutic Hypothermia

Hypothermia is neuroprotective in laboratory studies, improving survival and neurologic outcome. Much attention has been focused recently on moderate hypothermia (32–33°C) in adult and pediatric TBI based on the expected reduction of secondary injury, including raised ICP. However, current literature shows conflicting data on inducing hypothermia. It may be beneficial in selected cases of TBI.

Surgical Management

- *CSF drainage*: External ventricular drainage (EVD) can be extremely effective in controlling ICP. EVDs can be used both for ICP monitoring and therapeutic CSF drainage if ICP is elevated. In children, even removal of small amounts of CSF can result in a substantial reduction in ICP. However, EVD placement can be technically difficult when the ventricles are particularly small due to brain swelling. In this case, injury caused by several passes of the catheter to find the ventricle may outweigh the benefit. There is also a higher risk of causing a hematoma and infection.
- *Removal of mass lesions*: Initial CT head may reveal epidural, subdural, or intracerebral hematoma. The general principle is that lesions causing mass effect should be removed, however some small lesions can be safely managed conservatively. When the hematoma is intracerebral, this decision depends on the location. Hematomas that are discrete and fairly close to the surface are more amenable to surgical evacuation. Some surgeons may leave the bone flap open if there is considerable swelling of the brain even after the hematoma is removed. The key principle is that, if a hematoma is to be removed, this should be done as soon as possible. Hematomas may develop slowly and may not be evident on the initial scan or may be of smaller volume. Therefore, a low threshold should be maintained for obtaining repeat CT. Portable head CT may be useful in ventilated and critically ill patients.
- *Decompressive craniectomy*: Decompressive craniectomy for TBI remains a controversial. Several uncontrolled studies suggest that craniectomy may benefit children with refractory intracranial hypertension. The purpose of decompressive craniectomy is to remove a large part of the cranium to increase the volume available for cerebral swelling, preferably with dural augmentation as the dura similarly limits the volume. Several studies have demonstrated the clear and usually dramatic reduction in ICP following the procedure. After surgery, it is very important to avoid hypertension, as this may increase edema in the decompressed brain because of the changes in arterial-tissue pressure gradient and possibly impaired blood brain barrier.

CONCLUSION

Last five decades have witnessed tremendous advances in our understanding of the pathophysiology of cerebral edema and imaging modalities to detect cerebral edema, yet this has not made much impact in the management of elevated intracranial pressure. Currently management of primary pathology along with measures to reduce ICP and maintain CPP above 55–60 mm to prevent secondary ischemia remains standard practice.

REFERENCES

1. Monro A. Observations on the structure and function of the nervous system. Edinburgh: Creech and Johnson; 1823. p. 5.
2. Kellie G. An account of the appearances observed in the dissection of two of the three individuals presumed to have perished in the storm of the 3rd, and whose bodies were discovered in the vicinity of Leith on the morning of the 4th November 1821 with some reflections on the pathology of the brain. Trans Med Chir Sci. Edinburgh. 1824;1:84-169.
3. Avery RA, Shah SS, Licht DJ, Seiden JA, Huh JW, Boswinkel J, Ruppe MD, Chew A, Mistry RD, et al. Reference range for cerebrospinal fluid opening pressure in children. N Engl J Med. 2010;363(9):891-3. doi: 10.1056/NEJMc1004957.
4. Pollay M. Blood-brain barrier, cerebral edema. In: Wilkins RH, Rengachary SS (Eds). Neurosurgery, 2nd edn. New York: Mc Graw Hill Book Co., 1996. pp. 335-44.
5. Milhorat TH, Clark RG, Hammock MK. Experimental hydrocephalus gross pathological findings in acute and subacute obstructive hydrocephalus in the dog and monkey. J Neurosurg. 1970;32:390-9.
6. Milhorat TH, Clark RG, Hammock MK, et al. Structural, ultrastructural, and permeability changes in the ependyma and surrounding brain favoring equilibration in progressive hydrocephalus. Arch Neurol. 1970;22:397-407.
7. Doczi T, Szerdahelyi P, Gulya K, et al. Brain water accumulation after the central administration of vasopressin. Neurosurgery. 1982;11:402-7.
8. Pappius HM, OH JH, Dossetor JB. The effects of rapid hemodialysis on brain tissues and cerebrospinal fluid of dogs. Can J Physiol Pharmacol. 1967;45:129-47.
9. DiMattio J, Hochwald GM, Malhan C, et al. Effects of changes in serum osmolarity on bulk flow of fluid into cerebral ventricles and on brain water content. Pflugers Arch. 1975;359:253-64. doi:10.1007/BF00587383.
10. Katayama Y, Kawamata T. Edema fluid accumulation within necrotic brain tissue as a cause of the mass effect of cerebral contusion in head trauma patients. Acta Neurochir Suppl (Wien). 2003;86:323-7.
11. Milhorat TH. Classification of the cerebral edemas with reference to hydrocephalus and pseudotumor cerebri. Childs Nerv Syst. 1992; 8:301-6.
12. Bradley WG. In: Neurology in clinical practice, 5th edn. Pennsylvania, Elsevier Inc. 2008;2: 1698-9.
13. Nag S, Manias JL, Duncan J, Stewart. Pathology and new players in the pathogenesis of brain edema. Acta Neuropathol. 2009;118: 197-217.
14. Nag S. Pathophysiology of blood–brain barrier breakdown. Methods Mol Med. 2003;89:97-119.
15. Nag S. Structure and pathology of the blood–brain barrier. In: Lathja A (Ed). Handbook of neurochemistry and molecular neurobiology. Springer, New York, 2007. pp. 58-78.
16. Gopinath SP, et al. Jugular venous desaturation and outcome after head injury. J Neurol Neurosurg Psychiatry. 1994;57(6):717-23.

SUGGESTED READING

1. Daroff RB, Fenichel GM, Jankovic J. Bradley's neurology in clinical practice, 6th edn. Saunders Publication. 2012;1:1377-95.
2. Swaiman K, Ashwal S, Ferriero DM, et al. Swaiman's pediatric neurology principles and practice, 5th edn. Saunders Publication. 2012;2:1185-97.
3. Wheeler DS, Wong HR, Shanley TP. Pediatric critical care medicine, 2nd edn. Springer Publication. 2014;2:569-87.
4. Winn HR. Youmans Neurological Surgery, 6th edn. Saunders Publication. 2011;1:162-8.

CHAPTER 24

Sodium Dysequilibrium and the Brain Disorders in Children

Susan Uthup

INTRODUCTION

Disturbances in salt, water, acid-base and electrolyte balance are relatively common in children with neurological disorders like infections, tumors and head injuries. These disorders pose significant complexities in diagnosis and management. The neurological consequences are usually functional rather than structural and are usually reversible, particularly if effectively managed at an early stage. Since electrolyte disturbances are typically secondary processes, effective management requires identification and treatment of the primary disorder in addition to correction of the electrolyte abnormality.

PHYSIOLOGY OF SODIUM AND WATER BALANCE

Sodium is the major extracellular cation concerned with the maintenance of intravascular volume and cell integrity. The extracellular to intracellular sodium concentration gradient is maintained by the Na-K ATPase pump. Sodium reabsorption in kidneys occurs predominantly at the proximal convoluted tubule and is affected by sympathetic innervation, atrial natriuretic peptide (ANP) and brain natriuretic peptide (BNP). ANP and BNP cause natriuresis by direct effect on the inner medullary collecting duct as well as inhibition of renin and aldosterone. Under normal conditions, plasma sodium concentration is finely maintained within the narrow range of 135–145 mmol/L. Sodium and its accompanying anions, principally chloride and bicarbonate, account for 86% of the extracellular fluid osmolality (normal 285–295 mOsm/kg).

Water makes up 60% of the mass of the human body and moves freely between intracellular and extracellular fluid spaces as dictated by the movements of osmotically active particles. Water balance is monitored by osmoreceptors in the hypothalamus and baroreceptors. Baroreceptors include low pressure baroreceptors in the right atrium and great veins and high pressure baroreceptors in the carotid sinus. The two main mechanisms for controlling water balance are antidiuretic hormone (ADH) secretion and thirst. Increases in extracellular fluid (ECF) tonicity cause secretion of ADH from the posterior pituitary promoting free water reabsorption in the kidney leading to concentrated urine. Hypovolemia is also a potent stimulus for ADH release via the renin-angiotensin-aldosterone system. Normal regulation of sodium and water balance is shown in **Figure 24.1**.

The normal plasma osmolality (posm) is between 275 and 290 mOsm/kg. It is primarily determined by the concentration of sodium salts. The plasma osmolality is calculated using the following formula:

Serum osmolality = 2(Na) mEq/L + serum glucose (mg/dL)/18 + BUN (mg/dL)/2.8.

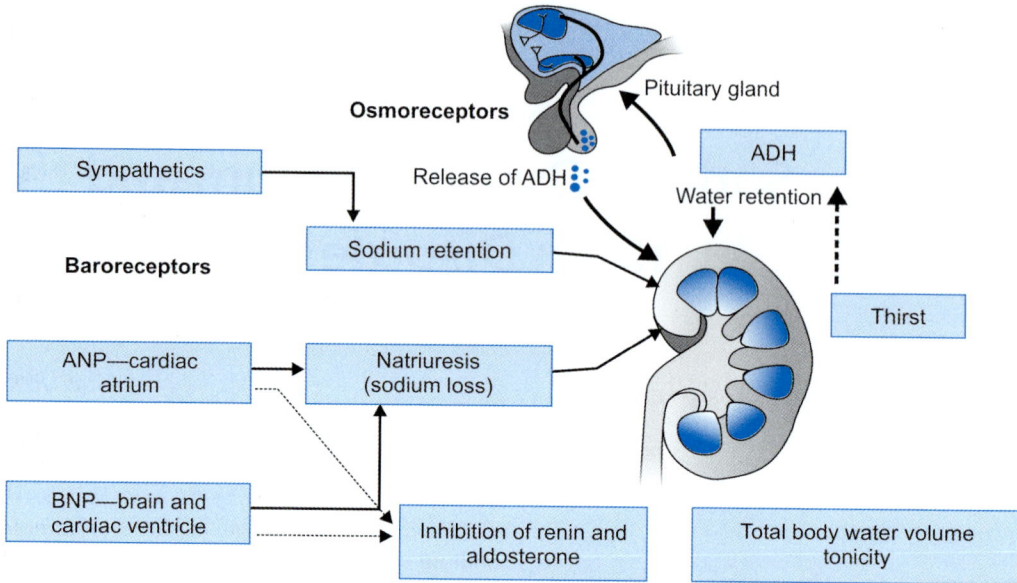

Figure 24.1 Normal regulation of sodium and water balance
Abbreviations: ADH, antidiuretic hormone; ANP, atrial natriuretic peptide; BNP, brain natriuretic peptide

Regulation of the plasma osmolality and sodium concentration is mediated by changes in water intake and water excretion. *This occurs via two mechanisms*:
1. Urinary concentration [via pituitary secretion and renal effects of antidiuretic hormone arginine vasopressin (AVP)].
2. Thirst.

Normally thirst and AVP release are stimulated by an increase in body fluid osmolality above the osmotic threshold (approximately 280–290 mOsm/L). An increased osmolality draws water from cells into the blood. Dehydration and deformation of specific cells in the brain activates the osmoreceptors or tonicity receptors that act like mechanoreceptors. On stimulation, they signal to other parts of the brain to initiate thirst and AVP release, resulting in increased water ingestion and urinary concentration, rapidly correcting the hypernatremic state.

DISORDERS OF SODIUM BALANCE

The disorders of sodium balance are actually disorders of water balance and are common in brain diseases especially in critically ill children. In brain injuries as well as diseases affecting the brain, there is organ cross talk that helps to maintain internal homeostasis **(Flow chart 24.1)**. However sodium imbalance is common in Neurological diseases especially in infections—meningitis encephalitis, brain tumors, trauma, hemorrhage and surgery.

IMPACT OF SODIUM BALANCE DISORDERS ON BRAIN

Hyponatremia and hypernatremia have profound impact on morbidity and mortality in neurological disorders. In acute hyperosmolar states (hypernatremia) there is loss of intracellular water with cell shrinkage. Initially cells will maintain the volume by retaining intracellular solutes like potassium. However, this adaptive mechanism is not efficient to maintain cell volume and shape. This is followed by gradual restoration of brain volume via the generation of nonelectrolyte osmotically active intracellular solute (Idiogenic Osmoles) which are synthesized within 48 hours. Cells thus achieve a relatively balanced state or equilibrium.

Flow chart 24.1 Brain injury and organ cross talk

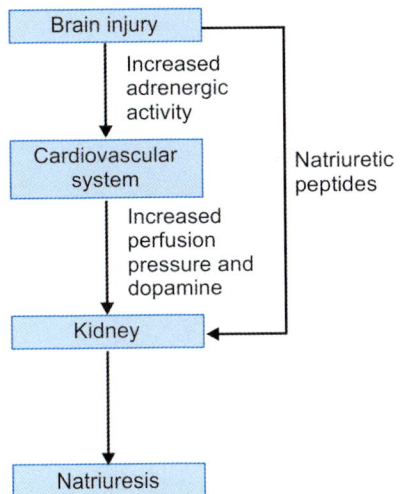

In the hypo-osmolar state (hyponatremia), there is cellular expansion which is corrected over time by the loss of intracellular solute like potassium initially. After 48 hours idiogenic osmoles synthesized by cells are extruded to maintain a new steady state. Total brain volume is therefore preserved by alterations in the intracellular milieu. Rapid correction in chronic hypo as well as hypernatremia (more than 48 hours) results in complications.

Symptomatology

Both hyponatremia and hypernatremia results in confusion, lethargy, convulsions and, finally, coma. They complicate CNS disorders and increase both morbidity and mortality.

HYPONATREMIA

Hyponatremia is the most frequent electrolyte disorder in critically ill children with neurological disorders. *Common causes of hyponatremia in CNS diseases include*:
- Syndrome of inappropriate antidiuretic hormone secretion (SIADH)
- Cerebral salt wasting syndrome (CSWS)
- Administration of hypotonic fluid (most common iatrogenic cause).
- Hyperglycemia or mannitol (translocational hyponatremia)
- Drug related hyponatremia (carbamazepine and oxcarbazepine).

If the measured serum osmolality exceeds twice the serum sodium concentration and azotemia is not present, suspect hyperglycemia or mannitol as the cause of hyponatremia.

Syndrome of Inappropriate Antidiuretic Hormone Secretion

Approach to hyponatremia is given in **Flow chart 24.2**.

The SIADH is characterized by high urinary sodium loss without corresponding loss of water, leading to a decrease in plasma osmolality. The urine is hypertonic. The most common causes are meningitis, encephalitis, brain tumor and, subarachnoid hemorrhage (SAH). SIADH has also been reported following spinal surgery. Plasma osmolality < 270 mOsm/kg with inappropriate urinary concentration (> 100 mOsm/kg) in a child with euvolemia suggests SIADH. Exclusion of hypothyroidism and glucocorticoid deficiency confirms the diagnosis. Treatment is by fluid restriction.[1]

Cerebral Salt-wasting Syndrome

Cerebral salt-wasting syndrome (CSWS) was first described by Peter, et al. in 1950.[2] It is defined by the development of excessive natriuresis and subsequent hyponatremia, dehydration in patients with intracranial disease. Subarachnoid hemorrhage (SAH) is one of the most common cause of CSWS. Other common causes are acute CNS disorders like septic, viral, and herpetic meningitis.[3-5] Cerebral salt-wasting syndrome is characterized by polyuria and natriuresis resulting in intracellular volume depletion and symptomatic hyponatremia. It usually develops in the first week following a brain insult. Its duration is usually brief and spontaneously resolves in 2–4 weeks. Sometimes it lasts for several months.

The cerebral salt wasting syndrome is due to renal sodium transport abnormality in intracranial diseases. The adrenal and thyroid functions are normal. It may be more appropriately termed renal salt wasting. The exact pathophysiology of

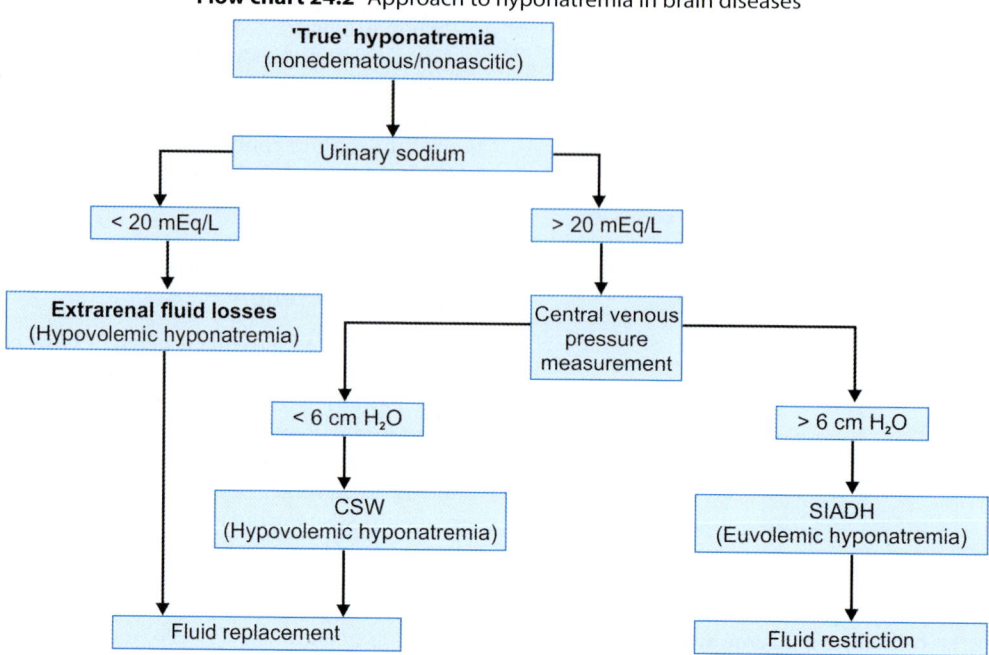

Flow chart 24.2 Approach to hyponatremia in brain diseases

CSWS is not known. Exaggerated renal pressure—natriuresis by increased activity of the sympathetic nervous system and dopamine release possibly results in urinary sodium loss. Another hypothesis involves the release of natriuretic factors ANP and BNP that cause natriuresis and hyponatremia. The decreased effective circulating volume activates baroreceptors, which increase antidiuretic hormone (ADH) secretion resulting in water conservation and return to an equilibrated state.[5] In contrast, SIADH primarily occurs due to an inappropriate rise in ADH secretion in the setting of euvolemia.

Differentiation of CSW from SIADH can be difficult as both can present with hyponatremia and concentrated urine with natriuresis. Failure to distinguish cerebral salt-wasting syndrome (renal salt wasting) from SIADH may lead to improper therapy. In SIADH fluid restriction is the treatment and this will exacerbate intravascular volume depletion and jeopardize the cerebral perfusion.

The following features may help in differentiating CSW from SIADH:

- *Urinary output:* Urine is relatively dilute and the flow rate is often high in cerebral salt-wasting syndrome. The urine is usually very concentrated and the flow rate is low in SIADH.
- Urinary sodium concentrations are typically elevated in cerebral salt-wasting syndrome and in SIADH (>40 mEq/L). However, 24 hour urinary sodium excretion is substantially higher than sodium intake in cerebral salt-wasting syndrome but generally equals sodium intake in SIADH. Therefore, net sodium balance (intake minus output) is negative in cerebral salt-wasting syndrome **(Table 24.1)**.[4]

An expectant and supportive management strategy is best adopted in asymptomatic patients with hyponatremia. Treatment is indicated in the presence of acute symptomatic hyponatremia. Rapid correction of hyponatremia, especially in the chronic setting can lead to neurologic sequel. This risk can be minimized by gradual correction of sodium deficit. The treatment should be targeted to the point of alleviation of symptoms rather than to the achievement of biochemical normality.[6-8]

Sodium Dysequilibrium and the Brain Disorders in Children

Table 24.1 Salient differentiating features of CSW from SIADH

Lab parameter	SIADH	CSW
Serum Na$^+$	< 135 mEq/L	< 135 mEq/L
Urine Na$^+$	> 25 mEq/L	> 40 mEq/L
Serum Osm	< 270 mOsm/kg	< 270 mOsm/kg
Urine Osm	> 300 mOsm/kg	> 300 mOsm/kg
Urine output	Oliguria	Polyuria
Central venous pressure	Normal/high	Low
Plasma ADH	High	Normal

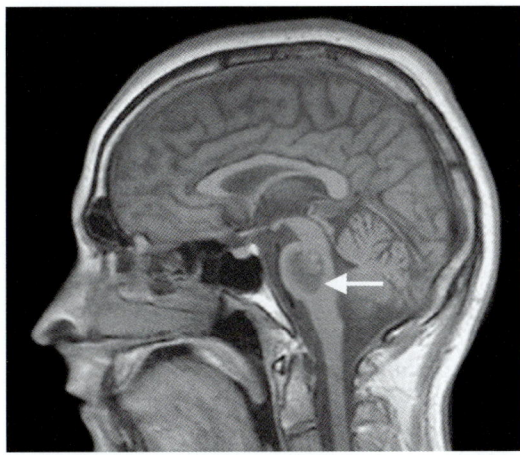

Figure 24.2 Central pontine myelinolysis

The appropriate management of SIADH is fluid restriction, initially to 1L per day. This usually results in a slow rise in sodium of 1.5 mmol/L/day. If supplemental intravenous fluid is required, 0.9% saline is the usual choice.

Best management of CSWS is fluid and sodium resuscitation with 0.9% saline. In acute symptomatic hyponatremia, hypertonic (3%) saline is recommended. If there is hypervolemia furosemide is given along with saline. In cases refractory to salt and fluid therapy, oral fludrocortisone 0.05–0.1 mg/day is given in combination with sodium chloride supplementation.

The dangers of rapid correction of hyponatremia are serious. Pontine and extrapontine myelinolysis **(Fig. 24.2)**, characterized by mutism, dysarthria and lethargy followed by spastic quadriparesis and pseudobulbar palsy occurs with rapid elevation of serum sodium levels. Risk factors for its development include malnutrition and liver disease. The risk of myelinolysis can be minimized by gradual correction of sodium deficit at a rate of less than 10 mmol/L/24 h. Close monitoring during treatment is mandatory. If over-rapid correction is suspected, desmopressin and water is given.[9,10]

HYPERNATREMIA

Hypernatremia is defined as serum sodium >145 mmol/L. It is relatively more common in neurologic and critically ill patients than in the general population. Hypernatremia indicates water depletion either due to inadequate water supplementation or excessive water loss.[5] Only rarely does it represent salt excess, such as ingestion of salt or infusion of saline or hypertonic fluids. Except in cases of uncontrollable diabetes insipidus, a hypernatremia can be maintained only if access to water is denied or thirst is impaired as in children with decreased level of consciousness. Osmotic diuresis due to urea may be also a cause of hypernatremia in critically ill patients.

Central diabetes insipidus (CDI) is due to failure of release of ADH from the hypothalamopituitary axis. It is characterized by the inability to concentrate urine and a large volume of inappropriately dilute urine is produced. There will be rise is plasma sodium, serum osmolality and progressive dehydration as more water is lost from the body as compared to sodium. Pituitary surgery is one of the common causes of CDI. Brain dead patients often develop severe CDI and is particularly relevant in the management of potential organ donors.

An abnormally high serum osmolality (> 305 mmol/kg) and serum sodium (> 145 mmol/L), in combination with an abnormally low urine osmolality (< 350 mmol/kg), reflecting the inability of the kidney to concentrate urine in an appropriate manner suggests the diagnosis of CDI.

A urine specific gravity (SG) of less than 1.005, in the light of raised serum sodium, points strongly to a diagnosis of CDI. Other causes of water diuresis, including prehospital and intraoperative volume resuscitation may also cause hypernatremia. Solute diuresis may also be caused by osmotic diuresis secondary to the use of mannitol or hypertonic saline for control of intracranial pressure, or hyperglycemia. Conscious patients with CDI are able to increase water intake and if this fails, or if urine output is greater than 4 mL/kg/h, parenteral or intranasal vasopressin may be administered. In the unconscious patient, fluid replacement is best achieved with either intravenous 5% dextrose or water via a nasogastric tube with concomitant DDAVP administration. Intranasal (DDAVP) is given in a dose of 5–40 μg/day (0.4–1.4 μg/kg/day) in 2–3 doses. Oral dose is 0.05 mg 2 times daily initially and effective dose range from 0.1–1.2 mg divided q8–12h. Restrict fluid intake as desmopressin may cause water intoxication and hyponatremia. If switching to PO from intranasal, start PO at least 12 hours after last intranasal dose. Desmopressin can be administered intravenously and subcutaneously 2–4 μ/day divided q12h or one-tenth the maintenance of intranasal dose.[10,11]

Rapid correction of hypernatremia may cause pulmonary and cerebral edema. A reduction in serum sodium concentration of 10 mmol/L/day is safe. A more rapid reduction is indicated only in acute symptomatic hypernatremia.

CONCLUSION

Sodium and water balance disorders affect the outcome of neurological disorders. Close monitoring of serum sodium must be carried out in all children admitted with neurological disorders for effective early interventions to improve the outcome.

REFERENCES

1. Schwartz WB, Bennet W, Curelop S. A syndrome of renal sodium loss and hyponatremia probably resulting from inappropriate secretion of antidiuretic hormone. Am J Med. 1950;23(4):529-2.
2. Peters JP, Welt LG, Sims EA, et al. A salt-wasting syndrome associated with cerebral disease. Trans Assoc Am Physicians. 1957;63:57-64.
3. Maesaka JK, Imbriano LJ, Ah NM, Hamathy E. Is it cerebral or renal salt wasting? Kidney Int. 2009;76(9):934-8.
4. Hardesty DA, Kilbaugh TJ, Storm PB. Cerebral salt wasting syndrome in postoperative pediatric brain tumor patients. Neuro Crit Care. 2012;17(3):382-7.
5. Bussmann C, Bast T, Rating D. Hyponatraemia in children with acute CNS disease: SIADH or cerebral salt wasting? Childs Nerv Syst. 2001;17(1-2):58-62. 25.
6. Moritz ML, Ayus JC. New aspects in the pathogenesis, prevention, and treatment of hyponatremic encephalopathy in children. Pediatr Nephrol. 2010;25(7):1225-38.
7. Albanese A, Hindmarsh P, Stanhope R. Management of hyponatraemia in patients with acute cerebral insults. Arch Dis Child. 2001;85(3):246-51.
8. Brimioulle S, Orellana-Jimenez C, Aminian A, Vincent JL. Hyponatremia in neurological patients: cerebral salt wasting versus inappropriate antidiuretic hormone secretion. Intensive Care Med. 2008;34(1):125-31.
9. Yee AH, Burns JD, Wijdicks EF. Cerebral salt wasting: pathophysiology, diagnosis, and treatment. Neurosurg Clin N Am. 2010;21(2):339-52.
10. Agha A, Thornton E, O'Kelly P, Tormey W, Phillips J, Thompson CJ. Posterior pituitary dysfunction after traumatic brain injury. J Clin Endocrinol Metab. 2004;89(12):5987-92.
11. Verkman AS. Aquaporins in clinical medicine. Annu Rev Med. 2012;63:303-16.

CHAPTER 25

Muscle Disorders: A Practical Approach

D Kalpana

Muscle diseases are a group of disorders in which there is a structural or functional abnormality of skeletal muscle. They can be hereditary, metabolic or acquired **(Table 25.1)**.[1] These disorders are relatively rare in children and often, identified relatively late. Accurate early diagnosis helps in prognostication and optimal rehabilitation; curative treatment (enzyme replacement therapy in Pompe's disase) in some, and aids in genetic counseling and prenatal diagnosis.

Common symptoms of neuromuscular disease may include infantile floppiness or hypotonia, isolated delay in motor milestones, feeding and respiratory difficulties, drooping of eye lids, ophthalmoplegia, abnormal gait and frequent falls, difficulty with climbing stairs or arising from the floor, and muscle pain, cramps or contractures. Muscle diseases can be distinguished from other disorders of the motor unit—including anterior horn cell disorders, neuromuscular junction disorders, and peripheral neuropathies—by characteristic clinical and laboratory features.

CLINICAL EVALUATION

In evaluating children with muscle weakness, the first step should be the anatomic localization of the lesion **(Table 25.1)**. A detailed history and focussed clinical examination help us to narrow down the differential diagnoses, so that there will be maximum yield from investigations. The second step is to identify whether it is due to a hereditary or acquired cause. The third step is to find out whether there is a definitive treatment. If not, try to provide optimal rehabilitation measures and adaptive equipment so that the child can use his/her functional abilities to the maximum. The final step should be an early, accurate genetic diagnosis, which is invaluable in genetic counseling and planning future pregnancies.

Table 25.1 Classification of myopathies[1]

Hereditary myopathies	Acquired myopathies
• Congenital myopathies	• Inflammatory myopathies
• Congenital myotonic dystrophy	• Drug induced (steroids, statins)
• Metabolic myopathies (Pompe's disease, McArdle's disease, carnitine deficiency)	• Toxic myopathies
• Mitochondrial myopathies	• Endocrine myopathies (Hypothyroidism, cushing's disease)
• Periodic paralysis	• Critical illness myopathy
• Muscular dystrophies	• Hypokalemia, hypocalcemia

Symptoms Pertaining to Muscle Disease

The most common presenting symptom is muscle weakness, which may affect specific groups of muscles in specific muscle diseases. Detailed enquiries should be made regarding the pattern of weakness. See **Table 25.2** for the functional assessment of muscle weakness by history.

Other symptoms include myalgia (muscle pain) which may be present in inflammatory myopathies (polymyositis and dermatomyositis), muscle cramps in glycogen storage disease type 5 (McArdle's disease), contractures in congenital muscular dystrophy and Emery Dreifuss muscular dystrophy (EDMD). Myotonia (impaired relaxation of muscle after voluntary contraction) manifests as difficulty in releasing the handgrip after a handshake, unscrewing a bottle top, or opening the eyelids after closing it tightly. Symptoms of myotonia is often absent in children with myotonic dystrophy, but the parents may have the signs and symptoms of myotonia, which should be enquired into.

Age of Onset and Progression of Symptoms[2]

Congenital myopathies, congenital muscular dystrophy and myotonic dystrophy and infantile onset Pompe's disease may be symptomatic from birth **(Table 25.3)**. Duchenne muscular dystrophy is often identified by 3–5 years. Most of the limb girdle muscular dystrophies and facioscapulohumeral muscular dystrophy (FSHD) present in the second decade. The tempo of the disorders with constant weakness can vary from: (1) acute or subacute progression in some inflammatory myopathies (dermatomyositis and polymyositis), (2) chronic slow progression over years (most muscular dystrophies), or (3) nonprogressive weakness with little change over decades (congenital myopathies). Congenital myopathies and congenital myotonic dystrophy may present with respiratory distress often requiring ventilation at birth. The weakness may improve significantly and then the disease runs a relatively static course. Glycogen storage diseases like McArdle's disease, channelopathies and carnitine deficiency may present with episodic weakness.

Family History

A detailed family tree should be completed to evaluate for evidence of autosomal dominant, autosomal recessive, and X-linked patterns of transmission **(Table 25.4)**. A history of consanguinity of parents is a clue for autosomal recessive disorders. Always ask for any weakness or disability in relatives rather than asking for "similar illness", specifically enquire about maternal uncles and grand maternal uncles' disability/death in X-linked recessive diseases like Duchenne muscular dystrophy and Becker muscular dystrophy.

Table 25.2 Functional assessment of muscle weakness[2]

Location	Symptoms of weakness
Facial	Inability to "bury eyelashes," "horizontal smile," inability to whistle
Ocular	Double vision, ptosis
Bulbar	Nasal speech, weak cry, nasal regurgitation of liquids, poor suck, difficulty swallowing, recurrent aspiration pneumonia, cough during meals
Neck	Poor head control
Trunk	Scoliosis, lumbar lordosis, protuberant abdomen, difficulty sitting up
Shoulder girdle	Difficulty lifting objects overhead, scapular winging
Forearm/hand	Inability to make a tight fist, finger or wrist drop
Pelvic girdle	Difficulty climbing stairs, waddling gait, Gower's sign
Leg/foot	Foot drop, inability to walk on heels or toes
Respiratory	Use of accessory muscles, paradoxical respiration

Muscle Disorders: A Practical Approach

Table 25.3 Age of onset of myopathies

Myopathies presenting at birth	Myopathies presenting in childhood
• *Congenital myopathies:* Central core disease, centronuclear myopathy, Nemaline (rod) myopathy, congenital fiber type disproportion • Congenital muscular dystrophy • Congenital myotonic dystrophy • Glycogen storage diseases • Carnitine deficiency	• Muscular dystrophies [DMD, BMD, LGMD, FSHD, Emery-Dreifuss muscular dystrophy, congenital muscular dystrophy (Ullrich and Bethlem)] • *Congenital myopathies:* Nemaline myopathy, centronuclear myopathy, central core • *Inflammatory myopathies:* Dermatomyositis, polymyositis (rarely) • Juvenile Pompe's disease • Mitochondrial myopathy • Periodic paralysis

Abbreviations: BMD, Becker muscular dystrophy; DMD, Duchenne muscular dystrophy; FSHD, facioscapulohumeral muscular dystrophy; LGMD, limb-girdle muscular dystrophy

Table 25.4 Myopathies and pattern of inheritance[2]

Autosomal-dominant
FSHD, LGMD, oculopharyngeal muscular dystrophy, myotonic dystrophy, periodic paralysis, paramytonia congenita, Thomsen's disease, central core myopathy

Autosomal-recessive
LGMD, metabolic myopathies, Becker's myotonia

Maternal transmission
Mitochondrial myopathies

X-linked
Duchenne's MD, Becker's MD, Emery-Dreifuss MD

Abbreviations: FSHD, facioscapulohumeral muscular dystrophy; LGMD, limb-girdle muscular dystrophy

Precipitating Factors[2]

A history of weakness, pain, and/or myoglobinuria that is provoked by exercise might suggest the possibility of a glycolytic pathway defect. Worsening of weakness with fever would be supportive of a diagnosis of carnitine palmitoyl transferase deficiency. Periodic paralysis is characteristically provoked by exercise and ingestion of a carbohydrate meal, followed by a period of rest.

Involvement of Other Systems[2]

Respiratory failure may be the presenting symptom of acid maltase deficiency, centronuclear myopathy, myotonic dystrophy, or nemaline myopathy. Cardiomyopathy is an early feature of Pompe's disease. It is also seen in Duchenne and Becker muscular dystrophy. Cardiac conduction defects are characteristic of myotonic dystrophy and FSHD. Hepatomegaly may be seen in myopathies associated with deficiencies in acid maltase (Pompe's), carnitine, and debranching enzyme. The presence of cataracts, frontal balding, and mental retardation strongly suggests the diagnosis of myotonic dystrophy. Heliotrope rash over the upper eyelids and Gottron's papules over the knuckles, clinches the diagnosis of dermatomyositis.

Distribution of Weakness, Atrophy/Hypertrophy

Most of the myopathies present with symmetrical proximal muscle weakness. Facial weakness and scapular winging suggests facioscapulohumeral muscular dystrophy (FSHD). Scapular winging is also seen in limb-girdle muscular dystrophy (LGMD) Type 2A (calpainopathy), Pompe's disease and sarcoglycanopathy. Distal myopathies may have profound atrophy of the anterior or posterior compartments of leg. Ptosis and ophthalmoparesis without prominent pharyngeal involvement is a hallmark of many of the mitochondrial myopathies. Ptosis and facial weakness without ophthalmoparesis is a common feature of myotonic dystrophy and FSHD **(Fig. 25. 1)**. Ptosis has diurnal variation in ocular myasthenia gravis and is often associated with diplopia. Bulbar weakness with dysphagia, drooling and recurrent aspiration is common in congenital myasthenia,

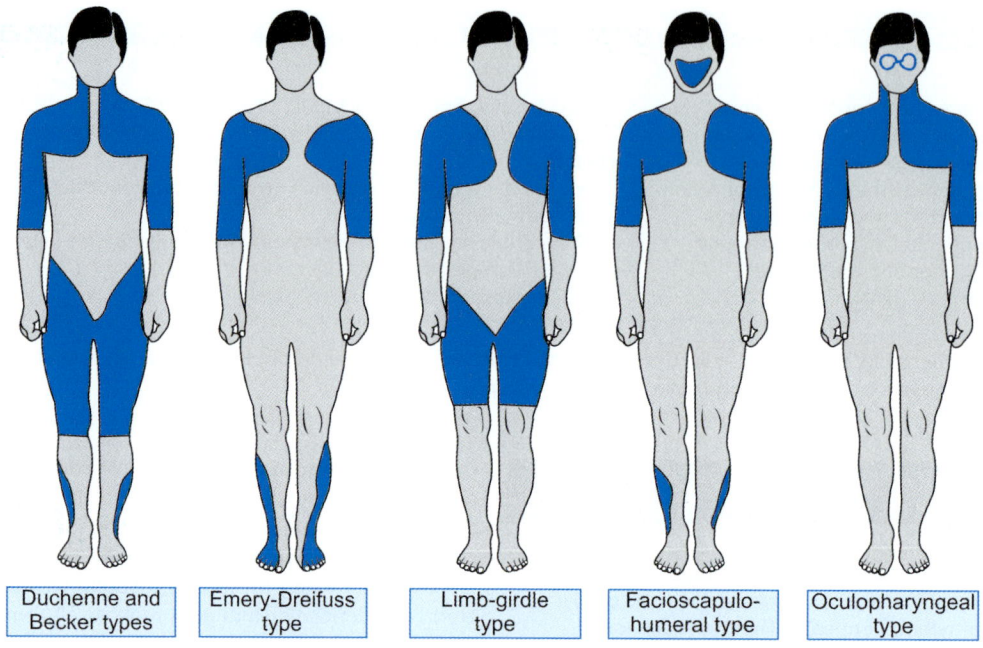

Figure 25.1 Pattern of muscle weakness in muscular dystrophies[1]

congenital myotonic dystrophy and some congenital myopathies.[3]

Calf muscle hypertrophy (pseudohypertrophy—the muscle fibers are replaced by fat and fibrous tissue) is seen in Duchenne, Becker, Sarcoglycanopathy and hypothyroidism (Kocher-Debré-Sémélaigne syndrome) and acid maltase deficiency (childhood type). The other muscles hypertrophied in Duchenne muscular dystrophy (DMD) include tongue muscles, deltoid, infraspinatus, brachioradialis, etc. In addition there is atrophy of quadriceps, pectoralis major, latissimus dorsi, etc. This selective atrophy and hypertrophy produces the characteristic Valley sign in DMD and Becker muscular dystrophy (BMD). In myotonia congenita there is generalized muscle hypertrophy (infant Hercules appearance).

DIFFERENTIAL DIAGNOSIS

When the infant presents with floppiness, we have to differentiate hypotonia due to central or syndromic causes from peripheral hypotonia.[3] History of prematurity, low APGAR score, neonatal encephalopathy and seizures may point to a central cause. Dysmorphic features may help in identifying Down syndrome, Zellweger syndrome, Prader-Willi syndrome, etc. (Prader-Willi syndrome children are born with a low birth weight and there may be failure to thrive initially. Obesity develops after the first year. Micropenis may be a clinical clue). Observe the degree of movement of the limbs, children with central hypotonia may be able to lift the limbs off the couch (floppy strong) whereas in lower motor neuron lesion (LMN), the limbs will be weak and lifting limbs against gravity is not possible (floppy weak) **(Table 25.5)**.

The floppy infant with a primary neuromuscular disorder typically presents as an alert baby who has paucity of movement, particularly proximal antigravity movement, and diminished or absent reflexes. The important causes of floppy baby due to peripheral hypotonia are anterior horn cell disease like SMA type 1, neuromuscular junction disorders like congenital myasthenia, and muscle disorders like congenital myopathies, congenital muscular dystrophy and congenital myotonic dystrophy. Involvement of facial

Table 25.5 Floppy infant: Differential diagnosis

	Central	Peripheral
Developmental delay	Global	Predominantly motor
Seizures	Common	Rare
Dysmorphic features	May be present	Absent
Spontaneous antigravity movements	Normal	Reduced
Ventral suspension	Lifts head up (extensor hypertonia)	Rag doll appearance
Vertical suspension	Scissoring	Floppy
Deep tendon reflexes	Normal or brisk	Decreased
Fasciculations	Absent	May be present
Respiratory muscle weakness	Absent	May be present

Table 25.6 Spinal muscular atrophy type 3 vs DMD

Spinal muscular atrophy type	Duchenne muscular dystrophy
Early prominent muscle wasting	Muscle wasting proportionate to degree of weakness
Early loss of DTR	DTR depressed, ankle jerk is retained till late
Muscle hypertrophy rare	Hypertrophy of calf muscle, deltoid, tongue, brachioradialis
Valley sign absent	Valley sign present
Tongue fasciculations and polyminimyoclonus present	Fasciculations absent
CPK: Normal or mildly elevated	Marked elevation
EMG: Neuropathic pattern	Myopathic pattern

Abbreviations: DTR, deep tendon reflexes; CPK, creatine phosphokinase; EMG, electromyography

muscles is characteristic of congenital myopathy, myasthenia and congenital myotonic dystrophy. Facial muscles are spared in SMA **(Table 25.6)**. Fasciculations of tongue, if present favors the diagnosis of anterior horn cell disease like spinal muscular atrophy. Intercostal muscle involvement is seen in spinal muscular atrophy, congenital myotonic dystrophy and certain congenital myopathies. Ptosis and ophthalmoplegia are seen in centronuclear myopathy, congenital myasthenia and mitochondrial myopathy. Short stature, cataract, baldness and history suggestive of myotonia in mother clinches the diagnosis of congenital myotonic dystrophy in the baby.

In a child with slowly progressive proximal muscle weakness, the important differential diagnosis is between anterior horn cell disease (spinal muscular atrophy type 2 or 3) and muscle disease (muscular dystrophy/myopathy). In spinal muscular atrophy, atrophy of muscles is more prominent, deep tendon reflexes will be lost early, and fasciculation of tongue or fine tremor of fingers (polymini myoclonus) may be seen **(Table 25.6)**.

In children with ptosis, ophthalmoplegia and bulbar weakness, neuromuscular junction disorders like myasthenia gravis or congenital myasthenic syndromes are an important diagnostic consideration.[4] The presence of diurnal variation of symptoms and fatigability on sustained muscle contraction points to the diagnosis of myasthenia. Here the weakness is purely motor and deep tendon reflexes are retained. Clinical improvement after neostigmine injection and repetitive nerve stimulation test helps in diagnosis.

INVESTIGATIONS

Creatinine Phosphokinase

The CPK is elevated in most patients with muscle disease, but may be normal in slowly progressive myopathies. The degree of CPK elevation can also be helpful in distinguishing different types of muscle diseases. Significant elevations of CPK (×10 times or more) is seen in muscular dystrophies, Pompe's disease and inflammatory myopathies, whereas it may be normal or mildly raised (2–3 times normal) in congenital myopathies.[3] Mild elevations of CPK can be seen in normal individuals and in spinal muscular atrophy. Enzymes such as aldolase, aspartate aminotransferase (AST), alanine aminotransferase (ALT) and lactate dehydrogenase (LDH) may be slightly elevated in myopathies.

Serum lactate is elevated in mitochondrial myopathies. While taking blood for CPK and lactate make sure that tourniquet is not applied, which may falsely elevate CPK and lactate.

Serum electrolytes, thyroid function tests, parathyroid hormone levels, vitamin D levels, and human immunodeficiency virus and serologic tests for collagen vascular diseases are other useful investigations.

Electrophysiologic Studies

Nerve conduction studies are typically normal in myopathies. Needle electromyography (EMG) examination shows absence of spontaneous activity, brief-duration, small-amplitude motor units and early, complete recruitment in myopathy. But the procedure is painful and often cannot be completed in most children. Inflammatory myopathies and metabolic myopathies like Pompe's disease may show fibrillation potentials. Demonstration of myotonia in mother, by the characteristic dive bomber sound on needle insertion, clinches the diagnosis of congenital myotonic dystrophy in the baby, as myotonia is often absent in young infants.

Muscle Biopsy

Muscle biopsy is a useful investigation in the diagnosis of muscle disorders. The selection of muscle is very important. Useful information is gained by selecting a muscle that is moderately involved by disease. Biopsy from a very weak muscle may show complete replacement by fat and fibrous tissue and if an uninvolved muscle is selected, normal result will be obtained. The ordinary H&E stain can show dystrophic changes in muscular dystrophy, it will be normal in congenital myopathies. Muscle tissue should be immediately frozen for histochemical and immune histochemical studies. Thus it is better to send the child to a specialized center for muscle biopsy. A well performed muscle biopsy narrows the differential diagnosis, so that appropriate genetic testing can be ordered. But when the clinical features clinch to a definite diagnosis, as in DMD, genetic testing can be sent without muscle biopsy.

MRI Brain

MRI brain may show characteristic abnormalities in congenital muscular dystrophy. In merosin deficient muscular dystrophy there will be symmetric white matter changes in brain, even though the baby is clinically asymptomatic. Pachygyria, polymicrogyria, cobblestone cortex and cerebellar cysts are seen in Fukuyama type of congenital muscular dystrophy and Walker Warburg disease.[5]

Molecular Genetic Testing[5]

The specific molecular genetic defect is now known for a large number of hereditary myopathies, and mutations can be identified by peripheral blood DNA analysis. Molecular genetic testing frequently eliminates the need for muscle biopsy. This technology is also extremely helpful for determining the carrier status and for performing prenatal testing. Genetic testing for DMD/BMD is widely available and cheap. For congenital muscular dystrophy, mitochondrial myopathy and LGMD, genetic panels are available, but are costly. For Pompe disease, dry blood spot assay is a good screening test, which must be followed by confirmation of acid alpha-glucosidase enzymatic activity in blood lymphocytes or other tissues (muscle or skin fibroblasts) or through gene sequencing.[5]

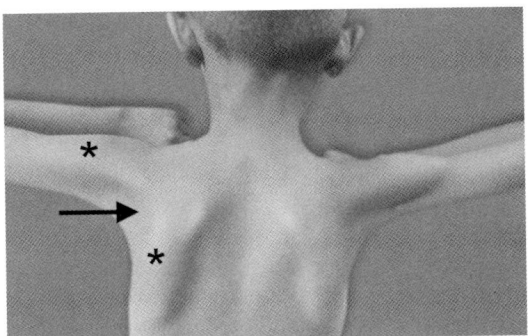

Figure 25.2: Valley sign in DMD. Note the valley (arrow) between hypertrophied deltoid and infraspinatus *(For color version, see Plate 5)*

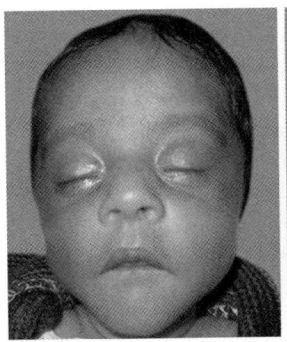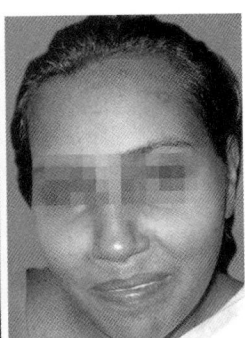

Figure 25.3 Baby with congenital myotonic dystrophy, note the myopathic facies, also note the frontal baldness of mother, she was short (148 cm) and had myotonia, previous baby was still born *(For color version, see Plate 5)*

Duchenne Muscular Dystrophy

The DMD is an X-linked disorder due to mutations in the dystrophin gene. Affected children usually present in their pre-school years with delayed gross motor milestones and inability to keep up with their peers in running and jumping; serum CK is usually markedly raised (10–100 × normal). The disease is characterized by progressive proximal weakness resulting in the Gower's sign, hypertrophy of calf muscles, deltoid and brachioradialis and, atrophy of pectorals, quadriceps and latissimus dorsi. The characteristic 'valley sign' is because of the hypertrophied deltoid and infraspinatus atrophy of latissimus dorsi. If untreated children lose independent ambulation by 13 years **(Fig. 25.2)**. Scoliosis and contractures, respiratory muscle weakness, cardiac conduction defects and cardiomyopathy are seen with progression of the disease. Becker muscular dystrophy is an allelic disorder (i.e. also due to mutations in the dystrophin gene), but patients have later onset and more variable progression and severity.

Limb-girdle Muscular Dystrophy

This is present with predominantly symmetrical proximal muscle weakness without facial involvement. The autosomal recessive types like sarcoglycanopathy and calpainopathy presents in the first decade.

Facioscapulohumeral Muscular Dystrophy

Involvement of face, proximal muscles of shoulder and peroneal muscles are involved. The weakness is often asymmetric. Asymmetric involvement of abdominal muscles result in positive Beevor's sign. FSHD is autosomal dominant and shows anticipation. There may be associated deafness in some.

Congenital Myopathies

The congenital myopathies usually present at birth or childhood with hypotonia and generalized weakness and a static or slowly progressive course. CK is usually normal or only mildly elevated. The presence of ophthalmoplegia, facial and bulbar involvement may help differentiate congenital myopathies from congenital muscular dystrophies, anterior horn cell disorders and early-onset peripheral neuropathies.

Myotonic Dystrophy

It is an autosomal dominant disorder characterized by hypotonia, weakness that may be proximally or distally predominant, ptosis, bilateral facial weakness, learning difficulties and myotonia on clinical examination and EMG **(Fig. 25.3)**. There are two genetic subtypes: myotonic dystrophy type 1 (DM1) is caused by an expanded CTG repeat in the dystrophia myotonicaprotein kinase gene, while type 2 (DM2) is caused by a CCTG expansion in the zinc finger protein 9 gene. Congenital myotonic dystrophy only occurs in DM1 and is associated with maternal transmission of an expanded trinucleotide repeat (usually with>1500 repeats). Patients present in the newborn period with hypotonia, talipes, bilateral facial weakness with a tented upper lip, open mouth and high arched palate. There may be a history of prematurity, reduced fetal movements and polyhydramnios. Respiratory insufficiency may be prominent and require mechanical ventilation. Reflexes are absent. The clinical course is characterized by motor and speech delay and a variable degree of learning difficulty. Clinical and EMG analysis of mother clinches the diagnosis, as myotonia is absent in infants.

MANAGEMENT

Specific treatment: Immunosupressant therapy with steroids and/or immune globulins is the mainstay of treatment in inflammatory myopathies like dermatomyositis. The treatment has to be continued for long periods (at least a year) to prevent relapses. Viral myositis responds very well to NSAIDs. Enzyme replacement therapy with alpha-glucosidase gives promising results in Pompe's disease. The treatment is very costly and has to be continued lifelong. Treatment modalities like antisense oligonucleotides, exon skipping and stem cell transplantation are in the experimental stage in DMD.

Supportive treatment: In most of the myopathies there is no definitive treatment. Moderate physiotherapy helps to prevent muscle atrophy and contractures. They should receive calcium and vitamin D supplements to prevent osteoporosis, obesity is to be avoided, as it will further impair mobility. Once the children lose ambulation, scoliosis develops rapidly, compromising respiration further. Nasal continuous positive airway pressure (CPAP) and noninvasive ventilation at night helps in ameliorating hypoxia due to respiratory muscle involvement.

Treatment with steroids (prednisolone 0.75 mg/kg/day or deflazacort 0.9 mg/kg/day) improves muscle strength and prolong the period of ambulation by at least 2 years in children with DMD. The treatment has to be started at least by 5 years of age. The children should be monitored for steroid side effects like obesity, osteoporosis, cataract, etc.

Genetic counseling and prenatal diagnosis: An accurate genetic or enzymatic diagnosis is absolutely essential in predicting the prognosis and identifying the recurrence risk in the family. Prenatal diagnosis is now possible with Duchenne muscular dystrophy, myotonic dystrophy, congenital muscular dystrophy, Pompe's disease, etc.

Summary: Muscle diseases even though rare, has to be recognized early. The recognition of the onset, progression, pattern of weakness helps to narrow down the differential diagnosis so that appropriate genetic or enzymatic diagnosis can be ordered. Early diagnosis helps in curative treatment, at least for a minority of cases and helps in predicting the prognosis and channelizing the optimal rehabilitation methods for the child. An accurate genetic diagnosis helps in reducing the chance of recurrence of the disease in the family.

REFERENCES

1. Barohn RJ, Dimachkie MM, Jackson CE. A pattern recognition approach to patients with a suspected myopathy. Neurol Clin. 2014;32(3):569-93.
2. McDonald CM. Clinical approach to the diagnostic evaluation of hereditary and acquired neuromuscular diseases. Phys Med Rehabil Clin N Am. 2012;23(3):495-563.
3. Jackson CE. A clinical approach to muscle diseases. Semin Neurol. 2008;28(2):228-40.
4. Walters RJ. Muscle diseases: mimics and chameleons. Pract Neurol. 2014;14(5):288-98.
5. Menezes MP1, North KN. Inherited neuromuscular disorders: pathway to diagnosis. J Paediatr Child Health. 2012;48(6):458-65.

CHAPTER 26

Ocular Movement Disorders in Children

M Madhusudanan

INTRODUCTION

Ocular motility disorders in children can occur secondary to dysfunction of oculomotor systems as in adults, due to lesions in the brainstem, the nerves, neuromuscular junction, muscles as well as in their supranuclear control pathways. This chapter deals with oculomotor movement disorders seen almost exclusively in children.

Transient Ocular Motor Disturbances of Infancy

A variety of benign, transient supranuclear eye movement disturbances can be seen in healthy infants. These include horizontal squints, tonic downgaze and upgaze, opsoclonus, skew deviations, and transient idiopathic nystagmus. Since each of these disorders can be due to various other serious neurological disease, it is mandatory to do relevant investigations to rule out these conditions, especially in older children.

Transient Neonatal Strabismus

The eyes of otherwise healthy, full-term neonates at birth are commonly misaligned. In one study of 1,219 neonates,[1] 48.6% had orthotropia, 32.7% had exotropia, 3.2% had esotropia, and 15.4% were indeterminate. Follow-up studies of these patients have shown that these transient heterotropias become orthotropic between 2 and 3 months of age, in the vast majority of children. This coincides with development of stereoscopic vision.[2] Unlike exotropia, which may be found transiently in the neonatal period, congenital esotropia does not manifest in the neonate, which usually appears after 6 weeks of age. When it is seen in the neonate, other conditions such as sixth nerve palsy and Möbius syndrome have to be ruled out. Moreover, the eyes of premature infants may transiently display exotropia with limited adduction, suggesting an immaturity of the medial longitudinal fasciculus in the premature infant. Large convergent movements of the eyes, producing esotropia,can often seen in the first 2 months of life.[3] These convergent eye movements resolve spontaneously, giving way to normal ocular alignment.

Transient Idiopathic Nystagmus

Transient idiopathic nystagmus can occur infants, often associated with other visual abnormalities like retinopathy of prematurity, coloboma and delayed visual maturation. This transient nystagmus is thought to indicate a fragile period of postnatal maturation of the ocular motor system.[4] It is also known that some infants with delayed visual maturation may exhibit transient nystagmus.[5]

Tonic Downgaze

Tonic downward deviation of the eyes can occur as a transient phenomenon in neonates and does not necessarily indicate underlying neurologic dysfunction.[6] When the infant is awake, both eyes are tonically deviated downward; however, during sleep, both eyes return to the midline. The intact vertical oculocephalic reflex is indicative of supranuclear dysfunction. It usually resolves within the first 6 months of life. The immaturity of the vestibular system has been postulated as the cause in these cases. These transient episodes of downgaze can be followed by abnormal body movements in some cases.[6]

Absence of eyelid retraction differentiates this benign, transient form of tonic downgaze from the "setting sun sign" associated with congenital hydrocephalus. The setting sun sign is due to a combination of lid retraction (Collier's sign) and tonic downgaze. Acquired hydrocephalus in older patients does not produce tonic downgaze. This probably suggests a specific susceptibility of the neonatal brain to the mass effect of hydrocephalus on midbrain pretectal area, leading to more severe upgaze palsy (causing the eyes to deviate downward) than is seen in older patients. In congenital hydrocephalus that is not caused by intraventricular hemorrhage, the setting sun sign responds quickly to reduction of intracranial pressure.

Similarly, paroxysmal downward deviations of the eyes have been described in neurologically affected infants by Yokochi.[7] This was thought to be due to cortical visual impairment in the brain damaged infants. The paroxysms spontaneously resolved with time in many of these infants. Episodic downgaze may be one of the presenting signs of Leigh's disease.[8]

Premature infants with intraventricular hemorrhages may show acute tonic downward deviation of the eyes, esotropia and upgaze palsy.[9] Similarly tonic downgaze in conjunction with esotropia can be in infants with periventricular leukomalacia, without intraventricular hemorrhage.[10] As with intraventricular hemorrhage, the tonic downgaze spontaneously resolves, and infants are usually left with an A-pattern esotropia with superior oblique muscle over action.

Tonic downgaze can also be seen in very ill patients with medial thalamic hemorrhage with altered consciousness, acute obstructive hydrocephalus or severe subarachnoid hemorrhage. An almost similar condition is V-pattern pseudobobbing, wherein the eyes show an abrupt arrhythmic, repetitive, downward and inward ocular jerks at a rate of 1 per 3 seconds to 2 per second followed by a slow, upward drift to primary position.[11] This is seen in patients with acute obstructive hydrocephalus. It differs from the ocular bobbing by the presence of a V-pattern, a generally faster rate, and associated pretectal, rather than pontine signs.

Tonic Upgaze

Tonic upgaze is less common than tonic downgaze, and it also tends to be more episodic. In the "benign paroxysmal tonic upgaze of childhood." described by Ouvrier and Billson,[12] there is episodic tonic conjugate upward deviation of the eyes that was relieved by sleep. These children had impaired downgaze in addition, with down beating nystagmus on attempted downgaze and apparently normal horizontal movements. The patients were otherwise neurologically intact, with the exception of mild ataxia. All these children eventually improved.

Similarly, episodic tonic upgaze have been reported in infants in the first few months of life and were most conspicuous when the infant was ill or fatigued. These episodes diminished with time.[13] It is possible that benign hereditary downbeat nystagmus and the syndrome of benign tonic upward deviation of the eyes with ataxia are variants of the same disorder. In several of these affected children, tonic upgaze has evolved into down beating nystagmus.[12] Intermittent episodes of upward ocular deviation may be a manifestation of oculogyric crisis or a seizure disorder, typically petit mal. Oculogyric crisis denotes a sustained, extreme, episodic upward rotation of the eyes, lasting several seconds, after which the eyes return to the horizontal position and the cycle repeats again.

Transient Vertical Strabismus in Infancy

Sometimes transient vertical deviation can be seen in the neonatal period.[14] Some infants showing this sign may subsequently develop large-angle esotropia typical for congenital esotropia or nystagmus compensation syndrome.[14] Whether this transient vertical deviation of the eyes is an early manifestation of dissociated vertical divergence and whether it is an early premonitory sign of developing congenital esotropia in uncertain.

Congenital Cranial Dysinnervation Syndromes

The congenital cranial dysinnervation syndromes comprise a group of disorders characterized by deficient innervation to the extraocular muscles and facial musculature.[15] Under this category are the congenital ptosis, congenital fibrosis of the extraocular muscles, Duane's syndrome and its variants, Möbius syndrome and horizontal gaze palsy with progressive scoliosis.[15] They present with varying degrees of ptosis and ophthalmoplegia from birth, together with signs of aberrant innervation.

Congenital Fibrosis Syndrome

Congenital fibrosis of the extraocular muscles (CFEOM) is characterized by the presence of congenital restrictive ophthalmoplegia, fixed downgaze, horizontal strabismus, ptosis and a compensatory backward tilting of the head.[16] In this disorder, the extraocular muscles and the levator muscles are variably replaced by fibrous tissue.[17] The disorder may be unilateral or bilateral and may be clinically limited to certain muscles in a given individual. The resultant ocular motility disorder depends on which of the extraocular muscles are affected. The inferior rectus muscle is most commonly involved, followed by the levator muscle and the lateral rectus muscle. In the presence of ptosis, inferior and lateral rectus muscle involvement may resemble unilateral or bilateral congenital oculomotor palsy. Rarely, all of the extraocular muscles are affected (generalized fibrosis syndrome). Restricted forms are more common. These include congenital fibrosis of the inferior rectus with ptosis, strabismus fixes, congenital unilateral enophthalmos with ocular muscle fibrosis and ptosis,[18] and the vertical retraction syndrome.

Patients with CFEOM may show rapid convergent movements of the eyes on attempted upgaze, simulating convergence retraction nystagmus. The diagnosis of CFEOM should therefore be suspected when "convergence-retraction" nystagmus is accompanied by ptosis rather than lid retraction. This disorder is thought to result from a supranuclear deficiency of elevation.[19] Since these patients with CFEOM, show multiple synkinetic eye movements, Brodsky et al.[20] suggested that this disorder is caused by failure of normal neuronal connections with the extraocular muscles to become established early in embryogenesis. A primary failure to establish normal neuronal connections with the extraocular muscles and levator muscle would predispose to neuronal misdirection, which innervates few of the muscle fibers and replacement of the remaining muscle by fibrous tissue.[20] This would explain the superimposition of synkinetic eye movements on a diffuse congenital ophthalmoplegia.

Duane's Retraction Syndrome

This is one of the most common congenital disorders affecting the brainstem ocular motor system. The condition is usually sporadic, but familial cases are recognized. Pathologically these cases show a variety of abnormalities, typically absence of the abducens nucleus and nerve with evidence of aberrant innervation of the lateral rectus or recti by branches from the oculomotor nerves. The condition is usually unilateral but bilateral affection is not uncommon. Most patients do not report visual symptoms and vision itself is usually normal. It is often an incidental finding in patients presenting with other neurological problems.

In this condition, there is limitation or absence of abduction, a variable degree of limitation of adduction and the adducting eye shows retraction of the globe, with narrowing of the palpebral fissure. In addition, adduction may be accompanied by some degree of vertical eye movement, typically upwards. In some cases, there may be other congenital defects in the nervous system as well as in the other systems.

Möbius Syndrome

Möbius syndrome is a rare congenital disorder characterized by congenital facial weakness with horizontal gaze palsy[21] or impairment of ocular abduction. This condition is often associated with cranial nerve palsies, orofacial or limb malformations, and musculoskeletal system defects. Affected children have mask-like facies, with the open mouth. The upper facial nerves are affected more than the lower facial nerves. The eyes may be straight, esotropic or, rarely, exotropic.[22] As in Duane syndrome, congenital ocular motor synkinesis may be responsible for the horizontal conjugate gaze paresis in some cases. Other cranial nerves affected are V, IX, and XII, producing feeding and sucking difficulties in the neonatal period.

Brown Syndrome

Brown syndrome, also known as Superior Oblique Tendon Sheath syndrome is a mechanical problem in which the superior oblique muscle/tendon is unable to lengthen due to contracture when the patient is asked look up in the adducted position. This makes looking up and in with the affected eye difficult. Brown syndrome may be present at birth (congenital) or begin later. It may be constant or intermittent.

Brown syndrome has to be differentiated from Monocular Elevation Deficiency, also known as Double Elevator Palsy. In this condition, there is an inability to elevate one eye in all fields of gaze, usually resulting in one eye that is pointed downward relative to the other eye. Double elevator palsy is caused by a paralysis of the inferior oblique and/or superior rectus muscles of the same eye. However, it can also result from restriction of the inferior rectus muscle on that side. Brown syndrome can be distinguished from double elevator palsy by its increasing limitation of elevation in the adducted position. Inferior oblique palsy can be differentiated from the Brown syndrome by the fact that there is no superior oblique over action in Brown syndrome. Moreover, a positive forced adduction test can differentiate the two.

Strabismus in Children with Neurological Dysfunction

Common neurologic disorders of children are frequently associated with strabismus. These include cerebral palsy, Down syndrome, myelomeningocele, and hydrocephalus. Ophthalmologic abnormalities are seen in 50–90% of children with cerebral palsy.[23] Children with cerebral palsy have a markedly increased incidence of strabismus,[24] which is usually a horizontal concomitant strabismus. This is often associated with vertical A-pattern strabismus. One of the unique feature of strabismus seen in cerebral palsy is transient fluctuation from esotropia to exotropia, which is termed dyskinetic strabismus.[25] The craniosynostosis syndromes can sometimes present with complex forms of horizontal and vertical strabismus.[26]

Visuo-vestibular Disorders

Visuo-vestibular eye movements refer to ocular abnormalities that presumably arise from unequal visual input to the two eyes. These conditions arise from unbalanced binocular visual input to the central vestibular system.[27] These consist of *latent nystagmus, dissociated vertical divergence, and primary oblique muscle overaction.* Since these visual reflexes are compensatory for a central vestibular imbalance, they are not associated with dizziness, oscillopsia, or other neurologic symptoms that are commonly seen in vestibular disease.

- *Latent nystgamus* (described along with nystagmus, later in this chapter)
- *Dissociated vertical divergence is* characterized by an upward drift of a covered or cortically suppressed eye[28]
- *Primary oblique muscle overaction* consists of bilateral over elevation or over depression of the adducting eye.

Neurologic Esotropia

A variety of prenuclear neurologic diseases are characterized by an esotropic deviation of the eyes. These include acute comitant esotropia, congenital cranial dysinnervation syndromes, exercise-induced diplopia, periventricular leukomalacia (with or without cerebral palsy), spasm of the near reflex, and thalamic esotropia.[29]

Anticholinergic drugs can produce esotropia as a side effect, (anticholinergic esotropia), a condition in which excessive accommodative effort leads to accommodative esotropia. Anticholinergic esotropia seems to be precipitated by increased convergence of the eyes due to the increased accommodative effort in children with an inherent tendency to develop esotropia.

Spasm of the Near Reflex

Spasm of the near reflex is characterized by intermittent episodes of miosis, convergence, and accommodation. Patients demonstrate variable esotropia associated with pupillary constriction. Patients with spasm of the near reflex may present with diplopia, blurred vision (especially for distant objects), or nonspecific ocular discomfort. The affected children may be erroneously misdiagnosed as having childhood esotropia, unilateral/bilateral sixth nerve palsy, horizontal gaze palsy, or ocular motor apraxia. Even though most cases are functional in nature, cases associated with organic disorders are occasionally reported, including head trauma, stroke, pretectal lesions, labyrinthine dysfunction, diphenylhydantoin intoxication, Wernicke's encephalopathy, metabolic encephalopathy and Fisher's syndrome.[30]

Spasm of the near reflex in infants and children should be distinguished from nystagmus blockage syndrome and from convergence substitution. The latter is seen in patients with congenital or acquired horizontal gaze paralysis (e.g. Möbius syndrome, multiple sclerosis), in which the patient substitutes a convergence movement for a lateral version movement while attempting to fixate an eccentric target.

Neurologic Exotropia

The differential diagnosis of constant exotropia includes cortical visual insufficiency, craniofacial synostosis, congenital cranial dysinnervation disorders (congenital fibrosis syndrome) and convergence insufficiency. Isolated infantile exotropia is very rare. Some cases of infantile exotropia are hereditary, showing an autosomal dominant inheritance pattern. However, the most common cause of neurologic exotropia is cortical visual insufficiency secondary to hypoxic-ischemic encephalopathy.[31]

Children with congenital homonymous hemianopia may develop a constant exotropia that helps to expand the existing visual field. Confrontation visual field testing can diagnose this situation. Congenital fibrosis syndrome is another condition which can cause exotropia (discussed above).

Convergence Insufficiency

Convergence insufficiency is a common condition characterized by:
- Diplopia or blurring at near
- Decreased convergence amplitudes
- A recessed near point of accommodation.

It is presumably caused by an inborn deficiency or acquired imbalance of vergence eye movements.[32] These patients complain of tearing, heavy lids, uncomfortable eyes, asthenopic symptoms, double vision on reading or doing near work. Convergence insufficiency is also reported in association with head trauma, neurodegenerative disorders, infarction, thyroid ophthalmopathy, myasthenia gravis, toxic agents, medications, and attention-deficit hyperactivity disorder (ADHD).[30]

Skew Deviation

Skew deviation refers vertical misalignment of eyes resulting from supranuclear derangements. The ipsilateral eye was hypotropic with caudal pontomedullary lesions and higher with rostral pontomesencephalic lesions. Skew deviation in children may be associated with a wide variety of conditions, including tumors, Chiari malformation, autoimmune disease, paroxysmal hemiparesis of childhood, and increased intracranial pressure.[30]

Horizontal Gaze Palsy in Children

Gaze palsy may reflect abnormalities of saccadic eye movements, and results from frontal lobe, fronto-mesencephalic saccadic pathway or in the gaze center in the pons. An infant or toddler with a VI nerve palsy may appear to have a gaze palsy when he or she adopts a compensatory head position to achieve binocularity and resists any gaze shift out of the zone of binocularity. This problem can be easily solved by putting a patch over the suspected paretic eye which leads to disappearance of the head turn in the case of VI nerve palsy, but not in gaze palsy.

Congenital bilateral paralysis of horizontal gaze has been reported with or without facial paralysis in Mobius syndrome (facial diplegia and sixth nerve palsy). The underlying defect has been speculated to be due to selective maldevelopment of the horizontal gaze center in the paramedian pontine reticular formation (PPRF) or the motor neurons and inter neurons in the abducens nuclei. Neuronopathic Gaucher disease can also be associated with isolated horizontal gaze palsy.

CHILDHOOD PATTERNS OF NYSTAGMUS

Congenital Nystagmus (Infantile Nystagmus Syndrome)[33]

Congenital nystagmus (CN) presents in the first few months of life. Congenital nystagmus may be present in patients with static encephalopathy or progressive neurodegenerative disorders. Congenital nystagmus most often is sporadic; however, there are also autosomal dominant, autosomal recessive, or x-linked cases.

CN appears as conjugate horizontal nystagmus and characteristically remains horizontal even in upgaze or downgaze. Even though the congenital nystagmus is classically pendular, it may acquire jerk quality at the extremes of gaze. Waveform is variable and there may be a rotary component. Pendular nystagmus can also be seen in acquired disorders; one useful differentiating point is that oscillopsia is not seen in congenital nystagmus, but is a very common complaint in acquired pendular nystagmus. Patients often adopt a head turn to place the eyes in the null position (position of gaze in which nystagmus is least and the visual acuity is the best). Visual fixation at a distance usually amplifies CN whereas convergence dampens nystagmus amplitude. CN is abolished in sleep. There are certain unique features of this nystagmus (1) there is increasing velocity slow phase that is easiest to identify on eye movement recordings (2) reversed optokinetic nystagmus i.e. The slow phase of eye movements moves in the direction opposite that of a rotating optokinetic stimulus.[34]

Congenital nystagmus may be seen in isolation or may be associated with strabismus (approximately 15% of patients with CN have concomitant strabismus). Since it may be associated with afferent visual system defects such as albinism, congenital stationary night blindness, it is important to exclude any afferent dysfunction; Occasionally, high astigmatism, strabismus, and accommodative dysfunction are seen with congenital nystagmus. Examination clues that help to diagnose a visual pathway lesion as responsible for the congenital nystagmus include a relative afferent pupillary defect, retinal abnormalities, or optic atrophy. Electrophysiologic testing (electroretinography, visual-evoked potentials) and neuroimaging may be helpful in select cases.

Patients may have a head tremor which, in some cases, improves visual acuity. Possible treatments include prism therapy to move a null point to the straight ahead position or to induce convergence and eye muscle surgery to move the null point into the straight ahead position. Botulinum toxin has recently been tried for congenital nystagmus as well.

Occasionally, congenital nystagmus may spontaneously resolve. In this situation, the congenital nystagmus is caused by an ocular motor form of delayed visual maturation. A monocular pendular nystagmus, particularly in childhood, may be caused by a lesion of the visual pathway, typically chiasmal glioma.

Latent Nystagmus (Fusional Development Nystagmus Syndrome)[33]

Latent nystagmus refers to a nystagmus induced by covering one eye. This appears very early in life and is a horizontal jerk nystagmus in the direction of the uncovered eye. In latent nystagmus, the eyes do not show any ocular motion, until one eye is occluded, eliminating binocular fixation. When one eye is occluded, nystagmus appears with the fast phase of the viewing eye beating toward the ear and away from the occluded eye and the slow phase of the viewing eye beating toward the nose. The slow phase reverses when the opposite eye is occluded. This condition is one where the visual acuity worsens by covering either eye as opposed to diplopia causing blurring of vision where visual acuity improves by closing either eye.

It is often seen in association with congenital esotropia, dissociated vertical deviation and/or congenital nystagmus. Should visual loss occur in one eye, the nystagmus will manifest constantly and is called manifest latent nystagmus.[34] It also may be present in children with strabismus and amblyopia. The nystagmus beats in the direction of the non-amblyopic eye, which is normally used for sight.

See-saw Nystagmus

See-saw nystagmus refers to an uncommon form of nystagmus with elevation and intorsion of one eye simultaneous with depression and extorsion of the other eye followed by a reversal of the cycle so that the eyes move like a See-saw.[35,36] The waveform may be of pendular or jerk type. The pendular form is seen most often with parasellar lesions such as pituitary tumors. Other causes include aplasia of optic chiasm and septo-optic dysplasia. Joubert syndrome is also a cause of this eye movement disorder. Lioresal and clonazepam may help lessen see-saw nystagmus.[37] See-saw nystagmus may occur in MS, Arnold Chiari malformation, syringobulbia, head trauma, or visual loss such as in cone–rod dystrophy. Patients with *congenital see-saw nystagmus* may show no torsional component or may have a reverse torsional component so that the elevating eye extorts and the depressing eye intorts.

In the jerk type of see-saw nystagmus, patients will display half of a see-saw cycle with a corrective quick phase (hemi *see-saw nystagmus*).[38] It typically occurs from a unilateral meso-diencephalic lesion involving the interstitial nucleus of Cajal. The torsional nystagmus seen in midbrain lesions may beat either to the right or left shoulder. Patients with visual loss alone may have see-saw nystagmus. Such patients will have normal neuroimaging.[39]

Spasmus Nutans

Spasmus nutans is characterized by the triad of:
- Torticollis
- Head nodding (2–3 Hz)
- Monocular or asymmetric nystagmus.[40]

The nystagmus is the hallmark, and the other two features may or may not be present.

Spasmus nutans is an intermittent, binocular, very small amplitude, high frequency (up to 15 Hz), primarily horizontal, pendular nystagmus.[41] The nystagmus may be dissociated or even monocular. It may be greater in the abducting eye, may have a vertical component, and may be more evident during convergence.

Onset of spasmus nutans is usually between the ages of 4 and 14 months and rarely up to 3 years. It typically lasts for several months but may last up to a few years. Patients with typical spasmus nutans do not usually have other neurologic abnormalities. However, there are a number of reports that document a similar nystagmus with parasellar and hypothalamic tumors.[42,43] If there is evidence of an afferent pupillary defect or optic pallor, or endocrinologic abnormalities including poor feeding or diencephalic syndrome, spasmus nutans may be a secondary phenomenon. It is recommended that all patients with spasmus nutans have neuroimaging. Spasmus nutans-like nystagmus and head movements have also been described in association with retinal diseases such as congential stationary night blindness,[44] and in spino-cerebellar degenerations.[45]

Idiopathic spasmus nutans requires no specific treatment, as the disorder usually remits spontaneously. However, careful follow-up by an ophthalmologist is mandatory as many children with idiopathic spasmus nutans will have amblyopia or strabismus in the eye with the nystagmus of greater amplitude. Refractive errors are also common. In some patients, subclinical nystagmus may persist up to the age of 12.[40]

Opsoclonus (Saccadomania)

Opsoclonus refers to an involuntary conjugate multidirectional saccades (saccadomania) that occur without an inter-saccadic interval.[46] The eye movement abnormality is often associated with eye blinking, facial twitching, myoclonus, and ataxia (Kinsbourne's 'dancing eyes and dancing feet'). Ocular flutter, a related disorder, refers to back-to back horizontal saccades without an inter saccadic interval. In this, there is no vertical or rotary component. The lack of an interval between the saccades distinguishes ocular flutter from square wave jerks. Ocular flutter has the same localizing value and differential diagnosis as opsoclonus.

Opsoclonus can occur as a paraneoplastic manifestation. Fifty percent of children with opsoclonus harbor a neuroblastoma, thus it is essential to exclude this tumor in any child with opsoclonus. Conversely, only 2% with neuroblastoma have opsoclonus.[47] Screening tests include urine Vanilylmandelic acid (VMA) and homovanillic acid (HVA) levels and magnetic resonance imaging of the thorax and abdomen. There may be a pleocytosis in the cerebrospinal fluid, and somatostatin receptor (octreotide) imaging may also be used.[48] This condition often responds to tumor removal along with adrenocorticotropic hormone (ACTH) or prednisone, but may also require other immune modulatory therapy such as gamma globulin or plasmapheresis in resistant cases. Relapses and corticosteroid dependence are common in opsoclonus associated with neuroblastoma, and some children have long-term neurologic deficits.

The other conditions where opsoclonus is seen in childhood include a benign, self-limited opsoclonus in neonates,[49] and opsoclonus associated with severe visual disturbances,[50] parainfectious cerebellitis, and encephalitis.

Nystagmus and Instability of Gaze Due to Diseases Affecting the Visual Pathways

Loss of vision due to disease of the anterior visual pathways causes instability of gaze. If the visual loss is binocular, there is nystagmus that has both horizontal and vertical components and changes direction over the course of seconds to minutes (wandering null point). The waveform of the slow phase is variable, being decreasing velocity, linear, or increasing velocity. These findings can be accounted by an abnormal gaze holding network (neural integrator). This abnormality is due to deprivation of visual inputs to the cerebellar or brainstem components of neural integrator.

Similarly, monocular visual loss may lead to instability of gaze that is most evident in the blind eye (monocular nystagmus of childhood). The eye will show low frequency bidirectional drifts which are more prominent vertically and unidirectional drifts with nystagmus occurring horizontally. The eye with nystagmus has decreased vision, an afferent pupillary defect, and optic atrophy. Monocular nystagmus of childhood is usually seen in benign conditions like profound amblyopia; however, it can be associated with optic nerve/chiasmal glioma and demands neuroimaging.

The Heimann-Bielschowsky phenomenon (HBP) is a monocular, vertical nystagmoid movement characterized by slow, coarse, pendular movements of variable amplitude. These movements may disappear when the vision is restored or they may persist in an eye with profound visual loss. The origin of these drifts is unknown but has been attributed to disruption of the fusional vergence mechanism or the monocular visual stabilization system.[34]

Congenital Ocular Motor Apraxia

The term oculomotor apraxia refers to conditions in which volitional saccades are defective, but reflex and random movements are preserved (i.e., the quick phases of vestibular or optokinetic nystagmus), suggesting that the lower motor neuron pathways are intact. In this ocular motility disorder, infants may first appear to be blind or have decreased peripheral vision because they have defective or absence of horizontal saccades to novel visual stimuli. Congenital ocular motor apraxia (COMA) is characterized by the selective absence of horizontal saccades with preservation of vertical saccades.[51] A prominent feature of this syndrome is large-amplitude horizontal head thrusting to achieve visual fixation. However, head thrusting need not always be present. Often initiating the sequence with an eyelid blink, patients move their heads rapidly towards a new visual target: then the eyes slowly refixate. A final correction in head position sometimes then occurs, as the eyes are maintained on target using the vestibulo-ocular reflex. In many instances the head thrusting and defective saccades spontaneously improve as the child gets older,[52] but the ocular motility disturbance may persist.

The head thrusts so characteristic of COMA appear when the baby acquires head and neck control (usually at 6 months). Hence this disorder is rarely diagnosed until late infancy. At an earlier age, blindness may be suspected due to failure to follow objects. Because infants "follow" an object with a series of small saccades, failure to pursue may be misinterpreted as a visual deficit. Evaluation of the vestibule-ocular response in such infants helps establish the diagnosis. Ocular motor apraxia is divided into congenital and acquired varieties. Although isolated COMA is usually sporadic, familial cases have been documented.[53]

Congenital ocular motor apraxia is observed in three main clinical situations:
1. In the "benign" or "idiopathic" variety of congenital ocular motor apraxia, there is no readily identifiable explanation for the disorder

and neuroimaging is normal. Although the neurological examination and intellect are usually normal, associated neurologic defects can be seen occasionally, which include hypotonia, motor and speech delay, and ataxia.[54] Many have infantile esotropia.

2. Some patients with congenital ocular motor apraxia have a non-progressive, non-inherited structural abnormality of the brain, caused either by a developmental anomaly or prenatal or perinatal insult. These include dysgenesis of the cerebellar vermis or corpus callosum, cerebellar hypoplasia, Dandy-Walker syndrome, grey matter heterotopias, and perinatal ischemia.

3. A variety of genetic disorders with multi-system involvement may present in infancy with congenital ocular motor apraxia. These include Joubert syndrome, Jeune's syndrome (nephronophthisis, asphyxiating thoracic dystrophy, retinal degeneration, and ataxia), and a subset of patients with Leber's congenital amaurosis, a retinal dystrophy.

While the ocular motor abnormalities tend to improve with age, most affected children show some degree of delayed motor, speech, or cognitive development.

REFERENCES

1. Nixon RB, Helveston EM, Miller K, et al. Incidence of strabismus in neonates. Am J Ophthalmol. 1985;100:798-801.
2. Sondhi N, Archer SM, Helveston EM. Development of normal ocular alignment. J Pediatr Ophthalmol Strabismus. 1988;25:210-1.
3. Horwood A. Too much or too little: neonatal ocular misalignment frequency can predict lateral abnormality. Br J Ophthalmol. 2003;87:1142-5.
4. Good WV, Hou C, Carden SM. Transient, idiopathic nystagmus in infants. Dev Med Child Neurol. 2003;45:304-7.
5. Bianchi PE, Salati R, Cavallini A, et al. Transient nystagmus in delayed visual maturation. Dev Med Child Neurol. 1998;40:263-5.
6. Wolsey DH, Warner JE. Paroxysmal downgaze in two healthy infants. J Neuroophthalmol. 2006; 26:187-9.
7. Yokochi K. Paroxysmal ocular downward deviation in neurologically impaired infants. Pediatr Neurol. 1991;7:426-8.
8. Mak SC, Chi CS, Chen CH. Mitochondrial encephalomyopathy presenting with clinical Leigh's disease: report of a case. Chung Hua I Hsueh Tsa Chih Taipei. 1991;47:54-8.
9. Tamura EE, Hoyt CS. Oculomotor consequences of intraventricular hemorrhages in premature infants. Arch Ophthalmol. 1987;105:533-5.
10. Brodsky MC, Fray KJ, Glasier CM. Perinatal cortical and subcortical visual loss: mechanisms of injury and associated ophthalmologic signs. Ophthalmology. 2002;109:85-94.
11. Keane JR. Pretectal pseudobobbing. Five patients with 'V'-pattern convergence nystagmus. Arch Neurol. 1985;42:592-4.
12. Ouvrier RA, Billson F. Benign paroxysmal tonic upgaze of childhood. J Child Neurol. 1988;3:177-80.
13. Ahn JC, Hoyt WF, Hoyt CS. Tonic upgaze in infancy: A report of three cases. Arch Ophthalmol. 1989;107:57-8.
14. Hoyt CS, Mousel DK, Weber AA. Transient supranuclear disturbances of gaze in healthy neonates. Am J Ophthalmol. 1980;89:708-13.
15. Gutowski NJ, Bosley TM, Engle EC. 110th ENMCC International Workshop. The congenital cranial dysinnervation disorders (CCDDs). Naarden, The Netherlands. 2002.pp.25-7. Neuromuscul Disord. 2003;13:573-8.
16. Traboulsi ET, Jaagar MD, Kattan HM, et al. Congenital fibrosis of the extraocular muscles: report of 24 cases illustrating the clinical spectrum and surgical management. Am Orthopt J. 1993;43:45-53.
17. Harley RD, Rodriguez MM, Crawford JS. Congenital fibrosis of the extraocular muscles. Trans Am Ophthalmol Soc. 1978;76:197-226.
18. Hertle RW, Katowitz JA, Young TL, et al. Congenital unilateral fibrosis, blepharoptosis, and enophthalmos syndrome. Ophthalmology. 1992;99:347-55.
19. Abeloos MC, Cordonnier M, Van-Nechel C, et al. Congenital fibrosis of the ocular muscles: a diagnosis for several clinical pictures. Bull Soc Belge Ophtalmol. 1990;239:61-74.
20. Brodsky MC, Pollock SC, Buckley EG. Neuronal misdirection in congenital ocular fibrosis syndrome: implications and pathogenesis. J Pediatr Ophthalmol Strabismus. 1989;26:159-61.
21. Goldschmit M. Further considerations about the ophthalmic features of the Möbius sequence, with data of 28 cases. Arq Bras Oftalmol. 2007; 70:451-7.

22. Cronemberger MF, de Castro Moreira JB, Brunoni D, et al. Ocular and clinical manifestations of Möbius syndrome. J Pediatr Ophthalmol Strabismus. 2001;38:156-62.
23. Arnoldi K, Jackson JH. Cerebral palsy for the pediatric eye care team: epidemiology, pathogenesis, and systemic findings. Am Orthopt J. 2005;55:97-105.
24. Levy NS, Cassin B, Newman M. Strabismus in children with cerebral palsy. J Pediatr Ophthalmol. 1976;13:72-4.
25. Buckley E, Seaber JH. Dyskinetic strabismus as a sign of cerebral palsy. Am J Ophthalmol. 1981;91:652-7.
26. Carruthers JD. Strabismus in craniofacial dysostosis. Graefes Arch Clin Exp Ophthalmol. 1988;226:220-3.
27. Brodsky MC. Visuo-vestibular eye movements. Infantile strabismus in three dimensions. Arch Ophthalmol. 2005;123:837-42.
28. Brodsky MC. Dissociated vertical divergence: a righting reflex gone wrong. Arch Ophthalmol. 1999;117:1216-22.
29. Spielmann AC. Convergence excess associated with neurological diseases: surgical treatment. J Fr Ophtalmol. 2006;29:432-7.
30. Brodsky MC. Complex ocular motor disorders in children. Pediatric Neuro-ophthalmology. Springer. 2010;7:309-82.
31. Brodsky MC, Fray KJ, Glasier CM. Perinatal cortical and subcorticalvisual loss: mechanisms of injury and associated ophthalmologic signs. Ophthalmology. 2002;109:85-94.
32. Arnoldi K, Reynolds JD. A review of convergence insufficiency: what are we really accomplishing with exercises? Am Orthopt J. 2007;57:123-31.
33. Eggenberger ER. Nystagmus and other abnormal eye movements. Continuum Lifelong Learning Neurol. 2009;15(4):200-12.
34. Leigh RJ, DS Zee. The neurology of eye movements, 3 edn., New York: Oxford Univ. Press; 1999.
35. Daroff RB. See-saw nystagmus. Neurology. 1965;15:874-7.
36. Nakada T, Kwee IL. Seesaw nystagmus: Role of visuovestibular interaction in its pathogenesis. J Clin Neuro-ophthalmol. 1988;8:171-7.
37. Carlow TJ. Medical treatment of nystagmus and ocular motor disorders. Int Ophthalmol Clin. 1986;26:251-64.
38. Halmagyi GM, Aw ST, Dehaene I. Jerk-waveform see-saw nystamus due to a unilateral mesodiencephalic lesion. Brain. 1994;117:789-803.
39. May EF, Truxal AR. Loss of vision alone may result in seesaw nystagmus. J Neuro-ophthalmol. 1997;17:84-5.
40. Gottlob I, Wizov SS, Reinecke RD. Spasmus nutans: A long-term follow-up. Invest Ophthalmol Vis Sci. 1995;36:2768-71.
41. Weissman RM, Dell'Osso LF, Abel LA, et al. Spasmus nutans: A quantitative prospective study. Arch Ophthalmol. 1987;105:525-8.
42. Antony JH, Ouvrier RA, Wise G. Spasmus nutans: A mistaken identity. Arch Neurol 1980;37:373-5.
43. Lavery MA, O'Neill JF, Chu FC, et al. Acquired nystagmus in early childhood: A presenting sign of intracranial tumor. Ophthalmology. 1984;91:425-35.
44. Lambert SR, Newman NJ. Retinal disease masquerading as spasmus nutans. Neurology. 1993;43:1607-9.
45. Kalyanaraman K, Jagannathan K, Ramanujam RA, et al. Congenital head nodding and nystagmus with cerebellar degeneration. J Pediatr. 1973;83:1023-6.
46. Digre KB. Opsoclonus in adults: Report of three cases and review of the literature. Arch Neurol. 1986;43:1165-75.
47. Pranzatelli MR. The neurobiology of the opsoclonus-myoclonus syndrome. Clin Neuropharm. 1992;15:186-228.
48. Posada JC, Tardo C. Neuroblastoma detected by somatostatin receptor scintigraphy in a case of opsoclonus-myoclonus-ataxia syndrome. J Child Neurol. 1998;13:345-6.
49. Hoyt CS, Mousel DK, Weber AA. Transient supranuclear disturbances of gaze in healthy neonates. Am J Ophthalmol. 1980;89:708-13.
50. Bienfang DC. Opsoclonus in infancy. Arch Ophthalmol. 1974;91:203-5.
51. Cogan DG. Congenital ocular motor apraxia. Can J Ophthalmol. 1966;1:253.
52. Prasad P, Nair S. Congenital ocular motor apraxia: sporadic and familial. Support for natural resolution. J Clin Neuro-ophthalmol. 1994;14:102-4.
53. Cogan DG. Heredity of congenital ocular motor apraxia. Trans Am Acad Ophthalmol Otolaryngol. 1972;76:60-3.
54. Harris CM, Shawkat F, Russell-Eggitt I, et al. Intermittent horizontal saccade failure ('ocular motor apraxia') in children. Br J Ophthalmol. 1996;80:151-8.

CHAPTER 27

Approach to a Child with Ataxia

TM Ananda Kesavan

Ataxia is a disorder of movement characterized by in coordination, lack of precision and speed of movement with inability to maintain balance. The most prominent feature is an abnormal wide based gait associated with lurching and staggering. It also includes abasia (unsteadiness of stance), asynergia (decomposition of complex movements into isolated, successive parts), dysmetria (abnormal excursions in movement), dysdiadochokinesia (impaired performance of rapid alternating movements) and impaired rebound response. The pathology causing ataxia can be anywhere in the cerebellum, or its connections with other parts of the nervous system.

PITFALLS IN THE RECOGNITION OF ATAXIA

The pediatrician sometimes uses the word ataxia for cerebella disorder alone; however it includes cases of sensory ataxia in which unsteadiness and poor coordination result from sensory loss especially of joint position sense rather than cerebella disconcertion. The problem of chronic ataxia in childhood differs in several ways from that of an adult. Development in the early years of life proceeds the rapid rate with dramatic equation of motor and social skills. A newborn baby or slightly older infant is not expected to perform motor tasks as sitting, crawling, standing, walking reaching and grasping which require coordination.

The motor difficulty imposed by ataxia usually delays the motor miles stones and this may be further delayed by any degree of mental retardation which often accompanies it. The child who is destined to become ataxic is often severely hypotonic in his earlier months thus it is very common for misdiagnosing the child with a neuromuscular disease.

Ataxia is first detectable when the child start to sit, he is observed to be abnormally unsteady when he tries to balance his head and body. The attempts for reaching and grasping objects are jerky and abortive. This 'physiological ataxia' is of limited duration in a healthy infant. Confusion may also arise when the child begins, to stand and to walk at a delayed age than normal. The frequent tumbling unsteadiness of a normal toddler should not be mistaken for ataxia. In some mentally retarded children who eventually outgrow their motor problems will have a persistent prolonged 'physiologically ataxia' but its eventual termination will clarify the situation.

HOW TO APPROACH TO CHILD WITH ATAXIA?

Chief Complaints

Swaying gait, inability to walk properly, unsteadiness in reaching out for objects and involuntary movements are the chef complaints.

Associated complaints like developmental delay, seizure, mental retardation often accompany. Regression of milestones and impairment of higher mental functions are seen in neurometabolic and neurodegenerative disorders.

Site of Lesion

Cerebellum

Ataxia is a disorder that specifically affects different parts of cerebellum, leading to characteristic spectrum of motor abnormalities. Midline cerebellar disease causes a disorder of stance and gait, truncal titubation, rotated postures of the head and disturbances in eye movement. These can be subdivided into rostral vermal lesions (abasia and gait ataxia) and caudal vermal lesions (nystagmus also). The disruption of the cerebellar hemisphere and dentate nuclei results in dysarthria, limb ataxia, hypotonia, intention tremor and abnormal eye movements.

Intermediate hemisphere lesions of interposed nuclei causes delayed rebound response, truncal titubation, abnormal rapid alternating movements, action tremor, oscillation of outstretched extremities and ataxia on finger-nose-finger test and heel-knee-shin maneuvers.

Cerebellar mutism is sometime seen after removal of vermian tumors and may result from bilateral involvement of the dentate-rubro-thalamic tracts. Cerebellar lesion may also be associated with clinical features suggestive of other intracranial structures.

Nonmotor manifestations of cerebellar disease can also occur. Cerebellar cognitive affective syndrome in which executive functions, spatial cognition, personality changes and language deficits are as the clinical picture has also been described.

Sensory ataxia: This is not very common in children. The gait is wide based and the child walks carefully looking constantly at the ground to get an idea about the position. There is difficulty in fine finger movement rather than reaching for objects. They do not experience dysarthria or visual symptoms. They may report other symptoms of peripheral nerve diseases such as parasthesias and numbness. Reduction of distal deep tendon reflexes, signs of posterior column lesion and positive Rhomberg's test can be elicited.

Frontal lobe: In bilateral frontal lobe lesions, child may have a gait disorder superficially resembling ataxia and may be indistinguishable from cerebellar ataxia.

Acute labyrinthitis: Acute onset of vertigo, nausea and vomiting with ataxia is suggestive of labyrinthitis.

Brainstem

In lesions of cerebellar tract involvement with in the brainstem, there is ataxia, but the main symptoms and signs are that of brainstem lesion.

Hysterical: Seen in an adolescent girl without much difficulty in sitting, but ataxic on standing. Nystagmus and dysarthria may be absent.

Age: The etiology of ataxia varies with age of onset of the disease. The particular age group and common causes are shown in **Table 27.1**.

Onset: Onset may be acute, subacute, chronic or episodic. The causes of ataxia based on mode of onset is given in **Tables 27.2 and 27.3**. A chronic condition may be acutely presented, e.g. a benign astrocytoma may acutely present after a bleeding. Pyruvate dehydrogenase deficiency may be precipitated by infection, stress and high carbohydrate meal leading to ataxia.

Acute ataxia with rapid improvement is seen in drug toxicity and acute postinfectious cerebellitis.

HISTORY

History of birth asphyxia will give a diagnosis of ataxic cerebral palsy while trauma will point to postcerebellar concussion syndrome.

History of otorrhea or tinnitus will help to making a diagnosis of labyrinthitis. History of diarrhea, steatorrhea, malabsorption or failure to thrive is a clue to diagnosis of abetalipoproteinemia. Many children presented with skin markers as the main complaints with or without ataxia as in von Hippel-Landau disease and ataxia telangiectasia.

History of contact with tuberculosis will point to tuberculous meningitis or abscess. History of fever

Approach to a Child with Ataxia

Table 27.1 Causes of ataxia related to age at onset

Age at onset	Acquired	Genetic
Infancy	Ataxic cerebral palsy, other intrauterine insults, congenital malformations	Inherited congenital ataxias, e.g. Joubert's syndrome, Gillespie's syndrome
Childhood	Infections like acute cerebellitis, abscess; posterior fossa vascular malformations; toxins such as anticonvulsants; immune related to neoplasm, e.g. opsoclonus – myoclonus	Ataxias related to " inborn errors of metabolisms "such as aminoacidurias, Wilson's disease, etc.; Friedreich's ataxia; ataxia with oculomotor apraxia; vitamin E deficiency syndrome; spino-cerebellar ataxia, episodic ataxia syndromes
Young adults	Infections such as HIV, posterior fossa mass lesions such as meningiomas, gliomas, abscess; congenital anomalies including vascular malformations, hypothyroidism; toxins such as anticonvulsants and alcohol; immune causes such as multiple sclerosis (MS)	Friedreich's ataxia; dominantly inherited spinocerebellar ataxia,; inherited tumor syndromes such as von Hippel – Landau syndrome

Table 27.2 Causes of acute and recurrent ataxia

Selected causes of acute ataxia	Selected causes of recurrent ataxia
Infection: • Acute cerebellar ataxia • Miller-Fisher syndrome • Cerebellar abscess • Viral encephalitis (brainstem) • Labyrinthitis *Toxins*: • Drug ingestion and toxicity *Vascular*: • Cerebellar hemorrhage • Posterior fossa subdural hematoma • Bleeding in a tumor *Others*: • Conversion hysteria	• Migraine • Benign paroxysmal vertigo • Genetic/metabolic disorders • Pyruvate decarboxylase deficiency • Carnitine acetyl transferase deficiency • Hartnup disease • Maple syrup urine disease, juvenile form • Ornithine transcarbamylase deficiency familial periodic ataxia • Ependymoma

Table 27.3 Causes of chronic ataxia

Chronic ataxia—nonprogressive	Chronic ataxia—progressive
• Head trauma • Ataxic cerebral palsy • Kernicterus • Congenital malformations • Cerebellar hemisphere hypoplasia • Cerebellar vermis aplasia/hypoplasia • Arnold-Chiari malformation • Basilar impression	• *Brain tumor*: Cerebellar astrocytoma, medulloblastoma, ependymoma, pontine glioma, frontal lobe tumor *Genetic* *Dominant*: Spinocerebellar degenerations *Recessive*: Abetalipoproteinemia, ataxia telangiectasia, Friedreich's ataxia, liposomal storage disease, Juvenile GM2 gangliosidosis, juvenile sulfatide lipidosis, Marinesco-Sjögren syndrome, Niemann-Pick variant, Refsum disease, mitochondrial disorders

and a rash is useful in case of acute cerebellitis and postinfectious encephalomyelitis. Viral infections leading to ataxia include: mumps, chickenpox, poliomyelitis, HIV infection, Epstein-Barr virus infection, ECHO virus and Guillain-Barré syndrome.

Common bacterial infection leading to ataxia are: typhoid fever, tuberculosis, pertussis, diphtheria, scarlet fever and postmeningitis.

History suggestive of migraine is common in adolescent girl with episodic ataxia. It is associated with headache, vertigo, ataxia, cranial nerve palsy and transient loss of consciousness.

History of drug intake can be elicited in selected cases. It is common in the age group of 1–4 years. Antiepileptic drugs (phenytoin, carbamazepine, phenobarbitone), antihistamines, antipsychotic drugs and piperazine will cause ataxia in children.

History has been elicited of seizure in congenital, degenerative and neoplastic disorders. Pseudoataxia is a condition where seizure will present as ataxia. Sometimes overdosage of anticonvulsants may be suspected in such condition. Myoclonus and seizures are prominent features of Ramsay-Hunt syndrome.

History suggestive of raised intracranial tension in the form of early morning headache, vomiting and neck stiffness will be there in a case of posterior cranial fossa tumor. The most common tumors include cerebellar astrocytoma, brainstem glioma, ependymoma and medulloblastoma. In ependymoma, there will be is history includes episodes of headache, vomiting, ataxia and nuchal rigidity lasting for days or weeks followed by periods of well-being. These intermittent symptoms are attributed to transitory obstruction of the fourth ventricle or aqueduct by a tumor acting in a ball valve fashion.

Recurrent sinopulmonary infection is common in ataxia telangiectasia.

Developmental history: In ataxic cerebral palsy and in congenital malformation, there will be developmental delay from birth, but ataxia may manifest by 6 months of age. In neurodegenerative and metabolic disorders, child will be normal at birth and later there will be deterioration. Associated mental retardation may also be there.

Immunization history: Many infectious disease will cause postinfectious ataxia, e.g. chickenpox, mumps, pertussis and diphtheria. Rarely vaccinations may produce demyelination, thus causing ataxia.

Family history: Many neurodegenerative and metabolic disorders are transmitted in an autosomal recessive fashion **(Table 27.3)**. Autosomal dominant mode of inheritance seen in olivopontocerebellar degeneration, episodic ataxia, spinocerebellar ataxia and mitochondrial myopathies.

X linked inheritance is seen in adrenoleukodystrophy, laber optic atrophy.

Family history of tuberculosis and other infectious disease should be looked for a try to elicit history of migraine may also run in the family.

Etiology: Various congenital, vascular, toxic, neoplastic and genetic causes are listed in **Table 27.4**. Of these the most important causes are acute postinfectious cerebellar ataxia, drug toxicity and neoplasm.

General examination: A detailed general survey will give certain physical findings which helps in diagnosis **(Table 27.5)**. Ophthalmological manifestations associated with ataxia are given in **Table 27. 6**.

Neurological examination: Certain neurological signs and symptoms that may help in the differential diagnosis of ataxia are given in **Table 27.7**.

INVESTIGATIONS

The investigations that have to be undergone are dependent on the suspected etiology. Appropriate and judicious investigation will save money and time. Specific investigations are needed in metabolic and degenerative diseases **(Table 27.8)**.

In the current age of molecular diagnostics, the gold standard is genetic testing. Genetic testing has an added advantage of providing information that can be used for genetic counseling. However, they are costly and not universally available. In new onset cases lacking specific presentation, a more comprehensive approach may be needed to identify the correct diagnosis.

Treatment: It includes medical and surgical treatment. Medical treatment again divided into symptomatic, supportive and specific treatment. Specific treatment is available for certain conditions

Approach to a Child with Ataxia

Table 27.4 Acquired and genetic causes of ataxia

Congenital defects	Ataxic cerebral palsy; congenital anomalies
Vascular	Cerebellar hemorrhage, Kawasaki disease, SLE, AVM
Infectious	Acute cerebellitis; postinfectious encephalomyelitis (HIV; infectious mononucleosis, mumps, typhoid fever, pertussis, diphtheria, scarlet fever, TB), cerebellar abscess
Toxic	Phenytoin, phenobarbitone, carbamazepine benzodiazepine, antihistaminie, piperazine, mercury, (5-FU); cytosine arabinoside
Neoplastic	Astrocytoma, gliomas, ependymomas, frontal lobe tumors, others (neuroblastoma, histocytosis, leukemic infiltration)
Immune	Multiple sclerosis; paraneoplastic syndromes; anti-GAD, gluten ataxia
Deficiency	Hypothyroidism, vitamin B_{12}, vitamin B_1 genetic disorders causing ataxia, vitamin E deficiency
Genetic disorders: Recessive	Friedreich's ataxia, ataxia telangiectasia, inborn error of metabolism, abetalipoproteinemia, Refsum disease
Dominant	Spinocerebellar ataxia, episodic ataxias, Machado-Joseph syndrome
X-linked	Adrenoleukodystrophy, Leber's optic neuropathy
Mitochondrial	NARP, MERRF, others including Kearns-Sayre syndrome and MELAS

Abbreviations: HIV, human immunodeficiency virus; TB, tuberculosis; SLE, systemic lupus erythematosus; AVM, arteriovenous malformation; 5-FU, 5-fluorouracil; GAD, glutamic acid decarboxylase; MELAS, mitochondrial encephalomyopathy, lactic acidosis, and stroke-like episodes; NARP, neuropathy, ataxia, and retinitis pigmentosa; MERRF, myoclonic epilepsy with ragged-red fibers

Table 27.5 Physical findings in ataxia

Systemic feature	Possible diagnosis
• Short stature	• Mitochondrial disease, early central nervous system (CNS) insults
• Failure to thrive	• Abetalipoproteinemia
• Kinky, colorless, friable hair	• Menkes disease
• Pellagra like skin lesion	• Hartnup disease
• Cervical lipoma	• Mitochondrial disease
• Telangiectasia over nose, ear	• Ataxia telangiectasia
• Organomegaly	• Gaucher's disease, Niemann-Pick disease, Wilson disease
• Hypogonadism	• Ataxia with hypogonadism
• Diabetes	• Holmes's ataxia, Friedreich's ataxia (FA)
• Spine and foot deformity	• Friedreich's ataxia, Charcot Marie-tooth disease
• Hematological malignancy	• Ataxia telangiectasia
• Sinopulmonary infections	• Cerebrotendinous xanthomatosis, lipid metabolic disorders
• Xanthomas, xanthelasmas	• Pyruvate dehydrogenase deficiency, Leigh encephalopathy, Joubert syndrome, organic acidemias
• Abnormal breathing pattern	
• Torticollis	• Medulloblastoma, basilar impression

like drug toxicity, Wilson disease, etc. **(Table 27.9)**. Treatment of seizure with anticonvulsants and ataxia with L-dopa will improve quality of life. Surgical treatments are available for early stages of neoplasms. Symptomatic improvement may be seen after surgery in case of hydrocephalus, Arnold-Chiari malformation.

SUMMARY

Ataxia in children is not uncommon. It may be due to a variety of causes, commonly including postinfectious cerebellitis, drugs toxicity, congenital malformation and posterior fossa tumors. Careful clinical evaluation and judicious investigation

Table 27.6 Ophthalmological manifestations associated with ataxia

Ophthalmic feature	Possible diagnosis
• Bulbar congestion • Bulbar telangiectasia • Papilledema • Aniridia • Optic atrophy	• Kawasaki disease • Ataxia telangiectasia • Posterior fossa tumor • Gillespie syndrome • Lober optic neuropathy, Friedreich's ataxia, Menkes disease, Pelizaeus-Merzbacher disease
• Cherry red spot • KF ring • Retinitis pigmentosa • Nystagmus/peculiar eye movements • Cataract • Bulging eye	• GM2 gangliosidosis • Wilson disease • Sea blue histocytosis, Bassen-Kornzweig syndrome, Refsum syndrome • In majority of ataxia, Marinesco-Sjögren syndrome • Wilson disease • Machado-Joseph disease

Table 27.7 Neurological signs and symptoms in ataxia

Neurological signs or symptoms	Possible diagnosis
Focal and lateralized brainstem deficits such as facial palsy, hemiparesis	Brainstem encephalitis, posterior fossa tumors, multiple sclerosis (MS), spinocerebellar ataxia (SCA)
Visual loss from optic atrophy or retinopathy	MS, Friedreich's ataxia (FA), mitochondrial diseases
Papilledema, headache	Posterior fossa tumors or ataxia as a "false localizing" sign
Large head	Hydrocephalus, Arnold-Chiari malformation
Neck stiffness/torticollis	Medulloblastoma, basilar impression
Internuclear ophthalmoplegia	Posterior circulation strokes, MS, some SCA
Gaze palsies	MS, strokes, SCA
Ptosis and ophthalmoplegia	Mitochondrial disease, sea-blue histiocytosis
Slow saccades and ocular apraxia	SCA ataxia, recessive ataxia with oculomotor apraxia
Downbeat nystagmus	Arnold-Chiari malformation, basilar invagination, SCA, episodic ataxia type 2 (EA-2), lithium toxicity
Spasticity, upper motor neuron (UMN) signs	Posterior circulation strokes, tumors/malformations compressing brainstem, MS, many SCAs, FA
Basal ganglia deficits	Many SCA, Wilson's disease, Fahr's disease, mitochondrial disease
Proprioceptive loss	B_{12} deficiency, other sensory ataxias, FA
Epilepsy	Ataxia associated with anticonvulsants, some idiopathic ataxias, SCA
Myoclonus	Mitochondrial, SCA of childhood onset, sialidosis, ceroid lipofuscinosis, Ramsay Hunt syndrome
Cognitive decline	MS, HIV, congenital, neurodegenerative

Table 27.8 Investigations in a case of ataxia

- Wilson disease
- Organic academia
- Pyruvate dehydrogenase deficiency
- Ataxia telangiectasia
- Drugs/toxin
- Neuroblastoma
- Abetalipoproteinemia
- Ataxia-oculomotor apraxia
- Adrenoleukodystrophy
- Mitochondrial myopathy
- Friedreich's ataxia
- USG, CT, MRI

- Serum copper and urine copper excretion
- Amino acid in urine and blood
- Lactate level
- Low IgA, IgE
- Blood level measurement
- HVA and VMA
- Vitamin E level, low cholesterol, acanthocytosis
- Low albumin level
- Long chain fatty acid
- Lactic acidosis, ragged red fiber
- ECG and echocardiogram
- Congenital brain malformation, tumors, degenerative disorders

Abbreviations: HVA, homovanillic acid; VMA, vanillylmandelic acid; IgA, immunoglobulin A; IgE, immunoglobulin E; ECG, electrocardiography; USG, ultrasonography; CT, computed tomography; MRI, magnetic resonance imaging

Table 27.9 Treatment of childhood ataxia

Disease	Treatment
• Ataxia with vitamin E deficiency • Bassen-Kornzweig syndrome • Hartnup disease • Episodic ataxia-type 2 • Mitochondrial defects • Multiple carboxylase deficiency • Pyruvate dehydrogenase deficiency • Refsum disease • Urea cycle defects • Ataxia telangiectasia • Migraine • Wilson disease • Labyrinthitis • Myoclonic encephalopathy • Pseudoataxia • Kawasaki disease • Posterior fossa tumor • Arnold-Chiari malformation • Basilar impression	• Vitamin E • Vitamin E, fat restriction • Niacin • Acetazolamide • Riboflavin, CoQ10, dichloroacetate • Biotin • Ketogenic diet, carbohydrate (CBH) restriction, biotin • Dietary restriction of phytanic acid • Protein restriction, thiamin • Coenzyme Q10 (Co Q10), vitamin E, treatment of infection • Flunarizine, chlorpromazine • D Penicillamin, zinc • Treatment of underlying cause • Prednisolone, ACTH • Sodium valproate, clonazepam • Intravenous immunoglobulin (IVIG) • Resection, shunt surgery • Surgical decompression • Decompression of foramen magnum

will help in the diagnosis in a majority of the cases. Specific treatment is available for few conditions and a majority of them will recover with symptomatic treatment.

BIBLIOGRAPHY

1. Bradly WG, Daroff RB, Fenichel GM, Jankovic J. Neurology in clinical practice—principles of treatment and management, 5th edn. Butterworth Heinemann, Elsevier; 2008.pp. 285-90.
2. Kliegman RM, Behrman RE, Stanton BF, Schor NF. Nelson Textbook of pediatrics, 19th edn. Saunders Elsevier. 2011.pp.2053-5.
3. Menkes JH, Sarnat HB. Child neurology, 6th edn. Philadelphia: Lippincott Williams and Wilkins, 2000.pp.189-95.
4. Swaiman KF, Ashwal S, Feriero DM. Pediatric neurology—principles and practice. 4th edn. Mosby Elsevier; 2006. pp. 1241-69.

Eye: A Window to Neurological Disorders

Mallika OU

INTRODUCTION

Eye can be considered as an extension of brain and hence the developmental abnormalities of eye and brain are often concurrent. Severe brain abnormalities are those involving abnormal closure of neural tube and are frequently associated with anophthalmia, microphthalmia and anterior segment cleavage abnormalities. Pupil is a window to the brain since we can see the optic nerve, which is part of the brain, directly. More than half of the intracranial tumors[1] present with ocular signs and symptoms like, papilledema, optic atrophy, nystagmus, oculomotor dysfunction, reduced visual acuity, filed defects, etc. Another point that needs special mention is the manifestations of systemic vascular diseases that is visualized in the retina because retina is the only area where blood vessels can be seen directly. A lot of neurodegenerative diseases and metabolic diseases can present in the ophthalmology department with ocular findings like clouding of cornea and cherry red spot. Ophthalmologist may be able to give a clue to reach a diagnosis.[2-4] Also ophthalmic findings may help in assessing the progression of the disease like Wilson's disease.[5]

PEDIATRIC NEURO-OPHTHALMOLOGY EXAMINATION

History should include maternal infections, prematurity and birth trauma. Suspected brain damage as in hydrocephalus and cerebral palsy should be noted. Family history of visual problems needs to be specifically asked.[1]

Visual Acuity[6-9]

Parental assessment of child's vision by asking questions like: Is the child able to see and recognize faces? and whether the child is fixing on parents face or not? Measurement depends on the age of the child:
- *Birth to 2 months*: Blink to light and fixing and following objects.
- *2-6 months*: Blink to threat, reach for objects, preferential looking and optokinetic nystagmus (OKN) drum and visual evoked response (VER)
- *6-18 months*: Preferential looking, OKN drum, VER and reach for candy beads.
- *18-36 months*: Preferential looking, OKN, VER, matching of Snellen characters with HOTV chart, Allen cards and reach for candy beads.
- *3-5 years*: Reach for candy beads, Allen cards, HOTV test, "E" game, and Snellen's chart.

Pupillary Examination

Presence of Marcus Gunn pupil has to be specifically looked for. Anisocoria is not a sign of severe unilateral retinal or optic nerve lesions.

Extraocular Motility

It is important in neurological diseases especially cranial nerve involvement.

Eye: A Window to Neurological Disorders

Nystagmus

This differentiates between ocular cause and neurological cause.

Visual Fields

Confrontation field examination is simple but automated perimetry is more accurate and can be performed in children beyond 6-7 years.

Color Vision

In children pseudoisochromatic plates like Ishihara's chart is used.

Fundoscopic Examination

It is done with indirect ophthalmoscope with 20 or 28 diopter lens. Peripheral retinal examination is not important in neuro-ophthalmic cases.

ANTERIOR SEGMENT ANOMALIES OF NEURO-OPHTHALMIC SIGNIFICANCE

Aniridia[10]

Typical presentation is an infant with nystagmus who appears to have absent irides or a dilated unresponsive pupil **(Fig. 28.1)**. Photophobia may be present. Ocular associations include anterior polar cataract, foveal hypoplasia and corneal opacification due to limbal stem cell deficiency. Systemic associations include WAGR complex of Wilms' tumor, aniridia, genitourinary malformations and mental retardation.

Coloboma of Iris

Typical coloboma of iris occurs in the inferonasal quadrant due to failure of closure of embryonic fissure **(Fig. 28.2)**. Typical coloboma may involve ciliary body, choroid, retina and optic nerve. Atypical iris coloboma occurs in areas other than inferonasal quadrant and is not associated with posterior uveal coloboma.

Iris Nodules

Lisch nodules **(Fig. 28.3)** are melanocytic hamartomas commonly associated with

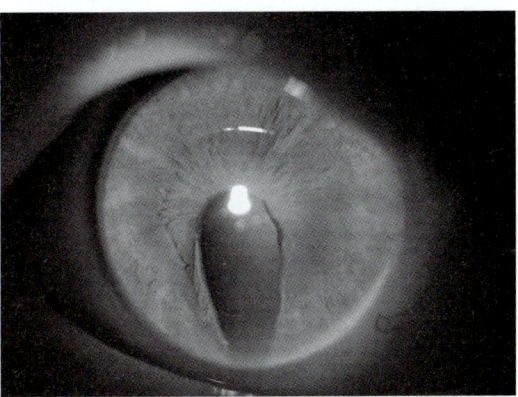

Figure 28.2 Iris coloboma
(For color version, see Plate 5)

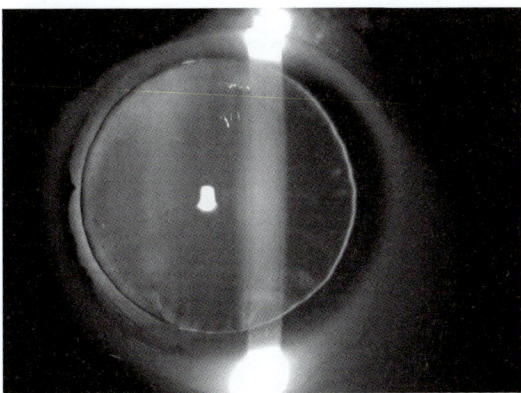

Figure 28.1 Aniridia
(For color version, see Plate 5)

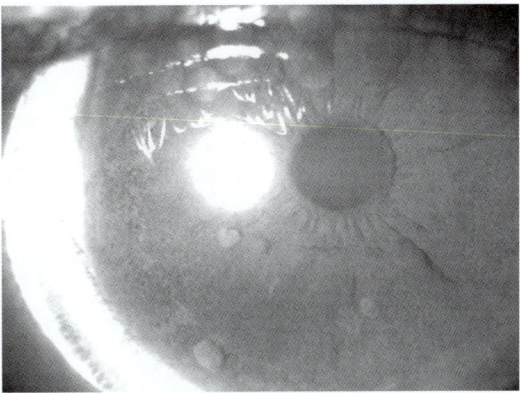

Figure 28.3 Lisch nodules
(For color version, see Plate 5)

neurofibromatosis type 1. These are raised and usually tan in color. It can vary in appearance significantly. By the age of 8 years Lisch nodules are present in approximately 80% of patients.

Iris Mamillations

It is seen more in neurofibromatosis type 1. They are not as diagnostic as Lisch nodules.

Brushfield Spots

These are hypopigmented spots seen in Down's syndrome.

Adie's Tonic Pupil

This can occur in children due to varicella zoster infection.

Horner's Syndrome

It is due to lesion at any location along oculo sympathetic pathway. Anisocoria is greater in dim light and is associated with mild ptosis. In congenital Horner's syndrome affected iris is hypochromic. Acquired Horner's syndrome in children is usually due to neuroblastoma affecting the sympathetic chain in the chest.

Congenital Iris Ectropion

It may be associated with neurofibromatosis and rarely with facial hemi hypertrophy and Prader Willi syndrome **(Fig. 28.4)**.

Iris Transillumination

Diffuse iris transillumination is characteristic of Albinism **(Fig. 28.5)**. Other features of Albinism include foveal hypoplasia, nystagmus, light sensitivity, high refractive errors, reduced central visual acuity, an abnormally large numbers of crossed fibers at chiasma precluding stereopsis and strabismus. There is characteristic deficit of pigments in the retina.

Abnormalities of Lens

Cataract

Causes of bilateral pediatric cataract **(Fig. 28.6)** includes hereditary conditions usually autosomal dominant, Downs' syndrome, Patau' syndrome, myotonic dystrophy, Lowe's syndrome, Alport's syndrome, metabolic disorders like Galactosemia, Fabry's disease, Wilson's disease, diabetes mellitus and maternal infections of TORCH group (toxoplasmosis, rubella, cytomegalovirus, varicella and syphilis).

Subluxated Lens

These are seen in systemic diseases like Marfan's syndrome, homocystinuria, Weill Marchesani syndrome, Sulfite oxidase deficiency. Syphilis and Ehlers-Danlos syndrome. In Marfan's syndrome lens is upwardly dislocated in 75% of cases. In homocystinuria downward subluxation is seen more often. The lens may dislocate into the anterior chamber with acute pupillary block glaucoma,

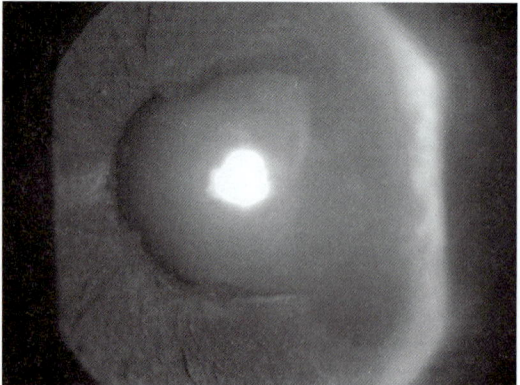

Figure 28.4 Congenital ectropion uvea with iris nodule
(For color version, see Plate 5)

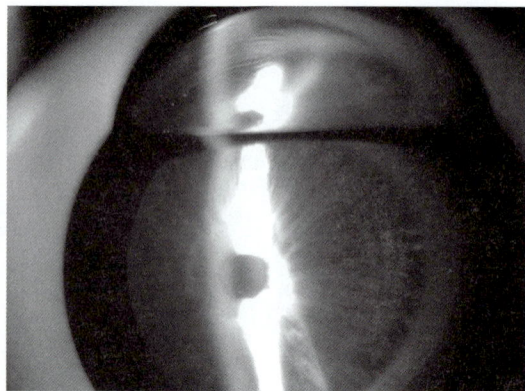

Figure 28.5 Iris transillumination defect
(For color version, see Plate 6)

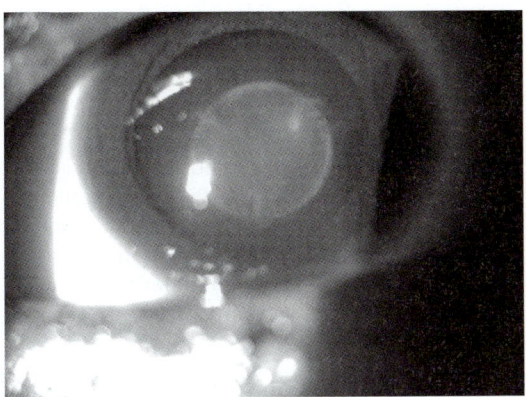

Figure 28.6 Congenital zonular cataract
(For color version, see Plate 6)

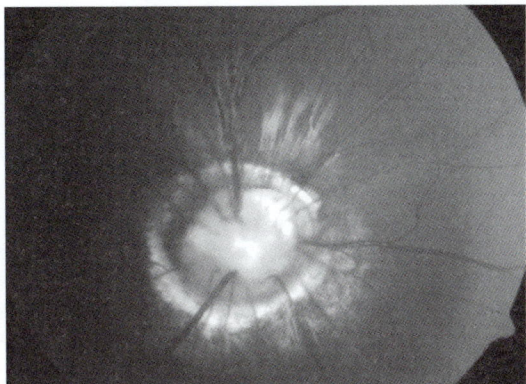

Figure 28.7 Morning glory syndrome
(For color version, see Plate 6)

a finding suggestive of homocystinuria. In Weill-Marchesani syndrome lenses are small and round (microspherophakia) and it can dislocate into the anterior chamber causing pupillary block glaucoma. In these cases a prophylactic laser peripheral iridotomy has been recommended.

POSTERIOR SEGMENT ABNORMALITIES OF NEURO-OPHTHALMOLOGICAL SIGNIFICANCE

Morning Glory Disc Anomaly[7,11-13]

This is caused by either an abnormal closure of embryonic fissure or an abnormal development of the distal optic stalk at its junction with primitive optic vessels. Clinically it appears as a funnel shaped excavation of posterior fundus that incorporates the optic disc **(Fig. 28.7)**. The surrounding retinal pigment epithelium is elevated with an increased number of blood vessels looping at the edge of the disc. Morning glory anomaly is associated with basal encephalocele in patients with midfacial abnormalities. Also they may have carotid circulation anomalies. Therefore magnetic resonance imaging and angiography of the brain should be performed in patients with morning glory anomalies.[4]

Coloboma of Optic Nerves[7,14,15]

It may be part of complete chorioretinal coloboma that involves the entire embryonic fissure or coloboma may involve only optic disc

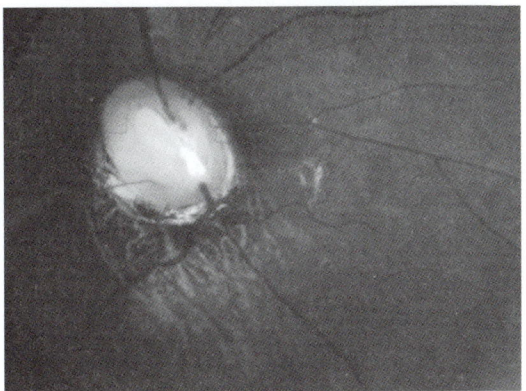

Figure 28.8 Coloboma of the optic nerve head
(For color version, see Plate 6)

(Fig. 28.8). Ocular coloboma may be associated with multiple systemic abnormalities like CHARGE association (Coloboma, Heart defects, choanal Atresia, mental Retardation, Genitourinary abnormalities and Ear abnormalities).

Tilted Disc Abnormalities[7]

Affected patients have myopic astigmatism and may show bitemporal hemianopia, which is typically incomplete and preferentially involves the superior quadrants **(Fig. 28.9)**. The hemianopia can be distinguished from a chiasmal lesion because the defect does not respect the vertical midline. It should be emphasized, however, that if a patient with tilted disc syndrome has a bitemporal hemianopia that respects vertical meridian, MRI of

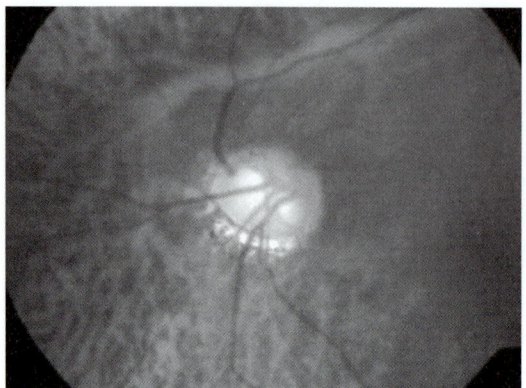

Figure 28.9 Tilted disc
(For color version, see Plate 6)

the brain is mandatory because congenitally tilted discs have rarely been reported with congenital and acquired suprasellar tumors.

Optic Nerve Hypoplasia[7,12,16]

Histologically they are characterized by a decrease in the number of optic nerve axons. Clinically the disc is pale or grey and smaller than normal. It may be associated with a yellow to white ring around the disc (Double Ring Sign). The vascular pattern is also abnormal. Children with bilateral optic nerve hypoplasia often present with congenital sensory nystagmus. Midline central nervous system abnormalities are sometimes associated with bilateral and unilateral optic nerve hypoplasia. Septo-optic dysplasia (de Morsier syndrome) denotes the association of optic nerve hypoplasia with absence of septum pellucidum, agenesis of corpus callosum, cerebral hemisphere abnormalities and pituitary gland abnormalities. Cerebral hemisphere anomalies like schizencephaly, periventricular leukomalacia or encephalomalacia occurs in approximately 45% of cases with optic nerve hypoplasia. It may also be associated with maternal ingestion of phenytoin, quinine and LSD as well as with fetal alcohol syndrome and maternal diabetes.

Optic nerve hypoplasia is now the most common congenital optic nerve anomaly encountered in pediatric ophthalmology practice. Many cases of optic nerve hypoplasia are undoubtedly misdiagnosed in the past. Some authors have suggested that drugs and alcohol abuse that have become more widespread in the recent years may be the cause for increased number of cases.

Growth hormone deficiency is the most common endocrinological abnormality associated with septo-optic dysplasia. Parents should be asked about the protracted neonatal jaundice (pointing towards hypothyroidism) and episodes of hypoglycemia in the neonatal period or during periods of illnesses (suggesting hypocortisolism).

Aicardi's Syndrome[17,18]

It is a cerebroretinal disorder associated with multiple depigmented 'chorioretinal lacunae' clustered around the optic disc.

Congenital optic disc anomalies including optic disc coloboma, optic nerve hypoplasia and congenital optic nerve pigmentation may accompany chorioretinal lacunae. The salient clinical features of Aicardi's syndrome are infantile spasm, agenesis of corpus callosum and chorioretinal lacunae.

Superior Segmental Optic Disc Hypoplasia (Topless Disc)

This is seen in approximately 10% of off springs if the mother has insulin dependent diabetes mellitus.

OPTIC ATROPHY[19]

Behr Syndrome

This presents in the first decade with visual loss, diffuse optic atrophy, spastic gait, ataxia and mental retardation (**Fig. 28.10**).

Wolfram Syndrome

It is also referred to as DIDMOAD syndrome (Diabetes Insipidus, Diabetes Mellitus, Optic Atrophy and Deafness). Presentation is between 5–21 years of age. It is characterized by diffuse and severe optic atrophy and systemic abnormalities apart from DIDMOAD, like anosmia, ataxia, seizures, mental handicap, short stature, endocrine abnormalities and elevated CSF protein.

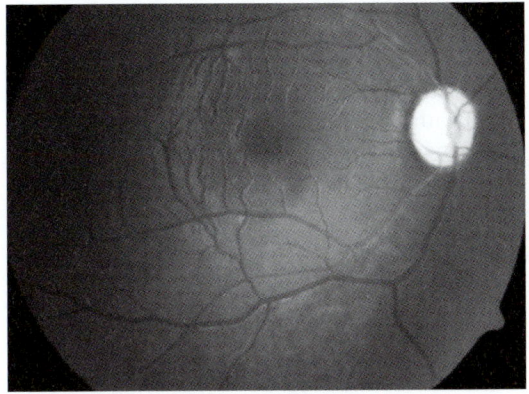

Figure 28.10 Primary optic atrophy
(For color version, see Plate 6)

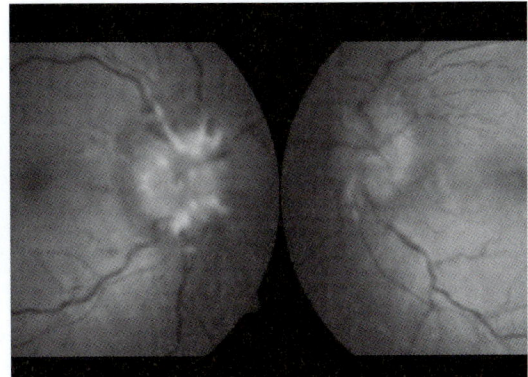

Figure 28.11 Papilledema
(For color version, see Plate 7)

Leber's Hereditary Optic Neuropathy[20]

It presents with acute or subacute severe painless loss of vision. Initially optic disc hyperemia with telangiectatic microangiopathy and later optic atrophy supervenes. Surprisingly the pupillary reactions remain brisk. Minor neurological abnormalities like exaggerated or pathological reflexes, mild cerebellar ataxia, myoclonus, tremor, movement disorders, seizures, muscle wasting, distal sensory neuropathy, motor neuropathy, auditory neuropathy and migraine had been described in Leber's hereditary optic neuropathy (LHON).

Optic disc should be carefully evaluated to rule out papilledema, optic neuritis, anterior ischemic optic neuropathy, and optic atrophy. It is not unusual for brain tumors to present with purely ophthalmological symptoms. Half of all the patients with brain tumors have ophthalmic signs and symptoms. These symptoms include loss of vision, optic disc changes (optic atrophy and papilledema), motility disorders (by involvement of third, fourth or sixth cranial nerves), exophthalmos, visual field defects, loss or desaturation of color vision and loss of somatic sensations (by involvement of fifth cranial nerve).

Things to Remember During Optic Disc Evaluation in a Suspected Case of Tumor

- Optic disc may be normal but may need perimetry if other features are suggestive of tumor.[8,21]
- Unilateral disc edema may be present in tumors of orbital apex and perimetry may be useful.
- Unilateral optic atrophy (indicating chiasmal or prechiasmal tumor) or bilateral optic atrophy (indicating tumors of chiasmal tract) warrants visual field examination.
- Bilateral optic disc edema or papilledema **(Fig. 28.11)** may be present in tumors of any location and immediate MRI of brain is warranted.
- If perimetry is normal MRI is needed if still there is clinical suspicion of tumors.
- In perimetry if there is nerve fiber pattern of defect, a prechiasmal tumor may be suspected and MRI of orbit will have to be ordered.
- If there is bitemporal hemianopia it is most likely a chiasmal tumor and need MRI of orbit and chiasmal region.
- If there is homonymous hemianopia, a retro chiasmal tumor is possible and MRI of brain is mandatory.

PHAKOMATOSIS

A group of disorders called phakomatosis[22] needs special mention since it involves retina and brain. The following conditions are included in phakomatosis group of diseases.

Tuberous Sclerosis or Bourneville Disease

It is a familial disease associated with anomalies of skin, eye, central nervous system etc. The astrocytic hamartomas are found in posterior pole involving the retina, optic nerve or both. The three classical findings called Vogt's triad are mental retardation, seizures and facial angiofibromas. All the findings are present in only 30% of cases with tuberous sclerosis.

Von Hippel-Lindau's Disease or Retinal Angiomatosis[23]

It is an autosomal dominant condition. This condition is associated with vascular tumors or hemangioblastomas of retina and CNS most often cerebellum. The hallmark of mature retinal tumors is a pair of markedly dilated vessels, both artery and vein, between the lesion and optic disc. This indicates significant arteriovenous shunting. Transudation of fluid into the subretinal space causes lipid accumulation, retinal detachment and loss of vision **(Fig. 28.12)**.

Sturge-Weber Syndrome or Encephalofacial Angiomatosis[24]

It consists of facial cutaneous angioma (port Wine stain) with an ipsilateral leptomeningeal vascular malformation that typically results in cerebral calcification, seizures, hemianopia, hemiparesis, and a highly variable degree of mental deficiency. Ocular involvement most commonly occurs in the form of increase number of well-formed choroidal vessels that give the fundus a uniform bright red or orange color, which has been compared to tomato catsup. Circumscribed choroidal hemangioma is another feature **(Fig. 28.13)**. Varying degree of increased conjunctival vascularity and abnormal episcleral vessels are also seen. Glaucoma is the most common and severe ocular complication that occurs in approximately 70% of cases.

Ataxia Telangiectasia or Louis-Bar Syndrome[25]

It is an autosomal recessive disorder that primarily involves the CNS particularly the cerebellum, ocular surface, skin and the immune system. Telangiectasia of the conjunctiva develops between 3-5 years of age. It was seen in 91% of cases in one study. Involvement is initially interpalpebral but away from the limbus, eventually becomes generalized. Recognition of ocular features is often the key to diagnosis of ataxia telangiectasia.

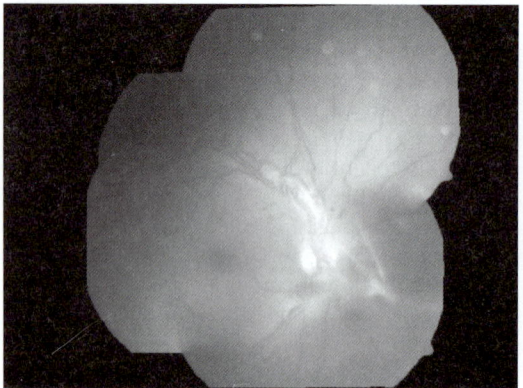

Figure 28.12 Retinal angioma in Von Hippel-Lindau's disease
(For color version, see Plate 7)

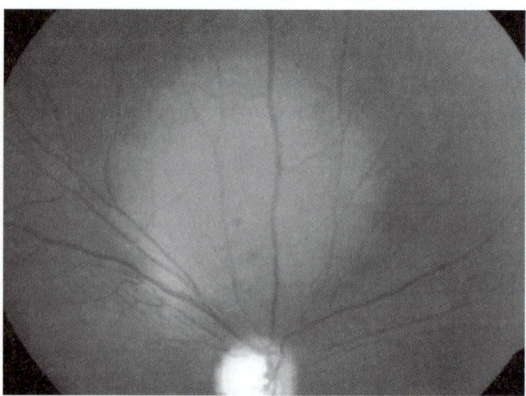

Figure 28.13 Circumscribed choroidal hemangioma
(For color version, see Plate 7)

This condition is thought to be the most common cause of progressive ataxia in early childhood. Truncal ataxia is usually noted in the second year of life, with subsequent development of dysarthria, dystonia and choreoathetosis.

Incontinentia Pigmenti or Bloch-Sulzberger Syndrome

This condition involves skin, brain and eyes. Ocular involvement occurs in at least one quarter to one third of cases, typically in the form of proliferative retinal vasculopathy that closely resembles retinopathy of prematurity. Abnormal arteriovenous connections, microvascular abnormalities and neovascularization develop at the junction of vascular and avascular retina. Rapid progression may lead to total retinal detachment and retrolental membrane formation or pseudoglioma within first few months of life.

Racemose Angioma or Wyburn-Mason Syndrome[26]

It is a non-hereditary arteriovenous malformation of the eye and brain, typically involving optic disc, retina and the midbrain. Ocular manifestations are unilateral and congenital, but may progress during childhood. The typical lesion consists of markedly dilated and tortuous vessels that shunt blood directly from arteries to veins. These vessels do not leak fluid. Vision in the affected eye may range from normal to markedly reduce. Intraocular hemorrhage and secondary neovascular glaucoma are the possible complications. No treatment is indicated for the primary lesion. Seizures, mental retardation, hemiparesis and papilledema may result from CNS lesion, which are frequently a source of hemorrhage, unlike hemangioma of Sturge-Weber syndrome.

METABOLIC AND NEURODEGENERATIVE DISEASES OF OPHTHALMOLOGICAL SIGNIFICANCE

This group of diseases can present with cherry red spot, retinitis pigmentosa, optic atrophy and corneal involvement.[4]

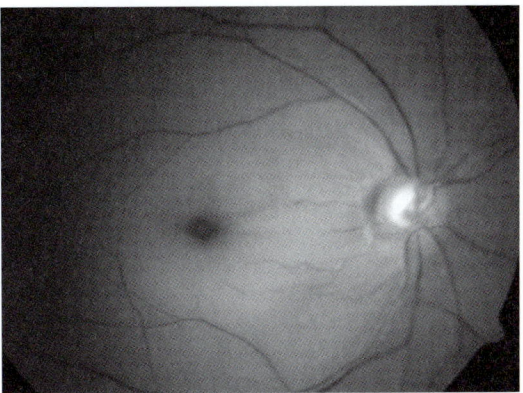

Figure 28.14 Cherry red spot
(For color version, see Plate 7)

Cherry Red Spot at the Macula[27,28] (Fig. 28.14)

It is a clinical sign seen when there is thickening and loss of transparency at the posterior pole of the fundus. The fovea is the thinnest part of retina, which is devoid of ganglion cell layer. It retains relative transparency allowing transmission of the vascular hue from beneath. This striking retinal lesion that is commonly seen in central retinal artery occlusion, is additionally a feature of a rare group of metabolic disorders called sphingolipidoses. The lipids accumulate in the ganglion cell layers of retina giving the retina a white appearance. As the ganglion cells are absent at the foveola this area retains relative transparency and contrasts with the surrounding opaque retina. As time passes the ganglion cells die and cherry red spot becomes less apparent. A late stage of the disease is characterized by degeneration of the retinal nerve fiber layer and consecutive optic atrophy.

Systemic Associations

- Tay-Sachs disease (Gm2 gangliosidosis type 1) or Infantile amaurotic familial idiocy. 90% cases have cherry red spot.
- Niemann pick disease—Incidence of cherry red spot is lower.
- Sandhoff's disease (Gm2 gangliosidosis type 2): It is identical to Tay-Sachs disease

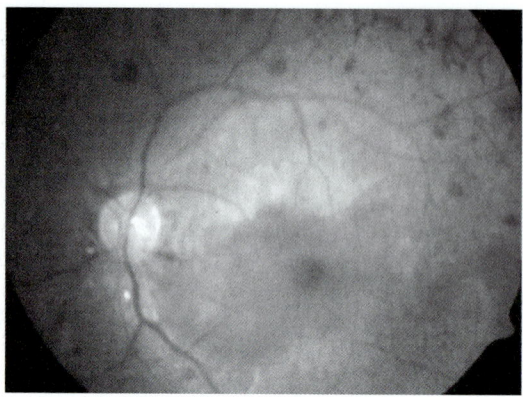

Figure 28.15 Retinitis pigmentosa
(For color version, see Plate 7)

- Generalized gangliosidosis (Gm1 gangliosidosis type 1)
- Sialidosis type 1 and 2 or Cherry red spot myoclonus syndrome. Here cherry red spot may be the initial finding
- Metachromatic leukodystrophy.

Retinitis Pigmentosa[9] (Fig. 28.15)

Bassen-Kornzweig Syndrome

It is caused by a deficiency of beta lipoprotein resulting in intestinal malabsorption. It is characterized by spinocerebellar ataxia, ptosis and progressive external ophthalmoplegia. Retinitis pigmentosa develops at the end of first decade of life. The pigment clumps are usually larger than the classic retinitis pigmentosa and are not confined to equatorial region. Early treatment with vitamin E may be beneficial for neurological disability.

Refsum's Syndrome or Heridopathia Atactica Polyneuritiformis

It is an inborn error of metabolism due to deficiency in the enzyme phytanic acid 2 hydroxylase resulting in accumulation of phytanic acid in the blood and body tissues. Pigmentary retinopathy develops in the second decade and is characterized by 'salt and pepper' fundus. Other ocular features are cataract, miosis, and prominent corneal nerves. Systemic features include polyneuropathy, cerebellar ataxia, deafness, anosmia, cardiomyopathy and ichthyosis. Early diagnosis can prevent blindness.

Kearns-Sayre Syndrome

It is a mitochondrial cytopathy associated with mitochondrial DNA deletion. Presentation is in the first or second decade of life with bilateral mild ptosis and progressive external ophthalmoplegia. Retinal findings are characterized by coarse pigment clumping affecting the central fundus. Systemic features include ataxia, fatigue, proximal muscle weakness, deafness, cardiac conduction defects, diabetes and short stature.

Bardet-Biedl Syndrome

Retinitis pigmentosa is severe and almost 75% patients are blind by the age of 20 years. It is associated with mental handicap.

Friedreich's Ataxia

Retinitis pigmentosa is common. Systemic features include childhood spinocerebellar ataxia, dysarthria, cardiomyopathy, deafness and diabetes mellitus.

OPTIC ATROPHY

It can occur in the following neurodegenerative disorders: 1. Tay-Sachs disease, 2. Sandhoff disease, 3. Krabbe disease, 4. Niemann-Pick disease, 5. Metachromatic leukodystrophy, 6. Adrenoleukodystrophy, 7. Ataxia telangiectasia, 8. Friedreich's ataxia.

CORNEAL INVOLVEMENT

This occurs in various forms in majority of lysosomal storage diseases. In mucopolysaccharidosis corneal clouding is a significant feature.

Mucopolysaccharidosis

Corneal clouding is present in all mucopolysaccharidosis except Hunter's and San Filippo's syndromes. Cornea is frequently affected by abnormal glycosaminoglycan metabolism.

This is because glycosaminoglycans form the ground substance in cornea.

Hurler's Syndrome (MPS1-H)

Diffuse corneal clouding occurs by the age of 3 years and the child presents with photophobia. Fine punctate corneal opacities predominantly involving the central cornea is present. Although keratoplasty can restore corneal clarity the visual acuity may be limited because of the optic nerve and retinal involvement.

Scheie's Syndrome (MPS1-HS)

Corneal clouding is progressive necessitating keratoplasty within the first decade.

Hunter's Syndrome

Usually corneal clouding is not clinically significant but detectable by slit lamp examination.

San Filippo's Syndrome (MPS III)

Corneal opacification is rare.

Marquio's Syndrome (MPS IV)

Diffuse corneal clouding occurs after 10 years of age.

Marateaux Lamy Syndrome (MPS VI)

Severe corneal clouding with increased corneal thickness develops within first few years of life, which necessitates keratoplasty.

Sly's Syndrome (MPS VII)

Only mild corneal opacities are present.

Mild corneal granularity and opacity is present in all mucolipidosis except mucolipidosis type IV or Berman's syndrome in which prominent and diffuse corneal clouding is present at birth or early infancy.

Fabry's Disease

It is an X-linked disease caused by deficiency of Alpha galctosidase A. Corneal involvement is

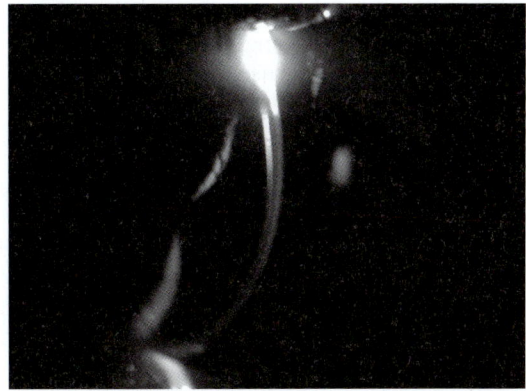

Figure 28.16 Kayser–Fleischer ring
(For color version, see Plate 7)

typical in both affected males and female carriers. The fine powdery opacities of corneal epithelium or sub epithelium usually develop in early infancy and are seen by retroillumination during slit lamp examination. They occur in a whorl like or vortex pattern called cornea verticillata. This is seen in the inferior part of cornea and do not affect vision.

Wilson's Disease

Kayser–Fleischer (KF) rings are an important diagnostic sign and management indicator **(Fig. 28.16)**. They are copper deposits in descemet's membrane first seen in gonioscopy in the upper and lower limbal edges. With time they extend to the full circumference of cornea and change color from yellow green gold to deep brown. Then it will be visible to naked eye. The ring may fade or disappear after treatment. KF ring may be also seen in primary biliary cirrhosis, familial cholestatic jaundice, neonatal liver diseases and multiple myeloma.

ABNORMAL OCULAR MOVEMENTS OF NEURO-OPHTHALMIC SIGNIFICANCE

Ocular motor apraxia or saccade limitation failure: This is characterized by impairment of voluntary saccadic movement with a relative preservation of reflex saccadic movements and quick phases of vestibular and optokinetic nystagmus. Infantile onset ocular motor apraxia is seen in infantile Gaucher's disease type 2 and 3, Krabbe's leukodystrophy, GM1 gangliosidosis and infantile Refsum's disease. Late onset ocular motor apraxia is seen in ataxia Telangiectasia, Huntington's disease and Wilson's disease.

Ocular dysmetria is a consistent over or under shooting of a saccade towards a target usually seen in cerebellar disease.

Ocular flutter consists of random conjugate to and fro horizontal saccades that disrupt fixation. It is seen in cerebellar disease.

Opsoclonus is a multidirectional ocular flutter. When it is associated with ataxia and myoclonus it is known as dancing eyes. It is seen in cerebellar diseases and occasionally associated with paraneoplastic syndrome in neuroblastoma.

Square wave jerks refer to small conjugate horizontal saccades away from fixation. It is seen in children with cerebellar diseases.

MATERNAL INFECTIONS OF NEURO-OPHTHALMIC SIGNIFICANCE

Common types of congenital infections called TORCHES (Toxoplasmosis, Rubella, Cytomegalic inclusion diseases, Herpes viruses infections, Epstein-Barr virus and Syphilis) have significant ophthalmic findings.[29,30]

Toxoplasmosis

Congenital infection can result in varying degrees of retinitis, intracranial calcification, microcephaly, hepatosplenomegaly, and developmental delay. The active area of retinal inflammation is usually cream colored with overlying vitritis. The area may be adjacent to an old flat atrophic scar, usually in the macula area. It is called satellite lesion **(Figs 28.17 and 28.18)**.

Rubella

Congenital rubella syndrome is a well-defined combination of ocular, otologic and cardiac anomalies along with microcephaly and variable developmental delay. Ocular abnormalities include nuclear cataract, glaucoma, microphthalmos, and retinopathy varying from subtle salt and pepper appearance to pseudoretinitis pigmentosa.

Cytomegalic Inclusion Disease

It is the most common congenital infection, occurring in 1% of infants. Congenital cytomegalovirus disease is characterized by fever, jaundice, hematological abnormalities, deafness, microcephaly and periventricular calcification. Ophthalmic manifestations of congenital cytomegalovirus infection include retinochoroiditis, optic nerve abnormalities, microphthalmos, cataract and uveitis. Retinochoroiditis usually presents with bilateral focal involvement consisting of areas of retinal pigment epithelium atrophy and whitish opacities mixed with retinal hemorrhages. Retinitis is usually progressive.

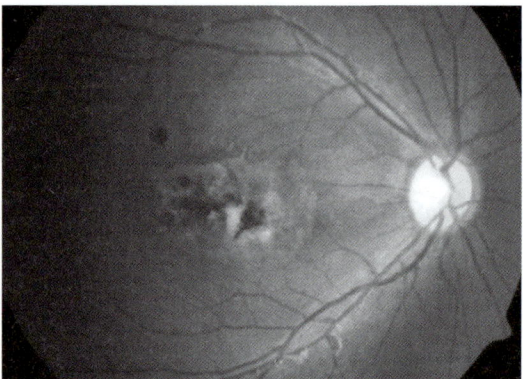

Figure 28.17 Toxoplasma scar at macula
(For color version, see Plate 8)

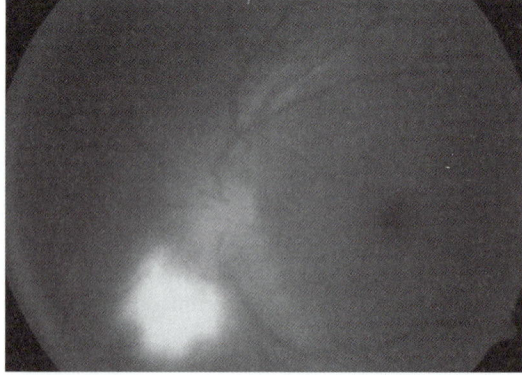

Figure 28.18 Active toxoplasma retinochoroiditis with headlight in fog appearance
(For color version, see Plate 8)

Herpes Simplex Infections

Ocular involvement in congenital infection includes conjunctivitis, keratitis, retinochoroiditis and cataract.

Syphilis

Chorioretinitis appears as a salt and pepper granularity of fundus. Bilateral interstitial keratitis is the classic ophthalmic finding in older children and adults.

Retinal Vascular Occlusive Diseases Associated with Neurological Diseases

Vasculitis or hypercoagulable status can lead to both retinal and cerebral vaso-occlusive events in young patients.

CONCLUSION

To conclude eye can be considered as a window to the neurological diseases. A proper ophthalmic examination may clinch or support a diagnosis with neurological manifestations. A timely diagnosis may be very helpful in preventing mental retardation and hence giving a good social life to them and their family.

REFERENCES

1. Repka MX. Brain lesions with ophthalmological manifetsations. In: Wright KW, Spiegel PH, Thompson LS (Eds). Handbook of Pediatric Neuro-Ophthalmology, 1st edition. Springer; 2006. pp. 255-89.
2. Buckly EG. Pediatric neuro-ophthalmological examination. In: Wright KW, Spiegel PH, Thompson LS (Eds). Handbook of Pediatric Neuro-Ophthalmology, 1st edition. Springer; 2006. pp. 62-85.
3. Philips PH, Broadsky MC. Congenital optic nerve abnormalities. In: Wright KW, Spiegel PH, Thompson LS (Eds). Handbook of Pediatric Neuro-Ophthalmology, 1st edition. Springer; 2006. pp. 204-47.
4. Borchert MS, Ying S. Neurodegenerative conditions of ophthalmic importance. In: Wright KW, Spiegel PH, Thompson LS (Eds). Handbook of Pediatric Neuro-Ophthalmology. 1st edition. Springer; 2006. pp. 324-71.
5. Basic and clinical science course, section 6: Pediatric ophthalmology and strabismus. American Academy of Ophthalmology; 2011-12.
6. Mc Keown CA, Davidson SL. The pediatric eye examination. In: Albert DM. Miller JW (Eds). Albert and Jakobiec's Principles and Practice of Ophthalmology, 3rd edition. Saunders. 2006;4:4133-43.
7. Schiefer U, Wilhelm H. Optic disc signs and optic neuropathies. In: Schiefer U, Wilhelm H, Hart W (Eds). Clinical Neuro-Ophthalmology. A Practical Guide,1st edition. Springer; 2007. pp. 101-27.
8. Leo Kottler B. Brain tumors relevant to clinical neuro-ophthalmogy. In: Schiefer U, Wilhelm H, Hart W (Eds). Clinical Neuro-Ophthalmology: A Practical Guide, 1st edn. Springer; 2007. pp. 171-84.
9. Kanski JJ. Clinical Ophthalmology: A Systematic Approach, 6th edition; 2007. pp. 663-94.
10. Nelson LB, Spaeth GL, Nowinski TS, Margo CE, Jackson L. Aniridia: A review. Surv Ophthalmol. 1984;28(6):621-42.
11. Ellika S, Robson CD, Heidary G, Paldino MJ. Morning glory disc anomaly: characteristic MR imaging findings. Am J Neuroradiol. 2013;34(10): 2010-4.
12. Kaur S, Jain S, Sodhi HB, Rastogi A, Kamlesh. Optic nerve Hypoplasia. Oman J Ophthalmol. 2013;6(2):77-82.
13. Lenhart PD, Lambert SR, Newman NJ, Biousse V, Atkinson DS Jr, Traboulsi EI, Hutchinson AK. Intracranial vascular anomalies in patients with morning glory disc anomaly. Am J Ophthalmol. 2006;142(4):644-50.
14. Maumenee IH, Mitchell TN. Colobomatous malformations of the eye. Trans Am Ophthalmol Soc. 1990;88:123-35.
15. Berk AT, Yaman A, Saatçi AO. Ocular and systemic findings associated with optic disc colobomas. J Pediatr Ophthalmol Strabismus. 2003;40(5):272-8.
16. Brodsky MC. Magnetic resonance imaging of colobomatous optic nerve hypoplasia. Br J Ophthalmol. 1999;83:753.
17. Apple DJ, Rabb MF, Walsh PM. Congenital anomalies of optic disc. Surv Ophthalmol. 1982;27(1):3-41.
18. Carney SH, Brodsky MC, Good WV, Glasier CM, Gribel ML, Cunnif C. Aicardi syndrome: More than meets the eye. Surv Ophthalmol. 1993; 37(6):419-24.
19. Lenaers G, Hamel C, Delettre C, Amati-Bonneau P, Procaccio V, Bonneau D, et al. Dominant optic atrophy. Orphanet J Rare Dis. 2012;7:46.

20. Behbehani R. Clinical approach to optic neuropathies. Clin Ophthalmol. 2007;1(3):233-46.
21. Hedges TR. Papilledema: its recognition and relation to increased intracranial pressure. Surv Ophthalmol. 1975;19(4):201-23.
22. Korf BR. Phakomatoses. Clin Dermatol. 2005; 23(1):78-84.
23. Chew EY. Ocular manifestations of Von Hippel Lindau disease: Clinical and genetic investigation. Trans Am Ophthalmol Soc. 2005;103:495-511.
24. Thomas Sohl KA, Vaslow DF, Maria BL. Sturge Weber syndrome: A review. Pediatr Neurol. 2004;30(5):303-10.
25. Perlman S, Becker Catania S, Gatti RA. Ataxia telangiectasia: Diagnosis and management. Semin Pediatr Neurol. 2003;10(3):173-82.
26. Rizzo R, Pavone L, Pero G, Chiarmonte L, Curatolo P. A neurocutaneous disease of sever course: Wyburn-Mason syndrome. J Child Neurol. 2004;19(11):908-11M.
27. Suvarna JC, Hajela SA. Cherry-red spot. J Postgrad Med. 2008;54:54-7.
28. Chen H, Chan AY, Stone DU, Mandel NA. Beyond the cherry-red spot: Ocular manifestations of sphingolipid-mediated neurodegenerative and inflammatory disorders. Surv Ophthalmol. 2014;59(1):10.
29. Mets MB, Chhabra MS. Eye manifestations of intrauterine infections and their impact on childhood blindness. Surv Ophthalmol. 2008; 53(2):95-111.
30. Stegman BJ, Carey JC. TORCH infections. Toxoplasmosis, other (syphilis, varicella-zoster, parvovirus B19), Rubella, Cytomegalovirus (CMV), and Herpes infections. Curr Womens Health Rep. 2002;2(4):253-8.

CHAPTER 29

An Approach to Children with Neurogenic Bladder Dysfunction

VT Haridas

Urinary bladder has a complex innervation with somatic and sympathetic systems and carries out dual functions of storage and emptying of urine. At least 25% of the clinical problems seen in pediatric urology are the result of neurologic lesions that affect the lower urinary tract function. Our increasing understanding of the neurophysiology of bladder coupled with advances in urodynamic techniques specifically designed for infants and young children have provided more accurate assessment of pediatric lower urinary tract disorders.

Neural control of bladder—sphincter unit in children is age dependant and hence much more variable and complex than those of adults. Of the various classifications of bladder dysfunctions the one proposed by International Children's Continence society in 1997 is well accepted **(Table 29.1)**.[1]

BASIC NEUROANATOMY AND PHYSIOLOGY

A thorough knowledge about the complex bladder innervations and regulation is essential to understand the pathophysiology of various conditions affecting the bladder.[2,3] Anatomically,

Table 29.1 Etiologic classification of bladder dysfunction	
A.	Derangement of nervous control • Congenital malformations of CNS—myelomeningocele, spina bifida occulta, caudal regression syndrome, tethered cord syndrome • Developmental disturbances—mental retardation, dysfunctional voiding, urge syndrome • Acquired conditions like—cerebral palsy, spinal cord trauma, transverse myelitis, multiple sclerosis, vascular malformations
B.	Disorders of detrusor and sphincteric muscle function • Congenital conditions like muscular dystrophy, neuronal dysplasia • Acquired conditions like chronic bladder distension, fibrosis of bladder wall
C.	Structural abnormalities • Congenital conditions like—bladder exstrophy, prune belly syndrome, epispadias, posterior urethral valve and other urethral anomalies • Acquired conditions—traumatic stricture or damage to sphincter or urethra
D.	Other unclassified conditions • Giggle incontinence • Hinmann's syndrome • Ochoa syndrome [urofacial syndrome]

the bladder is divided into a "body" or "dome" made of detrusor smooth muscle and the base, which includes the trigone and bladder neck that are intimately connected to the pelvic floor. The bladder outlet is controlled by two sphincters— the internal urethral (smooth muscle) sphincter in the bladder neck and proximal urethra and the external (striated muscle) sphincter of the membranous urethra. Lower urinary tract has sympathetic, parasympathetic as well as somatic nerve supply. The hypogastric nerve carries sympathetic fibers, the pelvic nerve carries the parasympathetic innervation, while the pudendal nerve carries the somatic innervations **(Fig. 29.1)**.

The sympathetic innervation to the lower urinary tract arises from the T11-L2 cord level, synapse in the inferior mesenteric and hypogastric plexuses and reaches bladder via the hypogastric nerves. The sympathetic stimulation release norepinephrine which acts through α-adrenergic receptors in the bladder neck and proximal urethra as well as β-adrenergic receptors in the bladder fundus. Alpha adrenergic stimulation closes the sphincter whereas the beta adrenergic stimulation inhibits and relaxes the detrusor muscles. The function of sympathetic innervations is to facilitate storage.

Parasympathetic supply arises from the detrusor nucleus at the S2–S4 cord level, passes through the pelvic nerves to cholinergic parasympathetic ganglia in the detrusor. Acetylcholine released by activation of these neurons produces detrusor contraction through M2 and M3 muscarinic receptor activation. Parasympathetic innervation in the proximal urethra causes nitric oxide to be released there which produces urethral smooth

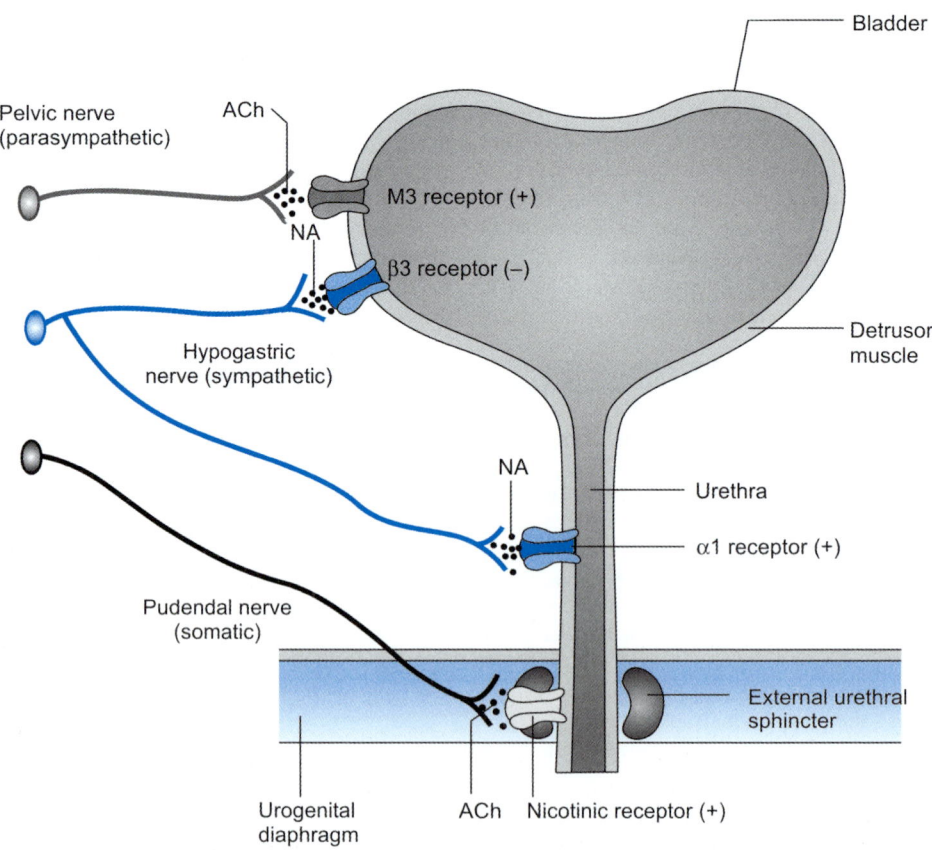

Figure 29.1 Innervation of lower urinary tract
Abbreviations: ACh, acetylcholine; NA, noradrenaline

muscle relaxation. Parasympathetic stimulation thus results in detrusor contraction and relaxation of the proximal urethra. The parasympathetic supply is activated during micturition.

Somatic innervation to the external urethral sphincter arises from the pudendal (Onuf's) nucleus at the S2–S4 cord level and passes through the pudendal nerve to the striated sphincter muscle. Voluntary centers in the cerebral cortex exert excitatory influence on the pudendal nucleus to produce external urethral sphincter and pelvic floor contraction which maintains continence. When one decides to void voluntarily this influence is lifted to produce urethral and pelvic floor relaxation which facilitates bladder emptying.

A dense sensory supply of small myelinated Aδ fibers and unmyelinated C fibers is found in the suburothelial and muscular plexuses which relays information about the bladder filling. Free sensory fiber endings extend through the urothelium into the bladder cavity and acts as transducers of physical and chemical stimuli. The Aδ fibers respond to bladder wall distention and trigger micturition, while C fibers respond to painful stimuli. Afferent fibers are carried through the pelvic nerves, relayed through sacral dorsal root ganglia to the dorsal horn of the spinal cord. The sensory information about bladder filling and tension is further transmitted rostrally to the PAG region which is important in the control of micturition.

Micturition is a complex phenomenon controlled and coordinated by various centers in the spinal cord, brainstem, subcortical centers and cerebral cortex. Cortical control areas in the supplementary motor area and cingulate gyrus as well as subcortical areas provide inhibitory influence on micturition at the level of the pons and excitatory influence on the external urinary sphincter. This allows voluntary control of micturition so that normally bladder evacuation can be delayed until an appropriate time and place to void are chosen.

The pontine micturition center (PMC, also known as Barrington's nucleus or M-region) is essential for the coordination of micturition. PMC modulates the opposing effects of the parasympathetic and sympathetic nervous systems on the lower urinary tract. PMC sends excitatory influence to the sacral spinal cord that produces detrusor contraction during emptying phase. Simultaneously thoracolumbar sympathetic outflow is inhibited producing internal urinary sphincter relaxation.[4] During bladder storage phase, PMC inhibits the sacral parasympathetic outflow leading to detrusor relaxation and simultaneously send excitatory influence to the thoracolumbar sympathetic centers producing internal urethral sphincter contraction. Experiments in lower animals have shown the presence of a group of neurons situated lateral to the PMC which inhibits voiding. This center is called L-region or lateral storage center. It is probable that such a center exists in human beings as well, but may not be anatomically well demarcated.

The PMC is under the direct excitatory influence of a group of neurons lying in the periaqueductal gray matter (PAG). PAG receives ascending sensory information from the bladder afferents. Higher centers in the hypothalamus, thalamus, the anterior cingulate cortex, insula, and prefrontal cortex has immense connections with PAG. They influence PMC indirectly through PAG. On voluntarily initiating micturition, the prefrontal cortex inhibition of the PAG is lifted and simultaneously the hypothalamus stimulates the PAG. The overall result is excitation of the PMC which produces voiding.

During the filling phase, the parasympathetic innervation of the detrusor is inhibited and the smooth and striated parts of the urethral sphincter are activated, thus preventing leakage of urine. This is a spinal reflex known as the 'guarding reflex'. The afferent impulses arise from the urethra and bladder wall and spinal interneurons in the sacral cord plays an important role. Some input from pontine storage center might facilitate sphincter reflexes. Suprasinal centers produce inhibition of the pontine micturition center, which results in enhancement of thoracolumbar sympathetic outflow with simultaneous suppression of sacral parasympathetic outflow to the lower urinary tract. These suprasinal centers also produce excitatory outflow through the pudendal nerve to produce external urethral sphincter contraction. The overall effect in normal bladder physiology is detrusor smooth muscle relaxation, bladder neck smooth muscle contraction, and external urinary sphincter skeletal muscle contraction that allow low pressure storage of urine in the bladder without leakage.

During the bladder emptying phase, the supraspinal centers' inhibitory outflow to the pontine micturition center is suppressed, resulting in reduction of thoracic sympathetic outflow with simultaneous enhancement of sacral parasympathetic outflow to the lower urinary tract.[4] The supraspinal centers' excitatory outflow through the pudendal nerve is suppressed producing external urethral sphincter relaxation. The overall effect in normal bladder physiology is detrusor smooth muscle contraction, bladder neck smooth muscle relaxation, and external urinary sphincter skeletal muscle relaxation that allow evacuation of urine stored in the bladder. The coordination between a contracting detrusor and a relaxing sphincter is lost in neurologic lesions especially those between the PMC and sacral cord. This detrusor sphincter dyssynergia can lead to obstruction in voiding and very high intravesical pressure leading to vesicoureteric reflux.

Maturation of Bladder Control

At birth, bladder is uninhibited and functions through reflex activities. Over the next 5–6 years the bladder control matures to the adult level **(Table 29.2)**.

Pathophysiology of Neurogenic Bladder

Many classifications have been used to group neurogenic bladder dysfunction. Each has their merits and clinical utility. These classifications may be based on urodynamic findings,[5,6] neurourologic criteria[7,8] or on bladder and urethral function.[9,10]

A popular classification of neurogenic bladder dysfunction based on the location of the neurologic lesions in the neural pathways is given below:

- Lesions above the pontine micturition center (e.g. cerebral palsy, brain tumor, pediatric stroke) producing an uninhibited bladder. The bladder empties when full even in socially inappropriate time. The voiding is complete and there is no residual urine.
- Lesions between the pontine micturition center and sacral spinal cord (e.g. Thoracolumbar spina bifida, traumatic spinal cord injury) producing an upper motor neuron bladder also called an automatic bladder. Voluntary control is lost, the bladder volume is low and there is a high incidence of detrusor sphincter dyssynergia and reflux uropathy.
- Sacral cord lesions that damage the detrusor nucleus but spare the pudendal nucleus producing a mixed type A bladder. Leads to a hypotonic bladder with large residual urine volume.
- Sacral cord lesions that spare the detrusor nucleus but damage the pudendal nucleus producing a mixed type B bladder, results in incontinence.
- *Lower motor neuron bladder*: Due to extensive damage of sacral cord or sacral nerve root injuries leading to an autonomic bladder. The bladder is totally denervated, is hypotonic and incontinent.

EVALUATION

The evaluation of a child with a neurogenic bladder includes a careful history of bladder and bowel habits, a thorough physical examination followed by relevant investigations. Symptoms due to lower urinary tract dysfunction may be broadly classified into storage symptoms and voiding symptoms

Table 29.2	Bladder control at various ages	
At birth	*Spinal reflex*	*Spontaneous, uninhibited micturition*
1–2 years	Frontal and parietal centers mature, bladder capacity increase	Bladder sensation appreciated, but micturition is still voluntary
3–4 years	Attains voluntary control of external sphincter when awake	Can postpone voiding
4–5 years	Cortical inhibition attained	Dry by night
More than 6 years	Can initiate micturition even if bladder is not full	Can initiate micturition in socially acceptable circumstances

An Approach to Children with Neurogenic Bladder Dysfunction

(Table 29.3). A careful history of bowel habits is equally important and must address the frequency of defecation and presence of fecal incontinence.

Abdomen should be palpated for a distended bladder or a loaded colon. A genitourinary examination should be done to look for developmental anomalies and dermatologic signs of urinary incontinence. The back should be examined for any congenital anomalies of the spine as well as any midline cutaneous markers such as dimples, hemangioma, nevus, or isolated tuft of hair. Asymmetry of the gluteal cleft may suggest abnormal sacral development. The anus is examined for sphincter tone and any evidence of fissures, skin tags, or hemorrhoids.

Investigations include urinalysis for infections, renal parameters to look for renal dysfunction, radiologic evaluation and urodynamic study.[11] An ultra sound examination of the abdomen and pelvis can easily detect developmental anomalies, signs of obstructive uropathy like hydronephrosis and post void residual urine.

URODYNAMIC STUDY OF BLADDER

Urodynamic studies (UDS) have revolutionized the assessment and management of pediatric neurogenic bladder in the last two decades. UDS is helpful in detecting, quantifying and in assessing the response to treatment. A computerized UDS lab carries out the tests as given in **Table 29.4**.

Bladder capacity in children above one year can be calculated using the Koff's formula—Bladder capacity [mL] = [Age [years] + 2] × 30. A normal bladder has good compliance and fills up to 200–300 mL without much increase in the pressure. Detrusor starts contracting after a particular level. The normal filling pressure should be <10 cm H_2O while the normal voiding pressure varies from 55 cm to 80 cm H_2O in boys and from 30 cm to 65 cm H_2O in girls. Detrusor over activity is considered an abnormal finding at any time. The examination findings are considered normal when there is an appropriate capacity, good compliant bladder, with no overactivity and normal innervation of

Table 29.3 Common symptoms of neurogenic bladder dysfunction

Symptoms due to abnormal filling	Voiding symptoms
• Increased day time frequency • Increased nocturnal frequency • Urgency • Urge incontinence • Stress incontinence • Mixed urgency and stress incontinence • Nocturnal enuresis • Continuous urinary incontinence • Situational incontinence—giggle • Abnormal bladder sensation—increased, decreased, absent	• Hesitancy • Straining • Slow stream • Splitting or spraying • Intermittent stream • Terminal dribble • Post-micturition dribble • Incomplete emptying

Table 29.4 Common tests used in urodynamics

- *Cystometry* helps to assess the bladder capacity, detrusor pressure, compliance, and bladder sensation
- *Uroflowmetry* evaluates the volume and flow rate of urine and helps in analyzing symptoms like hesitancy and intermittency
- *Residual urine volume* can be assessed using a post void USG or postvoid catheterization
- *Urethral pressure profile* studies the changes in urethral pressure during rest, micturition as well as maneuvers like cough and Valsalva's maneuver. Useful in analyzing incontinence as well as outlet obstruction
- *Pressure-flow micturition studies*
- *Video-urodynamic studies* simultaneous video recording using a radio-contrast dye and fluoroscopy helps in visually assessing detrusor contraction, vesicoureteral reflux and detrusor sphincter dyssynergia
- *Electrophysiologic studies* include sphincter EMG, pudendal nerve conduction study, pudendal somato sensory evoked potential [SSEP]—useful in assessing the integrity of local neural pathways

the sphincter with normal sacral reflexes and an increase in sphincter activity during filling and complete silencing during emptying. An upper motor neuron lesion is present when there is detrusor overactivity, a failure of the sphincter muscle to relax with a bladder contraction or leaking of bladder during filling. A lower motor neuron lesion is noted when there are no contractions of the detrusor muscle, denervation in sphincter EMG, no response in the sphincter to sacral reflexes during filling and voiding.

Urodynamic Study-based Functional Classification

With the advent of urodynamics it has become easier to assess the function of bladder during storage as well as voiding phase. Even subclinical abnormalities can be easily picked up, quantified and can be followed up. This has led to more practical classification of neurogenic bladder. The urodynamic study based classification accepted by International Continence Society (ICS) as well as the Madersbacher classification[12] accepted by European Association Urology (EAU) are gaining popularity **(Fig. 29.2)**. These classifications also help in planning therapy as the functional abnormalities are simplified down to practical problems like overactive or underactive detrusor, overactive or underactive urethra during storing or voiding phase.

Overactive bladder can be managed by having a fluid intake schedule aiming for 1000–1200 mL urine out put per day and drugs to reduce the detrusor contractions. Commonly used drugs are anticholinergics and tricyclic antidepressants. Nonselective anticholinergic agents like oxybutinin and selective agents like darifenacin or

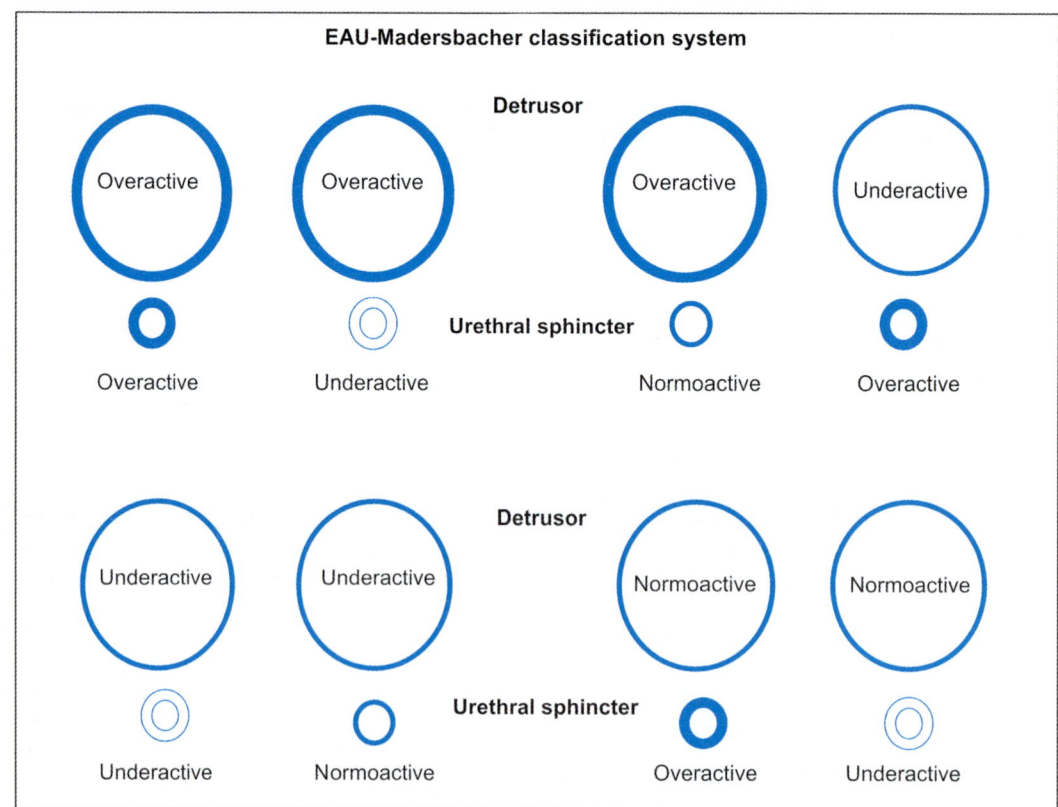

Figure 29.2 European Association Urology (EAU) classification of neurogenic bladder

solifenacin have been found to be useful. Tricyclic antidepressants like imipramine and amitriptyline have anticholinergic action on the detrusor muscles as well as alpha adrenergic action at the bladder neck and internal sphincter.[13] Injection of botulinum toxin in the detrusor muscles produces transient chemodenervation and reduce detrusor or overactivity lasting for 3–8 months.[14] Intravesical capsaicin instillation to reduce the hyperactivity of deafferented C fibers, sacral neuromodulation and augmentation of bladder capacity using cystoplasty are reserved for resistant cases of overactive bladder.

Alpha 1 receptor antagonists like terazosin, alfuzosin and doxazosin are used to reduce the high tone of a spastic sphincter. Benzodiazepines and baclofen which act through GABA-ergic inhibition have also been found to be useful. Botox injection to sphincter, sphincterotomy and urethral stents are reserved for those patients who fail to respond to pharmacological manipulation.

Drugs like duloxetine and pelvic floor exercises are found to be beneficial only in a minor subset of children with lax sphincter. Sling procedures may help these subjects to attain continence. Bladder neck closure and urinary diversion to colon has to be considered if the incontinence is intractable. Sacral cord stimulation and artificial urinary sphincter are emerging as promising therapeutic modalities for intractable incontinence.

Underactive bladder is of large volume and usually has high residual urine leading to recurrent UTI. Therapy with cholinergic drugs like bethanechol does not yield any significant clinical benefits. Clean intermittent catheterization (CIC) may be resorted to in these patients.

The concept of CIC introduced by lapides[15] four decades back has made a tremendous impact in the efficient management of complex neurogenic bladder dysfunction. The patient or caregiver is taught to catheterize the bladder 4–6 times a day. It is not a strictly aseptic procedure and hence the term 'clean'. Even though the subsequent urinalysis reveal significant bacterial colonization, clinically significant UTI are rare. CIC mimics the normal bladder physiology of storage phase for hours and intermittent voiding. CIC has been found useful to tackle complex problems like high detrusor pressure and reflux uropathy, recurrent UTI due to residual urine, bladder decompensation due to over distension, detrusor sphincter dyssynergia and spastic nonrelaxing sphincter.

COMMON PEDIATRIC NEUROUROLOGIC CONDITIONS

Bladder Dysfunction in Cerebral Palsy

More than one third of children with cerebral palsy present with dysfunctional urinary symptoms. Common symptoms include stress incontinence, frequency, urgency and difficulty in initiating micturition. Children with CP develops bladder control later than their normal counterparts. Cognitive abilities and IQ also can influence the attainment of bladder control. Neurogenic detrusor overactivity is observed in 70% of children with CP. As a result the functional bladder capacity is reduced and uninhibited contractions may result in incontinence. Detrusor sphincter dyssynergia is very rare in CP as the Pontine center and its connection with the spinal centers are intact.

Bladder Dysfunction in Spina Bifida

Incidence of spina bifida worldwide ranges from 0.3 to 4.5 per 1000 live births. Renal damage is an important cause for mortality and starts as early as the sixth month. The principal aims in the management of urological problems in spina bifida are:
- Preservation of renal function
- Achieve urinary dryness by school age
- Independence at an older age with respect to bowel and bladder care
- Maintain sexual and reproductive functions.

Presence of an overactive bladder and detrusor sphincter dyssynergia (DSD) increases the risk of renal failure and hence the assessment should be aimed to detect them at the earliest. Anal sphincter tone should be checked during the initial examination. A tightly closed anal sphincter may indicate an overactive pelvic floor and indirectly the possibility of DSD. The first UDS may be delayed till the second month, especially in children undergoing surgery in the neonatal period, as the pelvic floor behavior may change postoperatively.

All new born patients with spina bifida and suspected high bladder pressure are put on clean intermittent catheterization along with anticholinergics like oxybutinin to reduce the bladder activity and UTI prophylaxis with agents like trimethoprim. CIC is carried out initially by the care givers and subsequently by the child him/herself by the age of 8–9 years. CIC done properly at least 3 times a day has reduced the need for bladder augmentation surgery from 90% to less than 5%. The child is followed up yearly with UDS to look for bladder activity, capacity and compliance as well as USG to look for upper tract dilatation and renal development. If the bladder capacity is normal for age and the end filling detrusor pressure is less than 30 mL H_2O, the child may be followed up with regular CIC and anticholinergics. If the detrusor filling pressure is more than 40 cm H_2O and the voiding pressure is more than 100 cm H_2O and capacity is low surgical augmentation using ileocystoplasty or colocystoplasty may be considered.

Spina bifida patients with paralyzed pelvic floor are incontinent. Their detrusor pressure will be low, hence upper tract injury due to reflux is rare. Children need bladder neck surgery to attain continence. Transvaginal sling procedure in girls and transabdominal puboprostatic sling procedure in boys are the standard surgeries. Persistent leakage after sling surgeries can be tackled by injecting urethral bulking agents like silicon.

The timing for surgical procedure is determined by the type of bladder abnormality and magnitude. A surgical procedure may have to be performed even as early as by the third month of life in children with serious threat to the upper urinary tract.

Children with occult spinal dysraphism and sacral agenesis should undergo a MRI study of the spine as well as a UDS with sphincter EMG to assess the extent and nature of lesion. Almost equal incidence of upper and lower motor neuron lesions [35% vs 40%] are observed in these subjects.

Bladder Dysfunction in Acquired Myelopathies

Spinal cord injuries, demyelinating diseases like pediatric multiple sclerosis, vascular insults and infective myelitis are the main acquired myelopathies causing neurogenic bladder. The presence of severe motor deficits and disabilities often distracts the clinicians attention from the urologic dysfunction. Recurrent urinary infections and renal damage are the chief causes for morbidity and mortality in these unfortunate children and they should be addressed and managed during the acute stage itself.

Hinman's Syndrome

Also known as non-neurogenic neurogenic bladder is an acquired condition characterized by bladder—sphincter dyssynergia and poor emptying leading to decompensation and recurrent UTI. Urodynamic study shows a pattern classical of neurogenic bladder. Various mechanisms including occult spinal dysraphism, acquired psychological abnormality leading to voluntary sphincter disturbance and isolated bladder neuropathy have all been proposed. The management strategy is the same as for any other neurogenic bladder.

Nocturnal Enuresis

Primary nocturnal enuresis, a very common clinical problem in pediatric urology, usually results from a non-neurogenic dysfunction. Close observation and analysis have revealed that these children have multiple pathophysiologic mechanisms and hence need varying treatment strategies. A subset of these subjects have abnormally low antidiuretic hormone (ADH) secretion at night and will respond only to ADH replacement. Low bladder capacity and compliance, uninhibited bladder contractions, elevated arousal threshold leading to "heavy sleep" and psychological stress have all been found to play significant roles in the causation.

CONCLUSION

Neurogenic bladder dysfunction in children may result from congenital malformations like spina bifida as well as due to multiple acquired conditions like trauma and demyelinating diseases. Irrespective of the etiology, the basic principle in the management is to achieve a compliant bladder with adequate volume and low filling pressure which can empty intermittently. Judicious use of medications, techniques like CIC and surgical procedures can ensure a healthy upper urinary tract, longer life span and psychosocial well-being.

REFERENCES

1. Norgaard JP, van Gool JD, Hjalmas K, et al. Standardization and definitions in lower urinary tract dysfunction in children. International Children's Continence Society. Br J Urol. 1998;81 (Suppl 3):1-16.
2. Fowler CJ, Griffiths D, de Groat WC. The neural control of micturition. Nat Rev Neurosci. 2008;9: 453-66.
3. Wein AJ. "Lower urinary tract dysfunction in neurologic injury and disease," In: Wein AJ, Kavoussi L, Novick AC, Partin AW, Peters CA (Eds). Camppell-walsh vrology. Saunders, New York, NY, USA, 9th edition, 2007.pp.2011-45.
4. Dorsher PT, McIntosh PM. Neurogenic bladder. Adv Urol. 2012;2012:816274.
5. Lapides J. Neuromuscular vesical and urethral dysfunction. In: Campbell MF, Harrison JH. Urology. Philadelphia, PA, USA: WB Saunders; 1997.pp.1343-79.
6. Krane RJ, Siroky MB. Classification of neuro-urologic disorders. In: Krane RJ, Siroky MB (Eds). Clinical Neuro-Urology. Boston, Mass, USA: Little Brown; 1979.pp.143-58.
7. Hald T, Bradley WE. The Urinary Bladder: Neurology and Dynamics. Baltimore, MD, USA: Williams and Wilkins; 1982.
8. Bors E, Comarr AE. Neurological Urology. Baltimore, MD, USA: University Park Press; 1971.
9. Abrams P, Blaivas JG, Stanton SL, et al. Standardisation of terminology of lower urinary tract function. Neurourology and Urodynamics. 1988;7(5):403-27.
10. Wein AJ. Classification of voiding dysfunction: a simple approach. In: Barrett DM, Wein AJ (Eds). Controversies in Neuro-Urology. New York, NY, USA: Churchill Livingstone; 1984.
11. Fowler CJ, O'Malley KJ. Investigation and management of neurogenic bladder dysfunction. J Neurol Neurosurg Psychiatry 2003;74(Suppl 4):iv27-31.
12. Madersbacher HG. Neurogenic bladder dysfunction. Curr Opin Urol. 1999;9(4):303-7.
13. Yamaguchi O, Nishizawa O, Takeda M, et al. "Clinical guidelines for overactive bladder: guidelines" International Journal of Urology. 2009;16(2):126-42.
14. Schurch B, de Seze M, Denys P, et al. Botulinum toxin type A is a safe and effective treatment for neurogenic urinary incontinence: results of a single treatment, randomized, placebo controlled 6-month study. J Urol. 2005;174:196-200.
15. Lapides J, Diokno AC, Silber SJ, Lowe BS. "Clean, intermittent self-catheterization in the treatment of urinary tract disease". Journal of Urology. 1972;107(3):458-61.

CHAPTER 30

Brain Death in Children

TA Sheela

'Think of your child; then not as dead, but as living; not as a flower that has withered, but as one that is transplanted and touched by a divine hand, is blooming in richer colors and sweeter shades.'
—Richard Hooker

Brain death is the permanent cessation of the coordinated functions of the body as a whole. Its medical and legal aspects of determination have evolved over the past few years. Cardiopulmonary resuscitation and prolonged artificial support in advanced critical care maintain the vital functions for prolonged period of time even in presence of irreversible central nervous system (CNS) insults. It is more important to define brain death with greater precision in terms of timing and accuracy because of the increasing demand for organ transplantation worldwide and the awareness among people regarding the medical and ethical concerns related with organ procurement practices.

EVOLUTION OF CRITERIA FOR BRAIN DEATH

1967: The first US committee met to form a consensus opinion regarding the special criteria for the determination of brain death in infants and children.

1968: The Ad Hoc Committee from the Harvard Medical School published a report recommending the first neurological diagnostic criteria for determining brain death; with an objective to permit clinical transplant programs.[1]

1981: The National Conference of Commissioners on Uniform State Laws approved the Uniform Determination of Death Act. The UDDA provided the legal permission to procure vital organs after using only the brain death criteria to declare death.[2]

1995: Clinical guidelines were also established for adults by American Academy of Neurology. The consensus was that "these criteria may be in applicable in children under 5 years of age since the immature nervous system can survive significant periods of electro cerebral silence.[3]

1994: Transplantation of Human organ act—Government of India to streamline organ donation and transplantation activities.

1987: The clinical guidelines were first published in by the Task Force for the Determination of Brain Death in Children including pediatric organ donors.[4]

2011: Guidelines were revised under the auspices of the Society of Critical Care Medicine, the American Academy of Pediatrics, and the Child Neurology Society.[6]

DEFINITION OF BRAIN DEATH

An individual who has sustained either irreversible cessation of circulatory and respiratory functions or irreversible cessation of all functions of the entire brain including the brainstem is dead. A determination of death must be made in accordance with accepted medical standards.[2]

PROCESS FOR BRAIN DEATH DETERMINATION

Brain death in children most commonly develops following injury due to trauma or asphyxia. Pathogenesis is usually multifactorial with the end result being the irreversible loss of brain and brainstem function.[5,6] The diagnosis of brain death is primarily clinical.[5] The CNS of a child may be more resilient to certain types of injury and this should be considered when interpreting and confirming the diagnosis.[5] The revised guidelines include a consensus opinion regarding necessary clinical history, physical examination criteria, observation periods, and confirmatory laboratory tests required to determine brain death in children,[6,7] it also suggests minimum standards.

The three essential components diagnosis of brain death are irreversible coma, absence of brainstem reflexes, and apnea.[4]

DEMONSTRATION OF ABSENT CEREBRAL FUNCTION

It is essential to exclude the reversible medical conditions that can confuse the clinical assessment, which includes the following:[4]

Persistent Hypotension or Shock

Systolic blood pressure or mean arterial blood pressure (MAP) should be in an acceptable range, not 2 SDs below the mean values for the patient's age norm.

Hypothermia

Core body temperature should be maintained >35°C. Hypothermia, used as an adjunctive therapy for acute brain injury that reduces cerebral metabolic activity may confound the diagnostic assessment of brain death.[10]

Adequately re-warm with recording of 12 hours of normal temperature prior to performing brain death examination.

Severe Metabolic and Endocrine Abnormalities

Capable of causing metabolic encephalopathy-including glucose and electrolyte abnormalities, hypothyroidism, adrenal crisis, etc.

Central Nervous System Depressant Drug Intoxications

Barbiturates, opioids, anesthetic agents, sedatives, muscle relaxants, antiepileptic agents etc. Serum levels for these drugs should be performed if there is concern regarding recent ingestion or administration.

Nonconvulsive status epilepticus, SAH, brainstem lesions, liver or renal failure, sepsis, meningitis, brainstem encephalitis, etc. where a CNS catastrophe can occur.

The state of coma requires that the patient be unresponsive, must exhibit complete loss of consciousness, vocalization, and volitional activity; even to noxious stimuli. Decerebrate or decorticate posturing, seizures, shivering, response to verbal stimuli, and response to noxious stimuli not consistent with brain death.

ASSESSMENT OF BRAINSTEM REFLEXES

Pupillary Light Reflex

Cranial nerve II and III and midbrain.

No response to bright light. Size: Mid position (4–6 mm) to fully dilated (4–9 mm) consistent with brain death. Pin point pupil even if nonreactive indicates normal function of Edinger-Westphal nucleus in midbrain—not consistent with brain death.

Ocular Movements

Cranial nerve III, VI and VIII, midbrain, pons.

Oculocephalic reflex (doll's eye reflex)-(testing only when no fracture or instability of the cervical spine or skull base is apparent).

Oculovestibular Reflex

No deviation of the eyes to irrigation in each ear with 50 mL of cold water (tympanic membranes intact; allow 1 minute after injection and at least 5 minutes between testing on each side).

Facial Sensation and Facial Motor Response

No corneal reflex (cranial nerve III, V and VII and pons).

No grimacing to deep pressure on nail bed, supraorbital ridge, or temporomandibular joint (afferent V and efferent VII).

Pharyngeal and Tracheal Reflexes

- Gag and cough reflex (cranial nerve IX and X)
- No response after stimulation of the posterior pharynx
- No cough response to tracheobronchial suctioning.

Clinical Observations Compatible with the Diagnosis of Brain Death

Some complex movements originating from spinal cord or peripheral nerve may persist or pronounced in brain death[11] and these may get triggered by tactile stimuli. These should not be misinterpreted as evidence for brainstem function

Subtle, semirhythmic movements of facial nerve innervated muscles from denervated facial nerve.

Tonic neck reflexes: Passive neck flexion, may be accompanied by complex truncal and extremity movements, including adduction at the shoulders, flexion at the elbows and fingers, supination or pronation at the wrists, ("sitting up" type movements).

- Neck and abdominal muscle contraction or head turning to one side. These might be quite dramatic, often called a "Lazarus sign."[5,8]
- Triple flexion response with flexion at the hip, knee, and ankle when testing for a Babinski sign.
- Opisthotonic posturing, fasciculations of trunk and extremities, superficial abdominal reflexes.[4,9]
- Alternating flexion and extension of the toes with passive displacement of the foot (undulating toe sign).

APNEA TEST

Once the coma and absence of brainstem reflexes have been confirmed apnea test can be performed as the last part in the clinical examination.[4,13] It verifies the loss of rostral brainstem function and is conducted similar to adults. Positive test is the absence of respiratory effort in response to an adequate stimulus. A PCO_2 value of >60 mm Hg is usually considered an adequate stimulus as long as the patient's value was normal or a value 20 mm Hg above the baseline is sufficient. Testing can cause hypotension, severe cardiac arrhythmias, and elevated ICP. Therefore, it should be performed last in the clinical examination of brain death determination.[4,13] If the test is inconclusive consider confirmatory tests.

Conditions that invalidate the apnea test (such as high cervical spine injury) or raise safety concerns for the patient (high oxygen requirement or ventilator settings) are contraindications.

Technique for Apnea Testing (Fig. 30.1)

It should be performed in the setting of normal age appropriate physiologic parameters to be maintained like:[6]
- Normal of pH and $PaCO_2$
- Core body temperature of >35°C (95°F).

This should be achieved and maintained during examination and apnea test.[10,11] Hypothermia, being used as an adjunctive therapy for acute brain injury and following cardiac arrest[8] to protect the brain may confound the diagnostic assessment of death and can also delay the increase in $PaCO_2$ necessary to complete the apnea test.[12]

- Blood pressure appropriate for the age of the child.
- Correcting for factors that could affect respiratory effort.

The patient must be preoxygenated using 100% oxygen for 5–10 minutes before initiating this test. Intermittent mandatory mechanical ventilation should be discontinued once the patient is well oxygenated and maintain PCO_2. The patient can then be changed to a T piece attached to the endotracheal tube or a self-inflating bag valve system such as a Mapleson circuit connected to the ETT.[13]

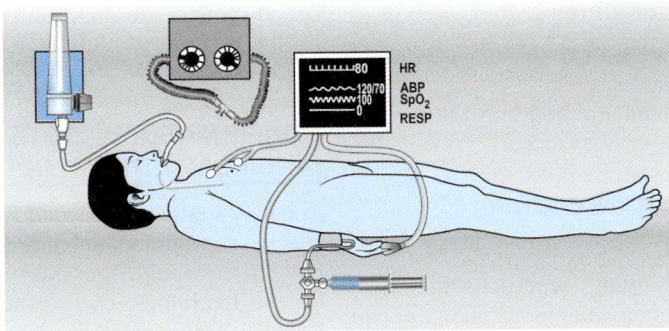

Figure 30.1 Apneic oxygenation. The patient is disconnected from the respirator while receiving pure oxygen via a catheter inserted into the endotracheal tube.[12]
Abbreviations: HR, heart rate; ABP, arterial blood pressure; SPO$_2$, oxygen concentration as measured by pulse oxymetry; RESP, respiration rate

Table 30.1 Age dependent observation period recommended for diagnosis of brain death		
Age	Hours between two examinations	Recommended number of EEGs
7 days–2 months	48	2
2 months–1 year	24	2
>1 year	12	Not needed

High gas flow rates with tracheal insufflation can promote CO_2 washout preventing adequate $PaCO_2$ rise during apnea testing. Continuous positive airway pressure (CPAP) ventilation has been used during the test.[4,13]

Continuous monitoring of heart rate, blood pressure, and oxygen saturation should be done for spontaneous respiratory effort throughout the entire procedure. If no respiratory effort is observed from the initiation of the apnea test to the time the measured $PaCO_2 \geq 60$ mm Hg and ≥ 20 mm Hg above the baseline level, the apnea test is consistent with brain death.

If oxygen saturations falls below 85%, hemodynamic instability limits completion of apnea testing, or a $PaCO_2$ level of ≥ 60 mm Hg cannot be achieved the child should be put back to the ventilator and medical management should be continued. Apnea testing should be discontinued allowing for adequate clearance before proceeding with these evaluations.[6]

INTERVAL OBSERVATION PERIOD

Assessment of neurologic function may be unreliable immediately following cardiopulmonary resuscitation or other severe acute brain injuries and evaluation for brain death should be deferred for 24–48 hours or longer or if there are concerns or inconsistencies in the examination.

The recommended observation period depends on the age of the patient and the laboratory tests utilized **(Table 30.1)**.[4]

The testing is not valid in neonates <7 days.
- *7 days–2 months*: Two clinical examinations and two EEG 48 hours apart
- *2 months–1 year*: Two clinical examinations and two EEG 24 hours apart
  Or two clinical examinations EEG and blood flow study
- *Age > 1 year–18 years*: Two clinical examinations 12 hours apart confirmatory study—optional.

2011 Updated Guidelines

- 24 hours for neonates (37 weeks gestation to term infants 30 days of age)
- 12 hours for infants and children (30 days to 18 years).[6]

NUMBER OF EXAMINATIONS AND EXAMINERS

The current committee supports the 1987 guidelines recommending the performance of two examinations. The examiners should be familiar with the clinical criteria in infants and children and the brain death examiner be someone other than the treating physician. Children being evaluated for brain death may be cared for and evaluated by medical and surgical specialists. The committee recommends that the best interests of the child and family are served if at least two different attending physicians participating in diagnosing brain death to ensure that (i) the diagnosis is based on currently established criteria, (ii) there are no conflicts of interest in establishing the diagnosis and (iii) there is consensus by at least two physicians involved in the care of the child that brain death criteria are met. The apnea test being an objective test, may be performed preferably by the attending physician who is managing ventilator care of the child.[6]

Repeat Clinical Assessment of Brainstem Reflexes

The examination as described above should be repeated in full and documented. When clinical circumstances prohibit completion of any steps in the clinical examination, these should be documented.

CONFIRMATORY TESTS (ANCILLARY STUDIES)

Ancillary studies are needed for patients in whom specific components of clinical testing cannot be reliably evaluated. These are neither a substitute for the neurologic examination nor required to establish brain death.[6,14]

Ancillary studies may be used:
- Incomplete components of the examination or apnea testing cannot be completed
- When there is uncertainty about components of the neurologic examination
- If a medication effect may be present
- Children under 1 year of age
- To reduce the inter-examination observation period and; as per institutional policy.

When ancillary studies are used, a second clinical examination and apnea test should still be performed and components that can be completed must remain consistent with brain death.[15]

Electroencephalography

Electroencephalographic documentation of electrocerebral silence (ECS) and the use of radionuclide CBF determinations to document the absence of cerebral blood flow remain the most widely used methods to support the clinical diagnosis of brain death in infants and children **(Figs 30.2A and B)**. Both of these studies remain accepted

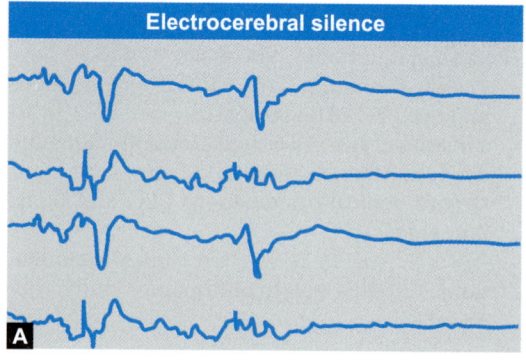
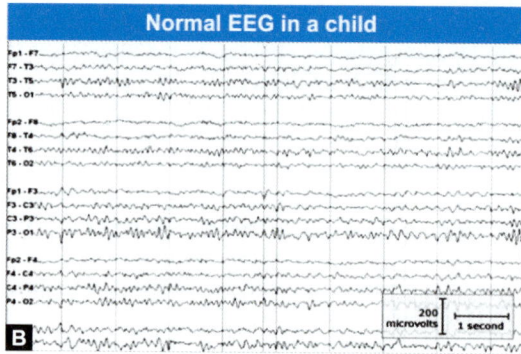

Figures 30.2A and B Normal electroencephalography and electrocerebral silence[15]

tests to assists with the determination of brain death in infants and children (**Flow chart 30.1**).

A valid electroencephalography (ECG) to confirm suspected brain death must be performed according to the accepted technical requirements, under conditions of normo-thermia and the absence of drug levels sufficient to suppress the EEG response.[5,14] Electrocerebral silence is present if no nonartifactual electric potential >2 mv is found during a 30 minute recording. EEG is strongly recommended as an essential part diagnosis in very young children. The advantage is wide availability

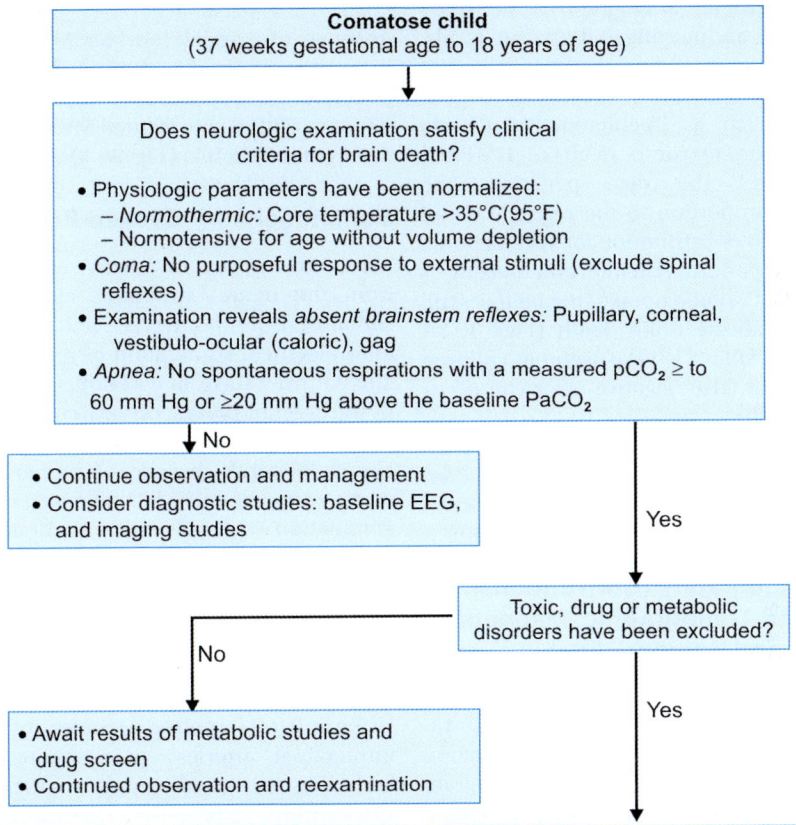

Flow chart 30.1 Algorithm to diagnose brain death in infants and children[6]

and low risk though potential confounders like artifacts in tracing, drug levels to suppress etc are there. EEG testing must be performed in accordance with standards established by the American Electroencephalographic Society.[15]

Nuclear Brain Scanning

Nuclear medicine scans are widely used as an alternative to cerebral angiography. The study is of low risk and are not affected by drug levels. Two–planar imaging using a radioactively-labeled substance that readily crosses the blood-brain barrier (such as Technetium-99m hexa methylpropyleneamineoxime [99mTc- HMPAO] is recommended.[16] The tracer penetrates the parenchyma in proportion to the regional blood flow and shows no redistribution for several hours making it easy to perform and interpret imaging.

The absence of isotope uptake (the hollow skull phenomenon) indicate brain death **(Figs 30.3A and B)**. HMPAO SPECT is very useful in children though occasional false negative error can occur with open sutures.[15]

Other ancillary studies are used to confirm brain death but not been studied sufficiently in children are: cerebral angiography, somatosensory brainstem evoked potentials, Doppler ultrasonography, etc.

Cerebral Angiography (Conventional, Computerized Tomographic, Magnetic Resonance, and Radionuclide)

Traditional gold standard among cerebral flow studies.[14] Demonstrates the absence of intra-cerebral filling at the level of the carotid bifurcation or Circle of Willis. A selective 4 vessel angiogram is done with the iodinated contrast medium under high pressure in both anterior and posterior circulations. A minimum 80 mm Hg of MAP should be assured. In brain death no perfusion other than occasional filling of the superior sagittal sinus is seen, that strongly recommend brain death **(Fig. 30.4)**.[16]

Magnetic Resonance Angiography

Absence of arterial flow on MRA supports the diagnosis of brain death. The specificity is uncertain and practically difficult in unstable patients. Diffusion weighted MRI is more sensitive to cerebral ischemia **(Fig. 30.5)**.

Somatosensory Evoked Potentials

These are waves of neural activity generated from the neural structures along the afferent somatosensory pathways, which are generated after electrical stimulation of a peripheral nerve. The pathway starts at a peripheral nerve, ascends by the brachial plexus, cervical cord, dorsal column nuclei, ventroposterior thalamus and sensory cortex bilateral absence of parietal to sensory cortex responses N19-P22 following median nerve stimulation is consistent with brain death. No reproducible waves of brain stem auditory evoked potentials are also diagnostic. These tests are having only limited utility as ancillary tests.[17]

Transcranial Doppler Ultrasonography

Using a 2 MHz pulsed Doppler instrument, the intracranial arteries are insonated bilaterally, including the middle and/or anterior cerebral

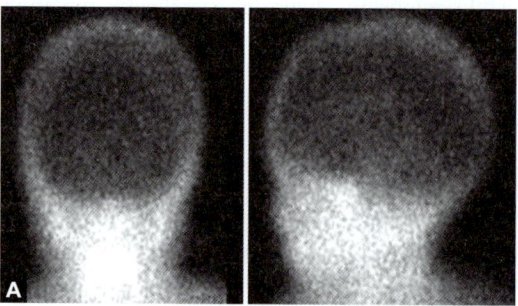
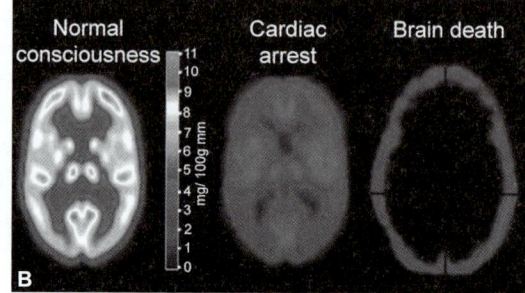

Figures 30.3A and B The hollow skull phenomenon of nuclear brain scanning *(For color version, see Plate 8)*

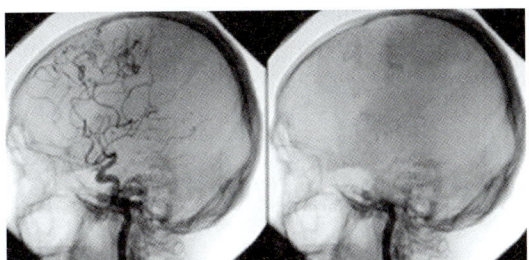

Figure 30.4 CT angiography showing normal and absent flow[16]

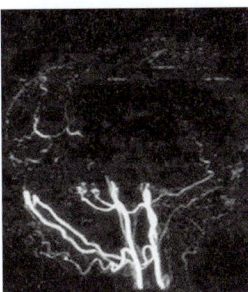

Figure 30.5 MRA showing almost absent blood flow[16]

arteries and the vertebral or basilar artery.[17] The absent diastolic or reverberating flow or small systolic peaks have been reported in brain death. It is safe, noninvasive and inexpensive bedside test but requires expertise.

SPECIAL CONSIDERATION FOR TERM NEWBORNS BABIES

The patent sutures and open fontanel resulting in less dramatic increase in intracranial pressure (ICP) after acute brain injury in newborns when compared to older patients. It is difficult to assess the level of consciousness as some of the brainstem reflexes may not be completely developed in critically ill neonate.

Recommendations for preterm <37 weeks have not been included.[6] Several of the cranial nerve reflexes like pupillary light reflex, oculocephalic reflex are not elicitable in babies less than 32 weeks of gestation.

Treatment with 100% oxygen during apnea test may inhibit the potential recovery of the respiratory effort. Profound bradycardia may precede hypercarbia and limit the apnea test. Ancillary studies are less sensitive. EEG activity is of low voltage and a greater chance of having a reversible ECS in this age group. Cerebral blood flow in viable newborns is extremely low due to reduced metabolic activity.

CERTIFICATION OF BRAIN DEATH

Brain death can be certified by a single physician privileged to make brain death determinations. However, before a patient can become an organ donor, New York State law requires that the time of brain death must be certified by the physician who attends the donor at his death and one other physician, neither of whom shall participate in the process of transplantation. This requirement ensures that all evaluations meet accepted medical standards, and that all participants can have confidence that brain death determination has not been influenced by extraneous factors, including the needs of potential organ recipients.[9,18]

Generally, both physicians should observe the patient, review the medical record, and note whether any additional information is required to make a definitive determination. Neither physician should certify brain death unless all aspects of the determination have been completed.

MEDICAL RECORD DOCUMENTATION

The medical record must indicate:
- Etiology and irreversibility of coma/unresponsiveness
- Absence of confounding factors; hypothermia, hypotension, hypoxia, significant metabolic derangement, significant drug levels
- Absence of motor response to pain
- Absence of brainstem reflexes during two separate examinations separated by at least 6 hours
- Absence of respiration with $pCO_2 \geq 60$ mm Hg, blood gas values should be documented at the beginning and end of the apnea test.
- Justification for and result of confirmatory tests if used.

Table 30.2 Clinical guidelines for determination of brain death in children[4]

- Clinical criteria
  - Unresponsiveness
    - Coma, and
    - Absence of motor responses to pain in all extremities
  - Absent brainstem reflexes:
    - Absence of pupillary responses to light and pupils at midposition with respect to dilatation (4–6 mm)
    - Absence of oculocephalic reflex
    - Absence of oculovestibular (caloric) responses
    - Absence of corneal reflex
    - Absence of jaw reflex
    - Absence of facial grimacing to deep pressure on supraorbital ridge, or temporomandibular joint
    - Absence of pharyngeal gag reflex
    - Absence of coughing in response to tracheal suctioning
    - Absence of sucking and rooting reflexes
  - Apnea (absence of respiratory drive at a $PaCO_2$ that is 60 mm Hg or 20 mm Hg above normal base-line values)
- Additional prerequisites
  - Presence of clinical or neuroimaging evidence of acute CNS catastrophe severe enough to explain the condition
  - Core temperature greater than 32°C (90°F)
  - No drug intoxication, poisoning, or neuromuscular blocking agents
  - Absence of systemic arterial hypotension
  - Absence of confounding medical conditions such as severe electrolyte, acid-base, metabolic or endocrine disturbances, and
  - Interval between two evaluations, according to patient's age:
    - Term to 2 months old, 48 hours
    - >2 months to 1 year old, 24 hours
    - >1 year to <18 year old, 12 hours
    - ≥18 years old, interval optional
- Confirmatory tests
  - Cerebral angiography
  - Electroencephalography
  - Transcranial Doppler ultrasonography
  - Cerebral scintigraphy
    - Term to 2 months old, 2 confirmatory tests (required)
    - >2 months to 1 year old, 1 confirmatory test (required)
    - >1 year to <18 years old, optional
    - ≥18 years old, optional

Source: Adapted from the American Academy of Pediatrics, Task Force on Brain Death in Children, and the American Academy of Neurology, Practice Parameters for the Clinical Diagnosis of Brain Death.

SUPPORTIVE CARE

Following the diagnosis of brain death the cardiorespiratory support can be withdrawn in accordance with hospital policies including those for organ donation. The concept of brain death is often difficult for families to come to term with when dealing with a tragic loss. The family should be treated with sensitivity and respect. The communication should be clear and concise to make them understand that once brain death has been declared their child meets legal criteria for death. Continuation of medical therapies including ventilator support is no longer an option unless organ donation is planned. If family members wish, they may be offered the opportunity to attend

Table 30.3 Comparison of 1987 pediatric brain death guidelines and the updated guidelines for determination of brain death in infants and children[6]

	1987 Task Force Recommendations	2011 Updated Guidelines
Waiting period before initial brain death examination	Not specified	24 hours following cardiopulmonary resuscitation or severe acute brain injury is suggested if there are concerns about the neurologic examination or if dictated by clinical judgment
Clinical examination	Required	Required
Core body temperature	Not specified	> 35°C (95°F)
Number of examinations	Two examinations Second examination not necessary in 2 months–1 year age group if initial examination, EEG and concomitant cerebral blood flow (CBF) consistent with brain death	Two examinations, irrespective of ancillary study results (if ancillary testing is being done in lieu of initial examination elements that cannot be safely performed, the components of the second examination that can be done must be completed)
Number of examiners	Not specified	Two (different attending physicians must perform the first and second exam)
Observation interval between neurologic examinations	Age dependent • 7 days–2 months: 48 hours • 2 months–1 year: 24 hours • >1 year: 12 hours (24 hours if HIE)	Age dependent • Term newborn (37 weeks gestation) to 30 days of age : 24hours • 31 days –18 years: 12 hours
Reduction of observation period between examinations	Permitted only for >1 year age group if EEG or CBF consistent with brain death	Permitted for both age groups if EEG or CBF consistent with brain death
Apnea testing	Required, number of tests ambiguous	Two apnea tests required unless clinically contraindicated
Final PCO$_2$ threshold for apnea testing	Not specified	≥ 60 mm Hg and ≥ 20 mm Hg above the baseline PaCO$_2$
Ancillary studies	Age dependent. 7 days–2 months—2 EEGs separated by 48 hours. 2 months–1 year—2EEGs separated by 24 hours CBF can replace the need for second EEG >1 year No testing required	Not required except in cases where clinical examination and apnea test cannot be completed. Term newborn (37 weeks – 30 days)- EEG and CBF less sensitive CBF may be preferred >30 days–18 years of age—EEG and CBF have equal sensitivity
Time of death	Not specified	Time of the second examination and apnea test (or completion of ancillary study and the components of the second examination that can be safely completed)

while the ventilator is disconnected. Supportive care may continue for hours to days with patience as the family makes decisions about potential organ donation.[5]

Though the concept of brain death is very useful in facilitating organ transplantation and accepted legally, it is not universally accepted. Objections regarding the idea of brain death exist at scientific, bioethical and religious levels as some patients continue to show integrative functioning such as control over free water homeostasis, EEG activity, temperature regulation, capacity to wound healing, variability of vital parameters in response to stimuli etc, though they meet the criteria for brain death.[5]

Surveys of prominent neurologic institutions have shown that there exists considerable variability in adherence to published guidelines and institutional policies regarding the examination and documentation of brain death **(Table 30.2)**.[18] The diagnostic criteria also varies among countries.[19]

According to 2011 update, there is a need to achieve a uniform approach to declare death in infants and children including neonates. It should also be incorporated into all hospital policies **(Table 30.3)**. The future directions strongly suggests that the development of a national database to track infants and children who are diagnosed as brain dead.[6,20]

"With increased experience of knowledge and development in the field of transplantation, there is a great need for the tissues and organs of the hopelessly comatose in order to restore to health of those who are still salvageable."[1]

—Henry K Beecher[1]

REFERENCES

1. Beecher H, Ad Hoc Committee of the Harvard Medical School to Examine the Definition of Brain-death. A definition of irreversible coma: Special Communication: Report of the Ad Hoc Committee of the Harvard Medical School to Examine the Definition of Brain Death. JAMA. 1968;205:337-40.
2. National Conference of Commissioners on Uniform State Laws. The Uniform Determination of Death Act 1981. Available from: URL: http://www.law.upenn. edu/bll/ulc/fnact99/1980s/udda 80.htm. Accessed May 5, 2008.
3. The Quality Standards Subcommittee of the American Academy of Neurology. Practice parameters for determining brain death in adults (summary statement). Neurology. 1995;45:1012-4.
4. American Academy of Pediatrics Task Force on Brain Death in Children. Report of special task force: guidelines for the determination of brain death in children. Pediatrics. 1987;80:298-300.
5. K Jane Lee. Brain Death. Nelson Textbook of Pediatrics. 19th edn. Section 63.1:304.
6. Nakagawa TA, Ashwal S, Mathur M, Mysore M, and the society of critical care medicine, section on critical care and section on neurology of the american academy of pediatrics, and the child neurology society. Clinical Report—Guidelines for the Determination of Brain Death in Infants and Children: An Update of the 1987 Task Force Recommendations. Pediatrics. 2011;128:e720–e740.
7. Willatts SM, Drummond G. Brainstem death and ventilator trigger settings. Anesthesia. 2000; 55:676.(PubMed).
8. Saposnik G, Maurino J, Saizar R, et al. Spontaneous and reflex movements in 107 patients with brain death. Am J Med. 2005;118:311.
9. Beckmann YY, Ciftçi Y, Seçil Y, et al. Fasciculations in brain death. Crit Care Med. 2010;38:2377.
10. Hutchison JS, Ward RE, Lacroix J, et al. Hypothermia therapy after traumatic brain injury in children. N Engl J Med. 2008; 358(23): 2447–56.
11. Hutchison JS, Doherty DR, Orlowski JP, Kissoon N. Hypothermia therapy for cardiac arrest in pediatric patients. Pediatr Clin North Am. 2008;55(3):529–44.
12. Lang CJG, Heckmann JG. Apnea testing for the diagnosis of brain death. Acta Neurol Scand. 2005:112:358–369. Blackwell Munksgaard 2005.
13. Lévesque S, Lessard MR, Nicole PC, et al. Efficacy of a Tpiece system and a continuous positive airway pressure system for apnea testing in the diagnosis of brain death. Crit Care Med 2006; 34:2213.

Pediatric brain death determination. Semin Neurol. 2015 Apr;35(2):116-24. doi: 10.1055/s-0035-1547540.

Epub 2015 Apr 3.Sciencehousestuffworks.com. www.sciencedirect.com/science/article/pii/s09877053140020.

14. Munari M, Zucchetta P, Carollo C, et al. Confirmatory tests in the diagnosis of brain death: comparison between SPECT and contrast angiography. Crit Care Med. 2005;33:2068. Commom confirmatory tests in Brain death. utswim.wordpress.com
15. Guideline three: minimum technical standards for EEG recording in suspected cerebral death. American Electroencephalographic Society. J Clin Neurophysiol. 1994;11:10.
16. Okuyaz C, Gücüyener K, Karabacak NI, et al. Tc99mHMPAO SPECT in the diagnosis of brain death in children. Pediatr Int. 2004;46:711.
17. Kuo JR, Chen CF, Chio CC, et al. Time dependent validity in the diagnosis of brain death using transcranial Doppler sonography. J Neurol Neurosurg Psychiatry. 2006;77:646.
18. Mathur M, Petersen L, Stadtler M, Rose C, Ejike JC, Petersen F, et al. Variability in pediatric brain death determination and documentation in Southern California. Pediatrics; 2008;121:988-993 pediatrics.aappublications.org by guest on May 2, 2015.
19. Wijdicks EF, Varelas PN, Gronseth GS, et al. Evidence based guideline update: determining brain death in adults: report of the Quality Standards Subcommittee of the American Academy of Neurology. Neurology. 2010;74: 1911.
20. Greer DM, Varelas PN, Haque S, Wijdicks EF. Variability of brain death determination guidelines in leading US neurologic institutions. Neurology. 2008;70:284.

Index

Page numbers followed by *f* refer to figure, *t* refer to table

A

Abetalipoproteinemia 205, 207, 209
Abscess 170, 205
    cerebellar 205, 207
    retropharyngeal 87
Academia, organic 30, 209
Acetazolamide 209, 224
Acid
    base imbalance 47
    disorders, organic 30
    fast bacilli 79
    maltase deficiency 188
Acidemia
    isovaleric 30
    methylmalonic 30, 31
    organic 207
    propionic 30
Acidosis 93, 155
    chronic 156
    lactic 30, 145, 170, 207, 209
Aciduria
    methylmalonic 30, 32*f*
    organic 29-31
Adenosine monophosphate 152
Adie's tonic pupil 212
Adrenoleukodystrophy 207, 209
    neonatal 56
Agenesis, cerebellar 15
Aicardi's syndrome 14, 56, 214
Aicardi-Goutières syndrome 39*f*
Alanine aminotransferase 190
Alport's syndrome 212
Alzheimer's disease 153
American Academy of Pediatrics 113, 119
Amino acid 209
Aminoaciduria 29, 205
Amniocentesis 19
Anal reflex 8
Andermann's syndrome 14
Anemia, severe malarial 93
Angiomatosis, encephalofacial 216
Aniridia 208, 211, 211*f*
Ankle jerk 8
Anorexia 161
Anticholinergics 52
Anticonvulsant therapy 175
Antidiuretic hormone 179, 180, 182, 230
    arginine vasopressin 180
Antiepileptic drug 26, 118, 123, 124, 145, 149
Antigen, types of 94*t*
Antitubercular drugs, recommended doses of 81*t*
Aphasia 60
    cerebellar 16
Apnea 145
    test 234
Apneic oxygenation 235*f*

Apoptosis 23, 54
Arachnoid cyst 19, 20*f*
Arachnoiditis 98
Arginase deficiency 39
Arginine 29
Argininosuccinate lyase 39
Arnold-Chiari malformation 205, 208, 209
Artemisinin based combination therapy 96
Arterial blood
    gas 24, 29
    pressure 235
Arteriovenous malformation 207
Artesunate 95
Aspartate
    aminotransferase 190
    transaminase 89
Asphyxia 32
Astrocytoma 207
    cerebellar 205
Ataxia 28, 106, 203, 207, 207*t*-209*t*
    acute 205*t*
    causes of 207*t*
    cerebellar 205
    childhood 209*t*
    chronic 205*t*
    oculomotor apraxia 209
    telangiectasia 52, 205, 207-209, 216
Atkin's diet 156
Atrophic cerebral hemisphere 50
Atrophy 187
Attention-deficit hyperactivity disorder 164, 197
Autoimmune encephalitis 71
Autosomal dominant 212
    epilepsy 117

B

Baclofen 53
Bacterial deoxyribonucleic acid 89
Bacterial meningitis 87, 89, 90, 105
Bardet-Biedl syndrome 218
Barrington's nucleus 225
Basal ganglia 107
    deficits 208
Bassen-Kornzweig syndrome 208, 209, 218
Bat-wing appearance 31*f*
Becker's muscular dystrophy 187, 188
Becker's myotonia 187
Behr syndrome 214
Benzodiazepines 128, 145
Biceps jerk 8
Biotin 30, 209
Birth trauma 32, 47
Bladder
    control 226

    dysfunction 229, 230
        classification of 223*t*
        urodynamic study of 2, 227
Bloch-Sulzberger syndrome 217
Blood 60, 88
    brain barrier 103
    level measurement 209
    pressure 174
        systolic 233
    volume, cerebral 167, 172*f*
Borrelia burgdorferi 60
Botulinum toxin injections 53
Bourneville disease 216
Brachioradialis jerk 8
Bradycardia 24, 145
Brain
    abscess 87, 105
    anomaly 56
    atrophy 104*f*
    congenital malformations of 47
    death 232, 234, 235*t*, 237, 240*t*
        certification of 239
    diseases 182
    disorders 179
    edema 172*f*
    energy metabolism 161
    hypertrophic dysplasia of 11, 18
    infarct 98
    injury 23, 24, 181
        traumatic 153, 170
    malformation, congenital 209
    natriuretic peptide 179, 180
    smooth 15*f*
    Trauma Foundation Guidelines 174
    tumor 52, 170
Brainstem 204, 205
    encephalitis 208
    reflexes 236
        assessment of 233
Brown syndrome 196
Brushfield spots 212
Bulbar
    congestion 208
    telangiectasia 208
Bulbo-spinal muscular atrophy 37

C

Cajal-Retzius cells 55
Calcium
    oxalate 156
    supplementation 156
Campylobacter jejuni 64
Carbamazepine 125, 126, 128, 145, 181
    benzodiazepine 207
Carbohydrate metabolism 28
Carbon monoxide 170
Carnitine
    acetyl transferase deficiency 205

deficiency 153, 185, 187
pamitoyl transferase deficiency 153
translocase deficiency 153
Cataract 208, 212
Central core
　disease 187
　myopathy 187
Central nervous system 87, 97, 103, 110, 145, 207, 232, 233
　immune-mediated inflammatory disorder of 59
Central pontine myelinolysis 183f
Centronuclear myopathy 187
Cephalocele 12
Cerebellar development, disorder of 11, 15
Cerebellum 204
Cerebral edema, types of 168
Cerebral palsy 24, 27, 34, 47, 48, 51, 51f, 52, 205, 229
　cerebellar 50
　choreoathetoid 50
　diplegic 48
　dyskinetic 24
　hypotonic 50
　mixed 50
　prevention of 52
　spastic hemiplegic 49
　types of 48f
Cerebral salt wasting syndrome 181
Cerebrospinal fluid 43, 79, 87-90, 167
　adenosine deaminase activity 80
Cerebrotendinous xanthomatosis 207
Charcot Marie-Tooth disease 207
Chédiak-Higashi syndrome 39
Chemotherapy, antituberculosis 81
Cherry red spot 28, 208, 217, 217t
Cheyne-Stokes respiration 6
Chiari malformation 15-17
Childhood epilepsy, treatment of 123
Chlorpromazine 209
Choriomeningitis, lymphocytic 88
Choroidal hemangioma 216t
Circle of Willis 238
Clobazam 135, 138
Clonazepam 209
Cob-Web appearance 88
Color vision 211
Coma
　pharmacological 177
　recurrent 27
Complex febrile seizure 111, 114
Confusion 77, 105
Conjunctivitis 106
Continuous positive airway pressure 235
Convulsions, multiple 93
Cornelia de Lange syndrome 56
Coronavirus 59
Corpus callosum
　agenesis of 13, 14f, 56
　lipoma 14
Cortical necrosis, cortical 145

Corticocerebellar fibers 50
Corticosteroids 68, 176
Cranial nerve 3, 6
　leave skull 4f
　lesions 105
　palsy 60, 77, 163
Craniorachischisis totalis 43
C-reactive protein 88, 89
Creatine phosphokinase 89, 189
Cremasteric reflex 8
Cryptococcal meningitis 105
Cryptococcoma 105
Cushing's disease 185
Cyst
　intraventricular 98, 99
　large 98
　lumps 98
　parenchymal 98
　spinal 98
Cysticercosis 97
　meningeal 98
Cysticercus cellulosae 98
Cysticercus recemosus 98
Cytomegalovirus 71
Cytosine arabinoside 207

D

Dandy-Walker
　malformation 18, 18f
　syndrome 15, 56
Dantrolene sodium 53
De Morsier syndrome 214
Deafness 214
Deep tendon reflexes 8, 9t, 189
Degenerative diseases 32
Dehydration 156
Dementia 28, 108
　dominant 33
Dengue virus 59
Depression 108
Dermal sinus, congenital 43
Dermatomyositis 187
Desanctis-Cacchione syndrome 33
Detrusor sphincter dyssynergia 229
Dextrose normal saline 144
Diabetes 207
　insipidus 183, 214
　mellitus 212, 214
Diarrhea 155
Diazepam 53, 146, 148
Dihydroartemisinin 95
Diphtheria 71, 112, 207
Diplegia 48
Diplopia 197
Dopamine 162
Double cortex syndrome 16f
Down's syndrome 188, 212
Dravet's syndrome 116, 117, 119, 120
Duane's syndrome 195
Duchenne muscular dystrophy 186-188, 191
Dyke-Davidoff-Masson syndrome 50
Dysostosis multiplex 33

Dysplasia 15, 58
　thanatophoric 56
Dystonia 28, 39
　musculorum deformans 39

E

Ectropion uvea, congenital 212f
Edema
　cerebral 145, 167, 170
　cytotoxic 171f
　hydrocephalic 168
　hydrostatic 168
　osmotic 168
　pulmonary 93, 145
　vasogenic 168, 169
Emery-Dreifuss muscular dystrophy 186
Encephalitis 73f, 87
Encephalomyelitis
　acute
　　disseminated 59, 71
　　hemorrhagic 60, 62
　postinfectious 207
　postvaccinal 59
Encephalomyopathy, mitochondrial 30, 207
Encephalopathy 23
　acute 28-30
　chronic 28, 32, 35, 36
　epileptic 116-118
　hepatic 170
　hypertensive 170
　hypoxic ischemic 23, 24, 145
　infantile epileptic 116, 117, 119
　myoclonic 116, 117-119, 209
　neonatal 24
　static 28, 32, 51
Endocrine system 145
Endotracheal intubation 173
Endotracheal tube 235f
Enzyme-linked immunosorbent assay 99
Ependymoma 205, 207
Epidermal nevus syndrome 56
Epilepsy 113, 114, 118, 123, 208
　juvenile absence 117-119, 125
　myoclonic 30, 118
　　astatic 117, 119, 120, 153
　progressive myoclonic 117
　severe myoclonic 119, 153
Epileptic syndrome 116, 117, 119, 125t
　types of 117t
Episodic ataxia 207
　syndromes 205
Epstein-Barr virus 59, 71
Erythrocyte sedimentation rate 60
Esotropia, neurologic 196, 197
Ethambutol 81
Euglycemia 175
European Association Urology
　Classification of Neurogenic Bladder 228f
Extracellular fluid 179
Extraocular muscle
　congenital fibrosis of 195

movement 5f
paralysis 5t

F

Fabry's disease 39, 212, 219
Facial
    nucleus 161
    palsy 7, 208
    sensation 234
Facies, role of 33f
Facioscapulohumeral muscular dystrophy 186, 187, 191
Fahr's disease 208
Fahr's syndrome 39
Fallacies 110
Familial
    basal ganglia calcification syndrome 39
    infantile seizures, benign 119
    neonatal convulsions, benign 116
    temporal lobe epilepsy 117
Febrile seizure 110-112, 114, 119, 164
    recurrent 113
    types of 111
Felbamate 125, 126
Fetal distress 23
Fever 60, 105, 106
Fibrosis
    meningeal 98
    syndrome, congenital 195
Filippo's syndromes 218
Floppy infant 189t
Fluid management 25
Focal cerebral lesions 108
Folic acid
    deficiency 43
    metabolism 43
Foot deformity 207
Foramen magnum 209
Fosphenytoin 147, 148
Foster-Kennedy syndrome 6
Friedreich's ataxia 205, 207-209, 218
Fukuyama muscular dystrophy 56
Fungal meningitis 88

G

Gabapentin 125, 126, 128
Galactosemia 212
Gamma-aminobutyric acid 162
    synthesis of 111
Gangliosidosis 218
Gastroenteritis, mild 119
Gastrointestinal tract 23
Gaucher's disease 207, 220
Gaze palsies 208
Genetic 111
    disorders 205
    testing 37
Genitourinary malformations 211
Gillespie's syndrome 205, 208
Glasgow coma score 173
Gliomas 205, 207
Global cerebral syndrome 108
Globus pallidus 161
    abnormalities of 31

Glomerular filtration rate 25
Glucose transporter deficiency 152, 153
Glutamate decarboxylase 162
Glutamic acid decarboxylase 207
Glutaric acidemia 30, 31f, 56
Gluten ataxia 207
Glycemic index 157
Glycogen storage diseases 187
Glycogenosis 153
Gram-negative meningitis 90
Granular layer 54
Growth retardation 161
Guillain-Barré syndrome 1, 64, 66t, 67t, 107

H

Hartnup disease 39, 205, 207, 209
Hashimoto's encephalitis 74
Hashimoto's encephalopathy 71
Hashimoto's thyroiditis 74
Head trauma 205
Headache 60, 77, 105, 106, 208
Heart
    failure, congenital 145
    rate 235
Heimann-Bielschowsky phenomenon 200
Hematoma, subdural 170
Hemimegalencephaly 19f
Hemiparesis 60, 77, 106, 208
Hemiplegia 48
Hemorrhage
    cerebellar 205, 207
    pulmonary 24
    subarachnoid 88, 181
Hepatitis
    A 71
    B 71
    C 59
    D 59
Hereditary spastic paraplegia 27, 33
Herniation syndrome 170, 171
Herpes simplex
    infections 221
    virus 59, 71, 115
Heterotopia 15, 57
    periventricular 56
Hexosaminidase A 37
Hinman's syndrome 230
Histidine rich protein antigen 94
Histocytosis 207
Holmes's ataxia 207
Homocystinuria 39
Homovanillic acid 199, 209
Hormone, adrenocorticotropic 118, 119, 200
Horner's syndrome 212
Human immunodeficiency virus (HIV) 59, 103, 107, 207
    encephalopathy 104, 104t
    infection 103, 105t, 108, 108t
    myelopathy 107
    virus 107
Hunter's syndrome 28, 219

Huntington's disease 220
Hydrocephalus 52, 82, 98, 208
Hygroma, subdural 19
Hyperammonemic crisis 39
Hyperbilirubinemia 47, 88
Hypercapnia 145
Hypercarbia 145
Hypercholesterolemia 155
Hyperglycemia 145, 181
Hyperlipidemia 153
Hypernatremia 183
Hyperparasitemia 93
Hyperpyrexia, management of 174
Hypertension 145
    malignant 170
    persistent pulmonary 25
    pregnancy-induced 23
    pulmonary 24
Hyperthermia 25, 145
    maternal 43
Hypertonic saline, administration of 176
Hypertriglyceridemia 155
Hypertrophy 187
    ventricular 39
Hyperuricemia 155
Hyperventilation 175
Hypocalcemia 185
Hypocarotenemia, secondary 155
Hypoglycemia 25, 93, 145
    transient 155
Hypogonadism 207
Hypohidrosis 134
Hypokalemia 185
Hypomagnesemia 155
Hyponatremia 83, 155, 173, 181, 182
    causes of 181
    translocational 181
Hypoplasia, cerebellar 20f, 56
Hypoproteinemia 155
Hyporeflexia 67
Hypotension 145
    persistent 233
Hypothermia 233
    therapeutic 177
Hypothesis, neurotrophic 55
Hypothyroidism 185, 188, 205
Hypotonia 33
Hypotonic fluid, administration of 181
Hypoventilation 173
Hypoxia 23, 145
    perinatal 47
    refractory 173

I

Idiopathic neonatal convulsions, benign 117
Immunosuppression, degree of 103
Immunotherapy 67, 148
Incontinentia pigmenti 56, 217
Indian Academy of Pediatrics 95
Infantile
    familial convulsions, benign 117
    nystagmus syndrome 198

seizures, benign 119
  spasms 117, 118, 119, 125
Inflammation, meningeal 98
Influenza 59, 71
Intermittent ataxic syndrome 39
Intracranial
  hypertension, benign 163
  pressure 27, 88, 167, 173, 175
    monitoring of 170
  tension, benign 87
Intrauterine
  growth restriction 47
  infection 11
Iris
  coloboma 211, 211*f*
  ectropion, congenital 212
  nodule 211, 212*f*
  transillumination 212, 212*f*
Iron 161
  deficiency 160, 161t, 162t
    anemia 160, 163
    neurologic sequelae of 162
Ischemia 23
Isoniazid 81, 84

J

Japanese B encephalitis 71
Jaundice 93
Joubert's syndrome 15, 16, 17*f*, 56, 205, 207
Juvenile myoclonic epilepsy 117-119, 121, 125

K

Kawasaki disease 207, 209
Kayser-Fleischer ring 219*f*
Kearns-Sayre syndrome 30, 207, 218
Keratitis 106
Kernicterus 205
Kernig's sign 105
Ketoacidosis 39
  diabetic 88, 170
Ketogenic diet 149, 151, 152, 155, 156, 157t, 209
  role of 151
Ketosis 29
Kidney disease, chronic 39
Kinky Menkes disease 56
Knee jerk 8
Kocher-Debré-Semelaigne syndrome 188
Koff's formula 227
Krabbe disease 38*f*

L

Labyrinthitis 204, 205, 209
Lacosamide 136
Lactic dehydrogenase 89
Lafora body disease 39, 153
Lamotrigine 125, 126, 128, 132, 138
Landau-Kleffner syndrome 116, 117, 153
Latent nystagmus 196, 198
Leber's optic neuropathy 207, 215
Legionella pneumophila 59

Leigh encephalopathy 207
Lennox-Gastaut syndrome 116-119, 125, 136, 153
Lens, abnormalities of 212
Leptospirosis 60
Lesch-Nyhan syndrome 28, 39
Leucopenia 24
Leukoencephalitis, acute hemorrhagic 60
Leukoencephalopathy, multifocal 107*f*
Leukomalacia, periventricular 51*f*
Levetiracetam 125, 126, 128, 132, 133, 138, 147, 148
Limb-girdle muscular dystrophy 187, 191
Lipid metabolic disorders 207
Lipoma, cervical 207
Liposomal storage disease 205
Lisch nodules 211*f*
Liver phosphorylase kinase deficiency 28
Lobar optic neuropathy 208
Lorazepam 146, 148
Louis-Bar syndrome 216
Low glycemic index diet 156
Lowe's syndrome 212
Lower cranial nerve palsies 6
Lower motor neuron bladder 226
Lumbar puncture 88, 112
Lungs 105
Lymphadenitis, cervical 87
Lymphopenia 60

M

Machado-Joseph
  disease 208
  syndrome 207
Magnesium infusion 149
Malaise 60
Malaria 92, 96
  cerebral 87, 92, 93
Maple syrup urine disease 30, 31, 170, 171*f*, 205
Marateaux Lamy syndrome 219
Marinesco-Sjögren syndrome 205, 208
Marquio's syndrome 219
Mass lesions, removal of 177
McArdle's disease 185, 186
Measles 59, , 71, 112
Meckel-Gruber syndrome 56
Medulloblastoma 205, 207, 208
Meningeal signs 60, 77
Meningiomas 205
Meningitis 78, 90, 105, 108, 170
  aseptic 89
  recurrent 90
  tubercular 77, 77t
  tuberculous 76, 82t
Meningocele 43
Meningoencephalitis 108, 170
Meningomyelocele 43
Menkes disease 207, 208
Mental retardation 27, 211
Mesial temporal sclerosis 115
Metabolic disorders 40, 205, 212
Metabolic myopathies 185, 187

Methyl mercury 56
Methylprednisolone, intravenous 149
Midazolam 146, 148
  infusion 148
Migraine 153, 205, 209
Miliary tuberculosis 76
Miller-Dieker syndrome 56, 57
Miller-Fisher syndrome 65, 68, 205
Mitochondrial
  defects 209
  disease 207, 208
  disorders 205
  myopathies 185, 187, 209
Möbius syndrome 195, 197
Monohydroxy metabolite 131
Mononucleosis, infectious 207
Monoplegia 48
Morning glory
  disc anomaly 213
  syndrome 213*f*
Motor
  axonal neuropathy, acute 64, 65
  deficit 47, 81
  weakness 60
Moyamoya disease 107*f*
Mucopolysaccharidosis 28, 33*f*, 36, 218
Multiple carboxylase deficiency 209
Multisystem disorder 37
Mumps 59, 71, 88, 112, 207
Muscle
  biopsy 190
  disease 33, 185, 186
  lengthening 52
  smooth 224
  weakness 186t
Muscular dystrophies 185, 187, 188*f*
  congenital 186, 187
  oculopharyngeal 187
Myalgia 60
Myasthenia gravis 67
Mycobacterium tuberculosis 105
  antigens 80
Mycoplasma pneumoniae 60, 64
Myelin formation 161
Myelitis, acute transverse 67
Myelomeningocele 43
Myoclonic epilepsy, benign 119
Myoclonus 208
  ataxia dementia syndrome 39
Myoglobinuria 145
Myopathies, classification of 185t
Myotonia 10
Myotonic dystrophy 56, 186, 187, 191, 212
  congenital 185, 187, 191*f*

N

N-acetylaspartate 62
Nasal
  continuous positive airway pressure 192
  meningoencephalocele 12*f*
National Family Health Survey 160
National Institute of Neurological Disorders and Stroke 114

Index

Nausea 105, 155
Neck stiffness 208
Neonatal
  convulsions, benign 117
  epileptic syndromes 116
  reflexes, persistence of 51
  seizures, benign 119
Nerve palsy 6
Nervous system
  infection 87t
  opportunistic infections of 104
Neural tube
  defects 42
  formation 54
Neuroblastoma 207, 209
Neurocysticercosis 97, 105
  classification of 98t
  treatment of 101
Neurodegenerative disorders 27, 28t
Neurofibromatosis 56
Neurogenic bladder 226
  dysfunction 223, 227t
Neuromuscular diseases 28, 56
Neuronal migration 54
  disorder 11, 14, 54, 56t
  treatment of 58
Neuro-ophthalmic significance,
  maternal infections of 220
Neuropathy, peripheral 27, 107, 108
Niacin 209
Niemann-Pick disease 207
Nitrazepam 53
N-methyl-D-aspartate 23, 71
  receptor-associated encephalitis 72
Nocturnal enuresis 230
Nonprogressive central motor
  disorder 34
Non-stress test 23
Nuclear palsy 6
Nutrition 7
Nystagmus 6, 93, 200, 208, 211
  childhood patterns of 198
  congenital 198
  downbeat 208
  optokinetic 210
  transient idiopathic 193

O

Obesity 44
Occipital epilepsy, benign 117, 118
Ocular
  motility disorders 193
  motor apraxia, congenital 200
  movement disorders 193
Oculomotor 77
  apraxia 205, 208
Oculovestibular reflex 233
Ophthalmoplegia 208
  internuclear 208
Opsoclonus 199
Optic
  atrophy 28, 208, 214
  primary 215f

nerve
  coloboma of 213
  head, coloboma of 213f
  hypoplasia 214
Optochiasmatic arachnoiditis 81
Ornithine transcarbamylase deficiency
  28, 39, 205
Orofacial digital syndrome 56
Osmotherapy 175
Osteopenia 156
Ovarian tumor 73f
Oxcarbazepine 125, 126, 128, 130, 131,
  138, 181

P

Pallidal hyperintensity, bilateral 32f
Pandysautonomia, acute 65
Panencephalitis, sub-acute sclerosing 153
Papilledema 6, 208, 215f
Paralysis, periodic 185, 187
Paramytonia congenital 187
Paraneoplastic syndromes 207
Paraparesis 67, 77
Parasite lactate dehydrogenase 94
Parenchymal calcifications 98
Parkinson disease 39
Paroxysmal vertigo, benign 205
Patau syndrome 212
Pediatric epilepsy, management of 137, 151
Pelizaeus-Merzbacher disease 208
Perisylvian syndrome, bilateral 15, 58
Pertussis 71, 112, 207
Phakomatosis 216
Pharyngio-cervical-brachial syndrome 65
Phenobarbitone 113, 125, 147, 148, 207
Phenylalanine 162
Phenylketonuria 162
Phenytoin 125, 126, 128, 146, 148, 207
Phosphoglycerate kinase deficiency 28
Photodermatitis 33f
Photophobia 77, 105
Phytanic acid 209
Piperaquine 95
Plantar extensor 8
Plasma acylcarnitine 29
Plasmapheresis 68
Plasmodium 92
  aldolase 94
  falciparum 60, 92, 94
  knowlesi malaria 92
  malariae 92
  ovale 92
  vivax 92
Pneumonia, aspiration 145, 173
Poliomyelitis 67
Polymerase chain reaction 89
Polymyositis 187
Polyneuropathy, acute inflammatory
  demyelinating 64
Polyradiculoneuropathy, acute
  inflammatory demyelinating 65
Polytherapy 124, 127

Pompe's disease 33, 185, 185-187
Pontine reticular formation 198
Porencephalic cyst 19f, 50, 53
Potter syndrome 56
Prader-Willi syndrome 188
Prednisolone 209
Pressure flow micturition studies 227
Primidone 125, 128
Propofol infusion 148
Protein
  energy malnutrition 87
  metabolic disorders 28
Pseudoataxia 209
Pseudo-bulbar palsy 49
Ptosis 208
  congenital 195
Pupillary light reflex 233
Pyramidal dysfunction, signs of 8
Pyrazinamide 81
Pyrexia 77
Pyrizinamide 84
Pyruvate
  carboxylase deficiency 153
  decarboxylase deficiency 39, 205
  dehydrogenase deficiency 39, 56,
    153, 209

Q

Quadriparesis 67
Quadriplegia 48
Quinine 96

R

Racemose angioma 217
Radial glial cells, role of 55f
Ramsay Hunt syndrome 208
Rasmussen's encephalitis 73, 117
Red blood cell 88, 94
Reflexes 3, 8
Refsum's disease 205, 207-209, 218
Renal
  failure, acute 145
  function 229
  impairment 93
  system 145
Respiratory system 145
Restless legs syndrome 164
Retinal
  angioma 216f
  angiomatosis 216
  vascular occlusive diseases 221
Retinitis 106
  pigmentosa 28, 208, 218, 218t
Retinopathy 208
Rett syndrome 153
Reye's syndrome 170
Riboflavin 209
Rifampicin 81, 84
Rubella 59, 71, 112, 220

S

Saccadomania 199
Salivary ducts, surgical transposition of 52

Salmonella typhi 60
San Filippo's syndrome 219
Sarnat and Sarnat staging 24
Scarlet fever 207
Scheie's syndrome 219
Sclerosis
    amyotrophic lateral 153
    multiple 61*t*, 205, 207, 208
    tuberous 56, 216
Sea-blue histiocytosis 208
Segawa syndrome 39
Seizure 26, 28, 60, 98, 106, 189
    atonic 120
    disorder 24
    genesis 98
    myoclonic atonic 118
    neonatal 125
Sensory
    ataxia 204
    axonal neuropathy 64, 65
    system 3
Septo-optic dysplasia 14, 214
Serotonin 162
Serum ammonia 29
Shock 24, 25, 67, 93, 233
Sialidosis 208
Sly's syndrome 219
Smith-Lemli-Opitz syndrome 56
Sodium
    balance disorders 180
    dysequilibrium 179
    valproate 209
Solitary cystic granuloma 97, 98, 99*t*
Spina bifida 229
    aperta 43
Spinal
    cord
        involvement 60
        lesion 33
    motor system examination 7
    muscular atrophy 37, 189, 189*t*
    stimulation 53
Spine 207
Spinocerebellar ataxia 205, 207, 208
Spinomotor system 3, 9
Status epilepticus 143, 145*t*, 146, 153
    classification of 143
    management of 148*t*
    nonconvulsive 144
Stenosis, aqueductal 19, 20
Steven Johnson syndrome 131
Strabismus 196
    transient
        neonatal 193
        vertical 194
Streptomycin 81
Stroke 107, 153, 208
    hemorrhagic 170
    ischemic 170
    pediatric 163
Sturge-Weber syndrome 216
Substantia nigra reticulata 161
Superficial reflexes 8, 8*t*
Sweating 145
Sylvian fissure 15, 15*f*, 19*f*, 31, 57*f*, 58
Syndrome of inappropriate antidiuretic hormone 25, 83
    secretion 170, 181
Syphilis 221
Systemic lupus erythematosus 207

T

Tachycardia 145
Taenia solium 97
Telangiectasia 220
Temporal lobe epilepsy 115
Tendo achilles spasm 53*f*
Tendon reflexes 50
Tetanus 71
    toxoids 112
Thomsen's disease 187
Thomson's score 24
Thrombocytopenia 24, 107
Tonic neck reflexes 234
Tonsillitis 87
Topiramate 125, 126, 128, 133, 134, 138
Torticollis 199, 207, 208
Toxic epidermal necrolysis 131
Toxoplasma
    encephalitis 105
    gondii 11
    retinochoroiditis 220*f*
    scar 220*f*
Toxoplasmosis 212, 220
Transcranial Doppler ultrasonography 238, 240
Tricarboxylic acid cycle 152
Triceps jerk 8
Triplegia 48
Trisomy 13,18, 21 56
Tubercular meningitis, treatment of 81
Tuberculin skin test 80
Tuberculoma 79, 105, 170
    intracerebral 83
Tuberculosis 76, 106*f*, 207
    encompasses tubercular meningitis 76
Tuberculous meningitis hydrocephalus, Vellore grading of 82
Tubular necrosis 145
Typhoid fever 207

U

Ulcers 106
Umbilical artery 24
Upper lobe pneumonia 87
Upper motor neuron 47
    lesions, signs of 8*t*
    signs 208
Upper respiratory infection 110
Urea cycle
    defects 28, 29, 32, 39, 209
    disorders 29, 39
Urethral pressure profile 227
Uric acid 39, 156
Urinary bladder 223
Urine
    copper excretion 209
    organic acids 29
Urolithiasis 156

V

Vagal nerve stimulation 130
Valproate 125, 128, 147, 148
Valproic acid 125, 126
Valsalva's maneuver 227
Vanillylmandelic acid 199, 209
Varicella zoster 71
    virus 59
Vasculitis 98
Vasopressin 89
Vein of Galen 21
    aneurysm 21
    malformations 21, 21*f*
Vellore grading system 82
Ventricular system, disorder of 11, 18
Viral
    encephalitis 205
    infections 59
    strain, neurovirulence of 103
Visceral reflexes 8
Vision impairment 106
Visual
    acuity 210
    deficits 105
    field 211
    loss 208
    problems 60
Vitamin
    B1 genetic disorders 207
    B12 207
    D 156
    E 209
        deficiency 205, 207, 209
        level 209
Vomiting 27, 39, 60, 105, 145, 155
von Hippel-Lindau
    disease 216, 216*f*
    syndrome 205
von Willebrand's disease 19

W

Walker-Warburg syndrome 56, 57
West Nile virus 67
White blood cell 88
White matter disorders 38*f*
Wilms' tumor 211
Wilson's disease 205, 207-209, 212, 219, 220
Wilson-Kayser-Fleischer ring 39
Wolfram syndrome 214
Wyburn-Mason syndrome 217

X

Xanthomas 207
Xeroderma pigmentosa 33*f*

Z

Zellweger syndrome 56, 188
Zinc deficiency 43
Zonisamide 125, 126, 136, 138
    phenobarbitone 126
Zonular cataract, congenital 213*f*